Transitional Age Youth and Mental Illness: Influences on Young Adult Outcomes

Editors

ADELE MARTEL
D. CATHERINE FUCHS

CHILD AND ADOLESCENT PSYCHIATRIC CLINICS OF NORTH AMERICA

www.childpsych.theclinics.com

Consulting Editor
HARSH K. TRIVEDI

April 2017 • Volume 26 • Number 2

ELSEVIER

1600 John F. Kennedy Boulevard • Suite 1800 • Philadelphia, Pennsylvania, 19103-2899

http://www.theclinics.com

CHILD AND ADOLESCENT PSYCHIATRIC CLINICS OF NORTH AMERICA Volume 26, Number 2
April 2017 ISSN 1056–4993, ISBN-13: 978-0-323-52398-1

Editor: Lauren Boyle
Developmental Editor: Kristen Helm

Child and Adolescent Psychiatric Clinics of North America (ISSN 1056-4993) is published quarterly by Elsevier Inc., 360 Park Avenue South, New York, NY 10010-1710. Months of issue are January, April, July, and October. Business and Editorial Offices: 1600 John F. Kennedy Boulevard, Suite 1800, Philadelphia, PA 19103-2899. Periodicals postage paid at New York, NY and additional mailing offices. Subscription prices are $316.00 per year (US individuals), $566.00 per year (US institutions), $100.00 per year (US students), $367.00 per year (Canadian individuals), $688.00 per year (Canadian institutions), $200.00 per year (Canadian students), $439.00 per year (international individuals), $688.00 per year (international institutions), and $200.00 per year (international students). International air speed delivery is included in all *Clinics* subscription prices. All prices are subject to change without notice. **POSTMASTER:** Send address changes to *Child and Adolescent Psychiatric Clinics of North America*, Elsevier Health Sciences Division, Subscription Customer Service, 3251 Riverport Lane, Maryland Heights, MO 63043. **Customer Service: 1-800-654-2452 (U.S. and Canada); 314-447-8871 (outside U.S. and Canada). Fax: 314-447-8029. E-mail:** JournalsCustomer Service-usa@elsevier.com **(for print support) or** journalsonlinesupport-usa@elsevier.com **(for online support).**

Reprints. For copies of 100 or more of articles in this publication, please contact the Commercial Reprints Department, Elsevier Inc., 360 Park Avenue South, New York, New York 10010-1710 Tel.: 212-633-3874; Fax: 212-633-3820, E-mail: reprints@elsevier.com.

Child and Adolescent Psychiatric Clinics of North America is covered in *MEDLINE/PubMed (Index Medicus), ISI, SSCI, Research Alert, Social Search, Current Contents,* and *EMBASE/Excerpta Medica.*

Contributors

CONSULTING EDITOR

HARSH K. TRIVEDI, MD, MBA
President and Chief Executive Officer, Sheppard Pratt Health System, Clinical Professor and Vice Chair of Psychiatry, University of Maryland School of Medicine, Baltimore, Maryland

CONSULTING EDITOR EMERITUS

ANDRÉS MARTIN, MD, MPH

FOUNDING CONSULTING EDITOR

MELVIN LEWIS, MBBS, FRCPSYCH, DCH

EDITORS

ADELE MARTEL, MD, PhD
Emeritus Medical Staff, Child and Adolescent Psychiatry, Ann & Robert H. Lurie Children's Hospital of Chicago, Health System Clinician, Department of Psychiatry and Behavioral Sciences, Northwestern University Feinberg School of Medicine, Chicago, Illinois

D. CATHERINE FUCHS, MD
Professor of Psychiatry and Behavioral Sciences and Pediatrics, Division of Child and Adolescent Psychiatry, Vanderbilt University Medical Center, Director, Psychological and Counseling Center, Vanderbilt University, Nashville, Tennessee

AUTHORS

LEE I. ASCHERMAN, MD
Department of Psychiatry and Neurobiology, Division of Child and Adolescent Psychiatry, University of Alabama at Birmingham, Birmingham, Alabama

OSCAR G. BUKSTEIN, MD, MPH
Vice Chair and Professor, Department of Psychiatry, Boston Children's Hospital, Harvard Medical School, Boston, Massachusetts

VIVIEN CHAN, MD
Chief of Mental Health Service, Student Health Center, University of California Irvine, Irvine, California; Associate Clinical Professor, Department of Psychiatry & Human Behavior, UCI Health, Orange, California; Behavioral Health Services, Children, Youth & Prevention Division, Center for Resiliency Wellness & Education (First Episode Psychosis), Orange County Health Care Agency, Orange, California

WINSTON W. CHUNG, MD
Vermont Center for Children, Youth, and Family, University of Vermont Medical Center, Burlington, Vermont

MARYANN DAVIS, PhD
Research Associate Professor, Director Transitions, RTC Systems and Psychosocial Advances Research Center, Department of Psychiatry, University of Massachusetts Medical School, Worcester, Massachusetts

CÉSAR G. ESCOBAR-VIERA, MD, PhD
Center for Research on Media, Technology, and Health, Health Policy Institute, University of Pittsburgh School of Public Health, Pittsburgh, Pennsylvania

D. CATHERINE FUCHS, MD
Professor of Psychiatry and Behavioral Sciences and Pediatrics, Division of Child and Adolescent Psychiatry, Vanderbilt University Medical Center, Director, Psychological and Counseling Center, Vanderbilt University, Nashville, Tennessee

JAMES J. HUDZIAK, MD
Professor of Child Psychiatry, Medicine, Pediatrics and Communication Sciences & Disorders, Director of the Vermont Center for Children, Youth, and Family, University of Vermont College of Medicine and Medical Center, Burlington, Vermont

TERRY LEE, MD
Associate Professor, Division of Public Behavioral Health and Justice Policy, Department of Psychiatry and Behavioral Sciences, University of Washington School of Medicine, Seattle, Washington

PATRICIA K. LEEBENS, MAT, MA, MD
Child, Adolescent, and Adult Psychiatry, Private Practice, New York, New York; Assistant Clinical Professor, Yale Child Study Center, Yale University School of Medicine, New Haven, Connecticut

JULIE LINKER, PhD
Assistant Professor of Psychiatry, Virginia Commonwealth University, Richmond, Virginia

CECILIA M.W. LIVESEY, MD
Clinical Associate, Department of Psychiatry, The University of Pennsylvania Health System, Philadelphia, Pennsylvania

ADELE MARTEL, MD, PhD
Emeritus Medical Staff, Child and Adolescent Psychiatry, Ann & Robert H. Lurie Children's Hospital of Chicago, Health System Clinician, Department of Psychiatry and Behavioral Sciences, Northwestern University Feinberg School of Medicine, Chicago, Illinois

MARGARET McMANUS, MHS
Co-Director, Got Transition, President, The National Alliance to Advance Adolescent Health, Washington, DC

WYNNE MORGAN, MD
Assistant Professor, Department of Psychiatry, University of Massachusetts Medical School, Worcester, Massachusetts

MARYLAND PAO, MD
Clinical & Scientific Director, National Institute of Mental Health, National Institutes of Health, Bethesda, Maryland

BRIAN A. PRIMACK, MD, PhD
Center for Research on Media, Technology, and Health, University of Pittsburgh School of Medicine, Pittsburgh, Pennsylvania

DEBORAH RIVAS-DRAKE, PhD
Associate Professor, Department of Psychology, School of Education, University of Michigan, Ann Arbor, Michigan

SCOTT M. RODGERS, MD
Professor and Chair, Department of Psychiatry and Human Behavior, University of Mississippi Medical Center, Jackson, Mississippi

ANTHONY L. ROSTAIN, MD, MA
Professor of Psychiatry and Pediatrics, Department of Psychiatry, Perelman School of Medicine, University of Pennsylvania, Philadelphia, Pennsylvania

JULIA SHAFTEL, PhD
Psychologist, Independent Practice, Lawrence, Kansas

BRIAN SKEHAN, MD, PhD
Child and Adolescent Psychiatry Fellow, Department of Psychiatry, University of Massachusetts Medical School, Worcester, Massachusetts

ARADHANA BELA SOOD, MD, MSHA
Professor of Psychiatry and Pediatrics, Virginia Commonwealth University, Richmond, Virginia

GABRIELA LIVAS STEIN, PhD
Associate Professor, Department of Psychology, University of North Carolina at Greensboro, Greensboro, North Carolina

GESA L. TIEMEIER, MD/PhD Program
Leiden University Medical Center, Leiden, The Netherlands

GERRIT I. VAN SCHALKWYK, MB,ChB
Child and Adolescent Psychiatry Fellow, Yale Child Study Center, Yale University School of Medicine, New Haven, Connecticut

FRED R. VOLKMAR, MD
Professor of Psychology, Irving B. Harris Professor of Child Psychiatry, Pediatrics and Psychology, Yale Child Study Center, Yale University School of Medicine, New Haven, Connecticut

PATIENCE WHITE, MD, MA
Co-Director, Got Transition, The National Alliance to Advance Adolescent Health, Professor of Medicine and Pediatrics, George Washington School of Medicine and Health Sciences, Washington, DC

EDWIN D. WILLIAMSON, MD
Training Director, Vanderbilt Child and Adolescent Psychiatry Fellowship Program, Assistant Professor of Psychiatry and Behavioral Sciences, Vanderbilt University, Nashville, Tennessee

Contents

Background

The transition from adolescence to young adulthood is a challenging time for many young people, given the multiple simultaneous demands placed by biological, psychological, and social forces that affect an individual's development. There are additional challenges when one is coping with ongoing or evolving mental health disorders. This article focuses on the demographics of transitional age youth, ages 16 to 26 years, in the United States, the unique characteristics of this developmental period, and how risk and resilience factors may affect the course of development and an individual's pathway to adulthood.

Over the past two decades, there have been substantial developments in the understanding of brain development and the importance of environmental inputs and context. This paper focuses on the neurodevelopmental mismatch that occurs during the epoch we term the 'transitional age brain' (ages 13–25) and the collateral behavioral correlates. We summarize research findings supporting the argument that, because of this neurodevelopmental mismatch, transitional age youth are at high risk for engaging in behaviors that lead to negative outcomes, morbidity, and mortality. We highlight the need to develop new, neuroscience-inspired health promotion and illness prevention approaches for transitional age youth.

Transitional age youth (TAY) are in a discrete developmental stage, different from both adolescents and mature adults. Serious mental illness can result in their delayed psychosocial development and morbidity. Systemic, provider, and individual barriers result in poor access to care for these youth, potentially impeding their transition to mature adulthood. Current strategies for TAY treatment include patient centered care, vocational and educational support, and shared decision making. There is a paucity of evidence-based practices to effectively treat this population or provide practice guidelines. The research required to do so should be a priority.

Successful transition from childhood to adulthood is context and culture dependent. This article reviews concepts of mental health and theoretic constructs of successful adulthood that suggest intentional policies and practices are developed with a specific vision of success. Parents, educators, mental health professionals, and policymakers need to be cognizant of their assumptions and essential roles in these processes. The early development of illness may disrupt and alter the timelines of different developmental milestones and trajectories. It is important to discuss what "success" looks like with transitional age youth and their family members, because treatment approaches may adapt accordingly.

Common Challenges

The progression from adolescence to adulthood is a time of tremendous change, characterized by issues of identity formation, autonomy, and shifting relationship dynamics. The family is embedded in all aspects of this transition and serves as both a protective support and a limiting factor, a complicated duality that raises psychological, ethical, and legal issues. This article discusses the influence of familial factors and provides assessment strategies for evaluating the family in relation to treatment of transitional age youth. It is increasingly evident that family engagement is a significant contributor to outcomes for transitional age youth seeking mental health treatment.

For transitional age individuals, social media (SM) is an integral component of connecting with others. There are 2 billion SM users worldwide. SM users may experience an increase in perceived social support and life satisfaction. Use of SM may facilitate forming connections among people with potentially stigmatizing mental disorders. However, epidemiologic studies suggest that increased SM use is associated with conditions such as depression, anxiety, and sleep disturbance. Future research should examine directionality of these associations and the role of contextual factors. It also will be useful to leverage SM to provide mental health care and surveillance of mental health concerns.

Youth transitioning to adulthood have unique developmental tasks that make them vulnerable to suicide. Brain development, life stressors, and psychological adjustments during the transition contribute to a high rate of suicidal gestures. To reduce the incidence of self-harm in this age group, a public health approach that identifies and reduces risk factors and enhances protective factors should be used. Institutions and employment arenas should consider structural supports to facilitate this transition of youth into adulthood, with a particular focus on youth with self-harm thoughts, and should provide education about suicide, evidence-based resources, and intervention programs to encourage help seeking.

Oscar G. Bukstein

Transitional age youth (TAY), developing from adolescence to adulthood, exhibit the highest level of alcohol and other drug use of any other age group. Risk factors mirror those for the development of problems and disorders in adolescents. Early screening of both college students and noncollege high-risk TAY in the community is critical to early and effective intervention. Brief interventions using motivational techniques are effective for many TAY, particularly for those in early stages of problem use on college campuses. Professionals in contact with TAY should be aware of evidence-based interventions and providers for substance use disorders in the community.

Deborah Rivas-Drake and Gabriela Livas Stein

Transitional age youth were born into a world that is becomingly increasingly diverse. Youth who are ethnic or racial minorities encounter cultural stressors, including acculturative stress and discrimination that undermine their health and mental health. Decades of research demonstrate that cultural assets can serve as risk-reducing and resilience-enhancing mechanisms among minority and immigrant youth. Cultural assets include the development of a healthy ethnic-racial identity and maintenance of cultural values. Practitioners should assess for culturally relevant stressors and incorporate cultural assets such as ethnic-racial identity and cultural values to support the mental health of these youth.

Special Populations

Terry Lee and Wynne Morgan

Transitional age foster youth do not typically receive the types of family supports their nonfoster peers enjoy. Many foster youth experience multiple adversities and often fare worse than nonfoster peers on long-term functional outcomes. Governments increasingly recognize their responsibility to act as parents for state dependents transitioning to adulthood and the need to provide services to address social/emotional supports, living skills, finances, housing, education, employment, and physical and mental health. More research is needed to inform the development of effective programs. Transitional age foster youth benefit from policies promoting a developmentally appropriate, comprehensive, and integrated transition system of care.

spectrum conditions, which are different from childhood-onset and early onset schizophrenia, and findings of psychotic-like experiences in the normal population. Taken from adult and childhood literature, clinical quandaries in accurate diagnosis, and treatment gaps in co-occurring, or sometimes confounding, conditions are discussed. Thoughts on the impact of schizophrenia on an emerging adulthood trajectory are offered. Recent best practices in the treatment of schizophrenia are consistent with a recovery-oriented model of mental health services for transitional age youth.

Model Programs

This article provides national data on the lack of transition preparation among youth with special health care needs, including those with emotional, behavioral, and developmental conditions. Consumer and provider transition barriers pertaining to inadequate transition support are summarized. In addition, current US transition goals are presented along with health professional recommendations on transition. The *Six Core Elements of Health Care Transition*, which are aligned with professional recommendations, are reviewed with practice-based lessons learned from quality improvement efforts. The article concludes with a discussion of transition evaluation needs and opportunities.

It is clear that environmental influences impact the structure and function of the human brain, and thus, thoughts, actions, and behaviors. These in turn influence whether an individual engages in high-risk (drugs, alcohol, violence) or health-promoting (exercise, meditation, music) activities. The developmental mismatch between cortical and subcortical maturation of the transitional age brain places college students at risk for negative outcomes. This article argues that the prescription of incentive-based behavioral change and brain-building activities simply make good scientific, programmatic, and financial sense for colleges and universities. The authors present University of Vermont Wellness Environment as an example.

Summary

CHILD AND ADOLESCENT PSYCHIATRIC CLINICS

FORTHCOMING ISSUES

July 2017
Early Childhood Mental Health: Empirical Assessment and Intervention from Conception through Preschool
Mini Tandon, *Editor*

October 2017
Pediatric Integrated Care
Gregory K. Fritz, Tami D. Benton, and Gary Maslow, *Editors*

RECENT ISSUES

January 2017
Health Information Technology for Child and Adolescent Psychiatry
Barry Sarvet and John Torous, *Editors*

October 2016
Substance Use Disorders, Part II
Ray Chih-Jui Hsiao and Paula D. Riggs, *Editors*

July 2016
Substance Use Disorders, Part I
Ray Chih-Jui Hsiao and Leslie Renee Walker, *Editors*

Preface

Transitional Age Youth and Mental Illness – Influences on Young Adult Outcomes

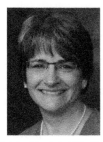 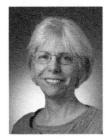

Adele Martel, MD, PhD   D. Catherine Fuchs, MD
Editors

The transition from adolescence to adulthood is characterized by developmental milestones in the areas of self-sufficiency, educational attainment, employment, contributing to a household, relationship changes, parenting, and positive community contributions. Achievement of these milestones involves gradually working through tasks central to this stage of life—separation-individuation, identity formation, and achieving intimacy.[1] It also involves adjusting to new situations, such as independent living, the work environment, the academic demands of post-secondary education, and changes in legal status. The transition to adulthood is a challenging stage of development for many young people.

For many of those youth and young adults diagnosed with a mental health condition before or during this life stage, the challenges of transitioning to adulthood are amplified.[2] Their psychosocial maturation in one or more aspects of development may be delayed or compromised, giving them a less consistent foundation to move through this transition.[3] The developmental period between late adolescence and young adulthood is a particularly vulnerable time for the new onset of major psychiatric disorders. The National Comorbidity Survey Replication Study[4] found that 50% to 75% of DSM IV–defined anxiety disorders, mood disorders, impulse control disorders, and substance use disorders emerge between the ages of 14 and 24, with substance use disorders showing a marked increase in prevalence in this age group. Among those with mental health disorders are young people with unique vulnerabilities and needs that further complicate this life transition. These include youth aging out of foster care, those transitioning from special education services, LGBTQ (lesbian, gay, bisexual, and transgender) youth, ethnic/racial minority youth, those with chronic medical illnesses, and youth with experiences in the justice system and the military. These transitional age youth (TAY) are at high risk for poor outcomes in young adulthood, which impacts them as individuals as well as their families and society as a whole.[5,6]

Child Adolesc Psychiatric Clin N Am 26 (2017) xiii–xvii
http://dx.doi.org/10.1016/j.chc.2017.01.001
1056-4993/17/© 2017 Published by Elsevier Inc.

childpsych.theclinics.com

The term *transitional age youth* (TAY) typically refers to the demographic spanning older adolescence (15-16 years) to young adulthood (24-26 years).[7] The lack of preciseness in part reflects that this cohort is characterized by psychosocial transitions, which are not uniformly accomplished by a specific age and are influenced by culture.[8] Physical maturation, including neurodevelopment, is also very individualized during this time period and influenced by genetics and environment.

It is critical to understand how adverse mental health and functional outcomes evolve during the transition to adulthood in order to identify points of intervention. It is also important to focus on factors contributing to resilience and to consider this life stage as a developmental opportunity to foster a positive and productive life course.[9-11] An individual's psychosocial capacities and trajectory into adulthood, including both vulnerabilities and strengths, are the result of a complex and dynamic interaction among biological processes, psychological factors, and sociocultural context over time. During the transition from late adolescence to young adulthood, there are "pervasive and often simultaneous contextual and social role changes"[10] as well as challenges and opportunities for self direction, new experiences, and new relationships. Although we recognize that efforts to promote wellness and prevent mental health disorders should begin long before the transition from late adolescence to young adulthood,[12] the impact of "more developmentally proximal influences"[10] on stability or change in a life pathway or in promoting resilience during the TAY period deserves more attention.[10,11]

Advances in developmental neuroscience and genetics also support the notion that the transition to the adulthood period offers considerable opportunity for intervention. Brain development continues well into the 20s, with reasoning, judgment, decision-making abilities, and impulse control still maturing. Extant evidence also points to considerable brain neuroplasticity, the ability of the brain to alter its structure in response to experience. Epigenetic research describes dynamic alterations in the transcriptional potential of cells in response to environmental experiences.[13,14] So, intentional and well-designed opportunities to practice self-sufficiency, problem-solving, setting priorities, and making choices during the transition to young adulthood may help facilitate movement to a more positive young adult trajectory.

Mental health treatment is one of many resources that can promote resilience. Despite evidence from multiple epidemiologic studies that the prevalence of the full range of psychiatric disorders in this age group is 20%, it is notable that the use of mental health treatment services and health services in general is low or declining during this transitional age period,[15,16] contributing to a lost opportunity for promoting resilience. Many reasons have been put forth to explain these findings including systems issues, provider issues, and TAY issues. It is important to recognize and address these potential barriers to treatment.

ROLE OF THE CHILD AND ADOLESCENT PSYCHIATRIST

In 2013, Wilens and Rosenbaum[7] referred to TAY as "A New Frontier in Child and Adolescent Psychiatry". Many child and adolescent psychiatrists (CAP) continue to work with TAY beyond their high school years as providers of direct clinical care, consultants to various systems, and/or administrators involved in designing and directing programs for TAY.[7,17] Some reasons they may choose to do such work are interest in this vibrant and challenging transitional age group, recognition of the significant unmet mental health needs of TAY, and a desire to provide continuity of care for their patients. To this work, CAP bring knowledge of developmental psychopathology, comfort with systems of care and working with families, and experience with disorders that present in childhood or adolescence and which can impact the transition to young adulthood.[18] Still, these CAP and others working with this cohort of young people need to enhance their understanding of the complex tasks, contexts, and contemporary pathways of this age group and their interface with brain development and ethics in order to ensure that structures, programs, and practices meet the developmental needs of TAY. Those CAP who do not see patients beyond the age of 18 also need enhanced knowledge and skills. They have important roles to play in promoting patient coping skills, autonomy, and independent management of their mental health needs and other daily living tasks as they help prepare their patients not only for transfer of care to new providers but also for their developmental transition to young adulthood.[8,19]

This issue of the *Child and Adolescent Psychiatric Clinics of North America* aims to bridge the current state of knowledge about risk, resilience, mental illness, and neurodevelopment during this transitional stage with the need for developmentally attuned and culturally competent strategies to engage and maintain TAY in treatment. Contributing authors are asked to discover and evaluate the emerging literature regarding the following: (1) the impact of this transitional stage on the trajectory of mental health and well-being, (2) the strength of the evidence for particular practices and programs on clinical outcomes in TAY, (3) best practices in planning and preparation for the transition to adulthood, and (4) how exploration of risk and resilience may guide nuanced care of individuals with the potential for supporting the TAY population in the successful navigation of their lives as young adults coping with mental illness.

We designed this issue to help CAP and other mental health professionals evaluate and enhance their knowledge, clinical skills, and attitudes in regards to TAY. The topic of *Transitional Age Youth and Mental Illness* is both broad and complex. In opting to approach the topic by predominantly focusing on risk, resilience, treatment engagement, and functional outcomes (as opposed to focusing on DSM-5 diagnostic categories or a specific cohort of TAY, such as college students), we made certain content choices. Topics or subpopulations of TAY not presented do not reflect lack of relevance or importance. And, though we edited this issue with a mindset to avoid repetition or overlap among articles, inevitably some concepts and literature are cited multiple times; this reiteration, in our minds, reflects not only the need for contributors to frame their individual topics but also the salience of the information.

This issue is divided into four sections. The first section serves as a foundation for understanding the transition from late adolescence to young adulthood as a unique developmental stage with potential and opportunities to influence life trajectories. Topics include demographics, epidemiology, normal development, neurodevelopment, and factors promoting risk and resilience in the context of contemporaneous life pathways for TAY. Authors highlight the possible impact of mental illness on psychosocial development and the unique service needs of TAY that extend beyond those of early adolescents and which are clearly different from those of adults. A thoughtful look at how we conceptualize success in young adulthood, especially as we treat heterogeneous patient populations, sets the tone for the remainder of the issue.

The second section reviews common challenges faced by clinicians when working with TAY that cross different diagnostic categories, different treatment settings, and different TAY environmental contexts. Contributing authors discuss involving parents/family in the treatment of TAY, the interface of social media with mental health, suicide, and substance abuse from the perspective of brain maturation, risk, and resilience, and trajectories across the TAY age range. Given the increasing diversity of this age demographic, in parallel with the US population, and the challenge of providing culturally competent care, the article on "Multicultural Developmental Experiences" is included in this section and serves as a bridge to the next section.

In the third section, we focus on several special populations of TAY. These groups or special populations have been selected to highlight certain themes or experiences, such as transitioning to/from institutions or systems, issues of diversity during transition, having experienced adversity during early development, and having difficulties with self-awareness and the perception of others. We include some diagnostic groupings here. Discussion of NAVIGATE, a comprehensive early treatment program for people with first-episode psychosis, provides a link to the final section of the issue.

In the last section, consisting of two articles, the focus is on model programs for supporting transition to adulthood. One article describes an approach to health care transition from pediatric- to adult-oriented models of care, including assessment of readiness for transition, which can be broadly applied in both medical and behavioral health care. The other article highlights the transition to college and a wellness approach based on what we know about brain development, making choices, and life experiences.

We would like to thank our authors, for their valued and thoughtful contributions, and Kristen Helm at Elsevier, for her guidance and support.

Adele Martel, MD, PhD
Department of Psychiatry and Behavioral Sciences
Northwestern University Feinberg School of Medicine
Ann & Robert H. Lurie Children's Hospital of Chicago
Child and Adolescent Psychiatry
225 East Chicago Avenue Box 10
Chicago, IL 60611, USA

D. Catherine Fuchs, MD
Professor of Psychiatry and Behavioral Sciences and Pediatrics
Division of Child and Adolescent Psychiatry
Vanderbilt University Medical Center
Director, Psychological and Counseling Center
Vanderbilt University
1601 23rd Avenue South
Nashville, TN 37212, USA

E-mail addresses:
adele.martel@gmail.com (A. Martel)
catherine.fuchs@vanderbilt.edu (D.C. Fuchs)

REFERENCES

1. Grayson PA. Overview. In: Grayson PA, Meilman PW, editors. College mental health practice. New York: Routledge; 2006. p. 1–20.

2. Davis M. Addressing the needs of youth in transition to adulthood. Adm Policy Ment Health 2003;30(6):495–509.
3. Davis M, Van der Stoep A. The transition to adulthood for youth who have serious emotional disturbance: developmental transition and young adult outcomes. J Ment Health Adm 1997;24(2):400–27.
4. Kessler RC, Berglund P, Demler O, et al. Lifetime prevalence and age-of-onset distributions of DSM-IV disorders in the National Comorbidity Survey Replication. Arch Gen Psychiatry 2005;62(6):593–602.
5. Copeland WE, Wolke D, Shanahan L, et al. Adult functional outcomes of common childhood psychiatric problems: a prospective, longitudinal study. JAMA Psychiatry 2015;72(9):892–9.
6. Martel A, Chenven M, Chan V. The mental health needs of transitioning youth and young adults: a public health priority. AACAP News 2014;45(5):191–2.
7. Wilens TE, Rosenbaum JF. Transitional aged youth: a new frontier in child and adolescent psychiatry. J Am Acad Child Adolesc Psychiatry 2013;52(9):887–90.
8. Oesterle S. Background paper: pathways to young adulthood and preventive interventions targeting young adults. In: IOM (Institute of Medicine) and NRC (National Research Council), editor. Improving the health, safety, and well-being of young adults: workshop summary. Washington, DC: The National Academies Press; 2013. p. 147–76.
9. Martel A, Derenne J, Chan V. Teaching a systematic approach for transitioning patients to college: an interactive continuing medical education program. Acad Psychiatry 2015;39(5):549–54.
10. Rutter M. Pathways from childhood to adult life. J Child Psychol Psychiatry 1989; 30(1):23–51.
11. Schulenberg JE, Sameroff AJ, Cicchetti D. The transition to adulthood as a critical juncture in the course of psychopathology and mental health. Dev Psychopathol 2004;16:799–806.
12. Sood AB, Hudziak J. Prevention of mental health disorders: principles and implementation. Child Adolesc Psychiatr Clin N Am 2016;25(2):xiii–xv.
13. Mychasiuka R, Metz GAS. Epigenetic and gene expression changes in the adolescent brain: what have we learned from animal models? Neurosci Biobehav Rev 2016;70:189–97.
14. Kandel ER. A new intellectual framework for psychiatry. Am J Psychiatry 1998; 155(4):457–69.
15. Copeland WE, Shanahan L, Davis M, et al. Increase in untreated cases of psychiatric disorders during the transition to adulthood. Psychiatr Serv 2015;66(4): 397–403.
16. Hower H, Case BG, Hoeppner B, et al. Use of mental health services in transition age youth with bipolar disorder. J Psychiatr Pract 2013;19(6):464–76.
17. Derenne J, Martel A. A model CSMH curriculum for child and adolescent psychiatry training programs. Acad Psychiatry 2015;39(5):512–6.
18. Sondheimer A, Martel A, Chan V. College student mental health. AACAP News 2012;43(4):188–9.
19. Martel A, Sood AB. Best practices and resources: national models for college student mental health. In: Sood AB, Cohen R, editors. The Virginia Tech Massacre—strategies and challenges for improving mental health policy on campus and beyond. New York: Oxford University Press; 2015. p. 93–125.

Background

Developmental Psychopathology
Risk and Resilience in the Transition to Young Adulthood

Patricia K. Leebens, MAT, MA, MD[a,b,]*, Edwin D. Williamson, MD[c]

KEYWORDS

- Transitional age youth • Risk • Resilience • Pathway to adulthood • Adolescence
- Development • Psychology • Psychiatry

KEY POINTS

- The group of young people in transition between adolescence and adulthood faces a unique set of developmental challenges and is deserving of study as a distinct cohort: transitional age youth (TAY).
- There are multiple factors that present risk or promote resilience in TAY; the effect of these factors varies by individual.
- There are variable pathways to young adulthood in the twenty-first century.
- One common theme for support of TAY is development of connections, including relationships and access to services.
- Resilience in TAY depends on a dynamic set of ecological, biological, and psychological factors.

Growth forward is in spite of losses and therefore requires courage and strength in the individual, as well as protection, permission, and encouragement from the environment.

—*Abraham Maslow[1]*

INTRODUCTION

The word transition derives from the Latin verb *transere* meaning "to cross" or "to go across." In some cases, like a bridge crossing a river to connect two parts of a roadway, the bridge may serve as a passageway to provide a successful continuation of a part of the roadway to another. For some, the transition from adolescence to

Disclosure Statement: The authors have nothing to disclose.
[a] Child, Adolescent, and Adult Psychiatry, Private Practice, 20 West 86th Street, Suite 1A, New York, NY 10025, USA; [b] Yale Child Study Center, Yale University School of Medicine, 230 South Frontage Road, New Haven, CT 06519, USA; [c] Vanderbilt Child and Adolescent Psychiatry Fellowship Program, Vanderbilt University, 1500 21st Avenue South, Nashville, TN 37212, USA
* Corresponding author. 20 West 86th Street, Suite 1A, New York, NY 10025.
E-mail address: patricia.leebens@gmail.com

Child Adolesc Psychiatric Clin N Am 26 (2017) 143–156
http://dx.doi.org/10.1016/j.chc.2016.12.001
1056-4993/17/© 2016 Elsevier Inc. All rights reserved.

childpsych.theclinics.com

young adulthood progresses smoothly, like a bridge crossing, with expected ripples of regression or distress when coping with new demands and new roles but, eventually, with overall effective adaptation to adult demands.

As in physics, transition may also refer to a more dynamic and potentially tumultuous process, such as the "change of an atom, nucleus, electron, etc., from one quantum state to another with emission or absorption of radiation."[2] Because of variations in cognitive and emotional maturity, levels of individual and parental psychopathology, differences in environmental supports or stresses, and other risk and resilience factors, negotiating this passage to adulthood may also be fraught with difficulty for many adolescents and their families, particularly those with past, ongoing, or evolving mental health disorders.[3–6]

DEMOGRAPHICS OF TRANSITIONAL AGE YOUTH

The developmental stage of transitional age youth (TAY) is not fixed in age but occurs as adolescence wanes and adulthood emerges, starting as early as 14 or 15 years for young parents and ending in the twenties or perhaps later given protracted schooling and delays to full-time employment (**Table 1**). As the population demographics in the United States change, so do the numbers for TAY. In 2012, there were 43 million people aged 15 to 24 years (48.7% female) in the United States, which made up 14% of the total population of the United States.[7] This population represents a great diversity of backgrounds, professions, and racial and ethnic groups. In 2015, 73.5% were white, 15.7% were African American, 1.5% American Indian or Native Alaskan, 5.4% Asian, 0.3% Native Hawaiian, and 3.6% 2 or more races. Nearly 22% of this population is Hispanic in ethnicity.[8] Looking ahead at changes to come, the US Census Bureau estimates that the percentage of Americans who are African American will grow by 30% and the percentage that are Hispanic will grow by 80% by 2060.[9]

In terms of activity and profession, a large proportion of the TAY demographic seeks postsecondary education. In 2014, the 18- to 24-year-old population in the United

Table 1		
Characteristics of transitional age youth in the United States		
Age Range of Group (y)	**Date of Study or Statistical Analysis**	**Characteristic Described**
15–24	2012	43 million TAY (14% of total United States)[7] 75% white, 21.7% Hispanic, 15.7% African American, 5.4% Asian, 1.5% Native American, 0.3% Hawaiian[8]
15–24	2012	1,222,199 births to TAY[20]
15–24	2015	57% of TAY in high school or college[11]
15–24	2016	20.5 million in college (50% of all college students)[10]
15–24	2015 1960	65.9% of HS graduates go to college 45% of HS graduates go to college[12]
25 or less	2015	572,293 active duty military[15] (43% are TAY)
18–24	2010	410,000 TAY incarcerated[18]
15–24	2010	10% of all TAY disabled (communicative, physical, mental)[23]
Not specified	2014	22,000 TAY aged out of foster care 36% of US population have college degrees, only 4% of those from foster care[26,27]

States reached approximately 31.5 million and 40% of this age cohort was enrolled in college. Total enrollment in degree-granting postsecondary institutions is expected to be 20.5 million in the fall of 2016. Of those 20.5 million, 15.5 million are expected to be between the ages of 14 and 29 years, and 12 million between the ages of 18 and 24 years. Essentially, the TAY demographic, even when using various age ranges, accounts for more than half of those to be enrolled in college.[10] The Bureau of Labor Statistics reported that in the fall of 2015, 57% of the nation's 15 to 24 year olds were enrolled in high school or college.[11] As for those graduating from high school, the New York Times recently reported that 65.9% of high school graduates go on to attend college. Although this is a slight decrease from the peak of 70.1% in 2009, the longstanding trend has been a steady increase from 1960, when roughly 45% of high school students attended college.[12] For some, attending college is a smooth part of the bridge to adulthood, whereas for others academic stresses and being away from home present challenges.

For some in this age group the main developmental task is achieving employment; however, the unemployment rate for TAY in the fall of 2016 was 8.1%, significantly higher than the average of the total population over 16, which was 4.9%.[13] For those who did find jobs, their median weekly earnings were less than the population as a whole, at $477 versus $791 per week.[14] Economic stressors can add to difficulty in transitioning to independence, whereas success at a job can reinforce development as an independent adult.

This age group also includes 572,293 active duty military 25 years and younger, 43% of all active duty members. In addition, there are 285,894 selected reserve members in this age group.[15] Time spent in the military for some creates a feeling of accomplishment and purpose, as well as leads to the acquisition of marketable skills and/or post-high school education. However, a tour in the military can also expose one to injury, to trauma resulting in post traumatic stress disorder, and to other medical and mental health illnesses. Although the numbers and percentages in the military have not changed over the last 2 decades, participation in war has increased as the United States has fought 2 major wars in Iraq and Afghanistan over the last 15 years. During those years, America has seen the greatest number of deaths and injuries in war since the Vietnam era. Since 9/11, 4683 Americans died in combat as of August 2016. Of those, 2433 were younger than 25 years. There have been a total of 32,799 service members wounded in combat, of all ages.[16] These deaths and injuries affect families, friends, coworkers, and classmates, with widespread ripple effects.

There are also a significant number of people incarcerated during this developmental stage. America saw a large increase in the incarcerated population over the last 50 years, from roughly 500,000 to more than 2 million incarcerated US residents in the current decade.[17] In 2010, there were 410,000 US residents in prison or jail between the ages of 18 and 24 years.[18] Roughly 2% of the adult population in the United States in 2014 was on probation or parole. Although the data are not available by age group, this accounts for 4.7 million US residents of all ages.[19] Time in the correctional system—in jail or on probation—presents risks related to abuse, trauma, and the challenges of finding work with a criminal record.

While navigating transitions of their own, from adolescence to adulthood, there are a significant number of TAY who are parents, as well. Data for the total number of parents living with their children in this age group are not available, but there are data on the number of births to mothers (see **Table 2**). Although there are fewer mothers in this age group now than 15 years ago, almost all of them are unmarried, presenting its own challenges for navigating developmental tasks.

TAY are generally thought of as physically healthy, with a lower rate of death than older adults. However, the Institute of Medicine report on "Investing in the Health and Well-Being of Young Adults,"[20] notes that young adults have high rates of obesity, as well

Table 2
Birth rates of unmarried women

Age Range of Group (y)	1994 (Live Births per 1000 Women)	2014 (Live Births per 1000 Women)
15–17	31.7	10.6
18–19	69.1	39.4
20–24	70.9	61.6

Births to Unmarried Women		
Age Range of Group (y)	1980 (Percent)	2014 (Percent)
15–17	61.5	95.7
18–19	39.8	86.0
20–24	19.3	65.7

Data from http://www.childstats.gov/americaschildren/tables/fam2a.asp and https://www.childstats.gov/americaschildren/tables/fam2b.asp. Accessed September 18, 2016.

as mental health and substance abuse issues. A 2014 Substance Abuse and Mental Health Services Administration (SAMHSA) study reports that one-fifth of young adults ages 18 to 25 had a mental illness in the past year, yet two-thirds of those did not receive treatment. Technological changes that contribute to increased sedentary occupations and pastimes also contribute to poor health. Prolonged transitions to adulthood isolate young adults from jobs and family life which, in turn, may decrease their participation in at-risk behaviors (drug and alcohol use, multiple sexual partners, poor lifestyle decisions).[20] Simultaneously, there is a significant portion of the population that lives with disability as classified by the federal government. In 2010, 10.2% of Americans ages 15 to 24 years had "any disability" (communicative, mental, or physical) according to the US census.[21]

Other marginalized groups that are subject to unique challenges are lesbian, gay, bisexual, and transgender (LGBT) youth and young adults. In a 2012 Gallup poll of 120,000 Americans, ages 18 to 29 years, 6.4% responded "yes" to the question, "Do you identify as lesbian, gay, bisexual or transgender?" Of these, 90.1% responded "no" and 3.5% refused to answer or replied "do not know."[22] Although consolidating sexual identity is a formative experience for some, discrimination and harassment is associated with higher dropout rates for LGBT students, presenting risks to normative development.[23]

TAY who are immigrants and children of immigrants are growing as a group. In 1990, there were roughly 8 million children younger than 18 years old in the United States with at least 1 immigrant parent, compared with 2014 when there were 17 million.[24] In addition to children of immigrants, in 2014 there were nearly 4 million immigrants in the United States between the ages of 15 and 24 years.[25] Challenges to TAY immigrants, particularly those without legal immigration status, include limited job and education opportunities, as well as access to health care services of all kinds, including mental health services.

Given the importance of family support and/or close relationships, it is no surprise that adolescents who age out of foster care have more difficulties with the transition to adulthood. In 2014, 22,000 young Americans aged out of foster care and entered this stage without the support of a family structure.[26] Navigating transition to college or a job without support from family has documented negative effects. Compared with the 36% of the general population who earn a 4-year college degree, only 4% of these youth who aged out of foster care were able to reach this same milestone.[27]

UNIQUE CHARACTERISTICS OF TRANSITIONAL AGE YOUTH
Body and Brain Changes

Driven by changes in the hormonal milieu in the adolescent, bodily changes include increased height and muscle mass; primary, and secondary sexual characteristics; and maturing internal organs (**Box 1**). These changes contribute to increased physical and sexual risk-taking, which may put the young adult into dangerous situations. TAY also have changes in brain neuroanatomy that impact their cognitive and emotional development. Synaptic pruning, which is very evident during this age, contributes to continued maturation of the basal ganglia and prefrontal cortex. However, these brain areas mature at different rates with the limbic system, governing reward-based drives, maturing earlier than the frontal lobes, which are related to processing, inhibiting, and decision making.[3,28] Fortunately, the prefrontal cortex continues to mature through the twenties, with improved executive functioning and lessened impulsive reactions to rewards. Changes in neurotransmitter levels during this age can affect psychiatric symptoms and responses to pharmacologic agents.[29] Exposure to toxins (ie, drugs, infections, extreme stress, or hypoxia) during preadolescence and adolescence can also affect adult functioning. For example, some adolescent exposure to marijuana may increase risk of psychosis in vulnerable youths.[3,29]

Social Changes

TAY also experience multiple changes in their social roles and legal status. Relationships with parents often change with the youth's push for separation and individuation. Relationships with peers and other adults outside of the family may intensify, causing strain in family relationships. The process of separation and individuation is particularly challenging for youths who immigrated to the United States or who are first-generation US citizens. The family may need the young person to stay attached to the family to help with English translation, to provide financial support for the family, and to help care for dependent family members. However, the young adult may have embraced the push for independence of the American culture, creating strain between the young adult and their family.

Increased independence and changes in legal status (eg, access to driving, drinking, tobacco, joining the military) may lead to new experiences and experimentation, which can contribute to individuation and growth or may increase risks such as substance use, impulsive sexual encounters, mismanagement of finances, traumatizing work, or training settings, which may alter the individual's mental health and course of development.

Box 1
Neurobiological features characteristic of transitional age youth stage of development

- Brain development incomplete: limbic areas (emotional or reward centers) develop earlier than frontal lobes (processing, inhibiting, judgment, decision-making).[3]

- Continued increase in synaptic density in prefrontal cortex: may lead to improved executive functioning and improved decisions making between ages 20 and 30.[50]

- Preadolescent and adolescent exposure to toxins (eg, drugs, hypoxia, stress, infection) can impact adult responses: adolescent marijuana exposure and increased risk of psychosis in vulnerable youth.[3,29]

- Continued myelination and extensive synaptic pruning: leads to maturation of affect, cognition (ie, abstract reasoning), and motor behavior.

- Changes in neurotransmitter levels and pharmacologic sensitivity: can affect onset of or changes in ongoing psychiatric disorders and response to psychotropic medications.

TRANSITIONAL AGE YOUTH DEVELOPMENTAL TASKS

The developmental tasks of TAY encompass many of the tasks of adolescence and young adulthood. Tasks such as forming one's own identity, separating from parents, and developing autonomy and intimacy are all central to this age group. Transition markers such as needing work and being available for work, starting a family, and engaging in civic roles may begin in this stage of life. At the same time, the context of life is crucial to determining how development unfolds during this stage. Whether one is living with one's parents, attending college, enrolling in the military, in jail, or on probation may be the determining factor of how development unfolds. The transition of late adolescents to young adulthood is also affected by one's race, ethnicity, location (urban vs rural), family background (eg, presence or absence of parental discord or divorce), education, socioeconomic status, and available community resources.[30,31] Going to college, getting a job, living independently, and having an intimate relationship and possibly children are all traditional developmental tasks but all require adaptation to new demands and new societal roles. An individualized approach that takes into account all of these factors while considering the developmental context is necessary to understanding the transition challenges of a young adult.

CONTEMPORARY TRENDS IN PATHWAYS TO ADULTHOOD

Changes in societal trends in recent years (ie, economic recessions, rising housing costs, evolving family structures with longer periods of education and lengthy delays until marriage) suggest that this developmental transition may be more protracted, more complex, and less linear (with returns to the family of origin or other adolescent supports for emotional and financial assistance) than previous generations.[30,31] Variability in the pathways to adulthood may continue throughout the twenty-first century, contributing to "less predictable and more precarious" transitions to adulthood for all late adolescents.[32] The impact of natural and man-made disasters in the beginning of the twenty-first century, which has often resulted in large numbers of displaced and traumatized individuals and families, has also highlighted the importance of appreciating resilience within a cultural and global framework.[33]

As the transition time between adolescence and adulthood has lengthened and become less standardized, it is less a mere passageway into adulthood milestones (ie, work, marriage, children) and more a unique time of development.[5] During this time, childhood and adolescent risk factors may magnify problems of functioning and interact with emerging psychiatric disorders, resulting in worse adult adjustment. For example, an adolescent with anxiety and attention deficit hyperactivity disorder (ADHD) who may have functioned well with a structured and well-supervised living environment, compliance with medication regimens, and loving support from parents, may see a decline in functioning in college when medication noncompliance, increased alcohol and drug use, and poor health practices lead to academic failure and worsened psychiatric outcomes. As Masten[33] notes, "risk factors are often related to one another: risk predicts risk." With a larger percentage of this age group going off to college than ever before, these challenges can be expected more frequently, particularly as TAY with special needs move away from home.

Likewise, children and adolescents with emotional and/or educational difficulties who have done well when provided with supportive home and school environments may not have become inoculated to stressful situations and may not have developed adequate and independent coping skills to help them manage the demands of independent living. Helping these adolescents transition successfully to adult demands may require ongoing support during higher education and employment while developing independent life skills. Ideally, this support is gradually lessened as the young adult demonstrates increased competence.

AGE OF VULNERABILITY

Changes in the young adult's hormonal milieu and neuroanatomy, along with the stress of changing demands and roles may contribute to their great vulnerability to psychiatric disturbances. Late adolescence and young adulthood is the most common age of onset of many psychiatric disorders. This transition, then, can be even more perilous for some adolescents because of the onset of or worsening of psychiatric disorders such as substance abuse, eating disorders, mood disorders, schizophrenia, persistent anxiety, continued effects of ADHD and learning disabilities (**Box 2**).

This is also a time of vulnerability because the evolving independence of the TAY may also interfere with the ability to acknowledge their difficulties and their need for help, to accept help when needed, to comply with treatment interventions, and to allow participation and communication between the treaters and parents. Because of the Affordable Care Act, many TAY may have access to medical and mental health care through their parents' insurance; however, some young adults may avoid mental health treatment, fearing their parents will see insurance claims for substance abuse treatment and/or mental health services. These issues may compromise the young adult's psychiatric stability just at a vulnerable time of transition to college, to the work world, or to a role as parent. Also, mental health services for TAY often do not address the specific needs or services for this population, and are often combined with services for adolescents or with older adults with chronic psychiatric disorders (**Box 3**).

Box 2
Psychiatric vulnerabilities in transitional age youth

- Childhood ADHD affect 6% to 9% of youth, but 75% of cases continue into adolescence and 50% of cases into adulthood.

- Childhood anxiety disorders increase likelihood of depression, post-traumatic stress syndrome, and substance use disorder (SUD) in adulthood.

- Rates of mood disorders and eating orders increase in TAY.

- Autism spectrum disorder affects 2% of children and adolescents but increase in male children ages 14 to 17 years.

- Three-fourths of adults with SUD have onset before age 25 years.

- Forty-seven percent of female patients and 62% of male patients with schizophrenia have onset before age 25 years.

- Homicide (mainly firearms) is second highest cause of death, whereas suicide is the third highest cause of death in 12 to 25 year olds. Unintentional injuries, mainly motor vehicle accidents, are first.

- More than 60% of young adults have had a psychiatric disorder by age 25 years.

- Young adults have the highest rates of sexually transmitted infections, including human immunodeficiency virus (HIV).

- Young adults have the highest rates of behavioral problems but the lowest perception of risk and least access to preventive care and treatment.

Data from Refs.[3,28,50]

Box 3
Mental health care in transitional age youth

- Transition of pediatric care to adult care is often difficult, confusing, or require individual TAY to initiate services

- 2014 Substance Abuse and Mental Health Services Administration (SAMHSA) study show one-fifth of TAY age 18 to 25 had mental illness in past year, but two-thirds had no treatment

- Current MH Services for TAY are often fragmented and lumped with older adults or younger adolescents

- 2012 Study report that 17% of TAY ages 16 to 24 were neither in school nor working, with decreased access to special education and/or mental health care

- TAY more likely to be noncompliant with treatment and/or with seeking help, particularly if barriers

- Confidentiality issues can compromise needed family involvement in treatment

Data from Refs.[3,20,28]

DEVELOPMENTAL PSYCHOPATHOLOGY

Understanding the unique developmental challenges and strengths of TAY, as well as their vulnerabilities, helps clinicians appreciate the complex impact of the passage to adulthood on an individual's developmental tasks as they interact with mental health issues. Recent research in developmental psychopathology helps mental health practitioners understand the interactions between the individual and his or her environment that affect mental health development.[5] This area of study provides an integrative framework to comprehend the relationships between normal and abnormal mental health development[34,35] and "individual differences in adaptation and development over the lifespan."[33]

Rather than describing mental illness as a specific entity that resides in an individual, this framework looks at the dynamic interaction between "intraindividual and extraindividual contexts."[35] **When** positive or deleterious circumstances arrive in an individual's life, or **when** signs or symptoms of abnormal development occur, and **how** these interact with past events and present internal or external situations may ultimately predict and/or affect future functioning.

The work of Eric Kandel[36] and others studying epigenetics, or the study of mechanisms controlling gene expression during an organism's development, demonstrate that experiences in life can produce sustained changes in behavior by altering gene expression, potentially worsening or easing the impact of a psychiatric disorder. For example, early childhood abuse may have negative impact on an adolescent's eventual occupational and psychosocial adjustment; however, an adolescent's above-average intelligence, his or her individual determination, an appropriate school placement, and support from a functional and caring parent may ameliorate the potential negative consequences of the abuse and may contribute to a positive adult outcome.

Early research in developmental psychopathology began by focusing on risk factors correlated with an increased probability of a negative outcome or maladjustment in an individual or groups of individuals.[33,35] Researchers focused on factors present in the child, family, and environment to understand factors that might lead to poor or compromised outcomes. Low birth weight, family violence, harsh parenting, homelessness, family history of mental illness, poverty, and poor health practices all became identified as risk factors contributing to maladjustment in adulthood.[33]

Studies of risk looked at the timing of exposure to risk, the degree of exposure to risk factors, the cumulative impact of multiple risk factors, and the impact of multiple risk factors over multiple developmental periods.[35] The Adverse Childhood Events (ACE) study looked at the impact of childhood traumas and a stressful environment on the later development of significant medical problems (eg, hypertension, obesity, diabetes), which led to premature aging and an early death for some.[37]

As this field matured, studies of risk revealed that not all children or adolescents exposed to known risk factors had the same negative outcome. Differences in outcome led to a realization that some individuals are more resilient than others. Aspects of one's individual biology (eg, higher intelligence, overall better physical health, greater brain plasticity) as well as psychosocial protective factors (eg, competent parenting, strong social network, safe living environment) contribute to the individual's resilience.[35] Predictors of resilience focused on the "triad of protective factors," which were characteristics of the individual (intelligence quotient [IQ], temperament), the family (predictable, effective parenting), and the environment (safe neighborhood, effective school).[38]

For most studies of risk and resilience, a better outcome was described as competence in 3 main areas: academic achievement, conduct (rule-abiding), and peer social acceptance and friendship.[39] A classic longitudinal study from the 1990s followed over 200 elementary children (90 boys, 114 girls; 27% racial minorities) for 10 years. Four important results emerged: (1) competence is related to psychosocial resources; (2) good resources are less available among children growing up with adversity; (3) if good resources are available, competence outcomes are good, even with chronic and severe stressors; and (4) children who have limited competence are stress-reactive, have longstanding adversity, and have low resources.[39]

Masten[40] has recently summarized a short-list of resilience factors in young people and/or their environment, based on 50 years of resilience research. Most important of these factors are (1) attachment and close relationships with others; (2) effective caregivers; (3) intelligence and problem-solving skills; (4) self-control, planfulness, and emotion regulation; (5) motivation to succeed; (6) self-efficacy; (7) effective schools; (8) effective neighborhoods; and (9) faith, hope, or belief that life has meaning.

Programs to support these resilience factors in children and adolescents, as well as their caretakers and communities, are being devised to encourage and support healthy development, particularly in populations at risk. Recent research demonstrates that programs that focus on promoting competence and success in children who may be at risk for behavioral or psychiatric disorders are much more effective than programs focused on reducing problems or deficits.[33] Because "competence begets competence,"[33] a smooth passageway to adulthood for many adolescents must begin with building competence and successes early on. Ideally, these youth develop strengths and strategies from coping with stress, along with supportive relationships, that help with a successful passage into adulthood.

Recent scholars describe resilience as a "dynamic process by which individuals adapt successfully to an adverse experience."[33] Resilience is not simply the outcome of the sum of protective factors minus risk factors. As a dynamic process, protective factors in a developmental stage that seem instrumental to a child's resilience, may contribute to worsening outcomes in another developmental stage. For example, attentive parents who provide much support and oversight for their ADHD or learning disabled child may help improve his or her functioning at home and in high school. However, these same parental behaviors may be detrimental to a young adult who has difficulty in college because of an inability to structure his or her own life to meet every day demands. Such young adults who have a failure to launch may require family therapy with their parents to alter the parental behavior to help stimulate growth and development in their child.[4] Recent resilience research has indicated that stress-inoculation or exposure to moderate amounts of stress may be necessary for developing effective coping skills to manage adversity.[33]

Pathways to Adulthood of Youth with Mental Illness

Early studies of childhood psychopathology raised questions about what contributions, if any, early psychiatric difficulties may play in the development of adult psychiatric illnesses. Recent longitudinal studies of children have increased opportunities to study possible connections between early childhood behaviors or possible prodromal symptoms and adult psychiatric disorders, as well as the impact of exposures or events during the transition to the new developmental stage. Costello and colleagues[41] in the Great Smoky Mountains Study, with a 20-year follow-up of school age youth, found that 60% of those with childhood psychiatric disorders had reported adverse outcomes (in health, legal, financial, or social areas) compared with 20% of those with no childhood mental health disorders. In an earlier study in New Zealand, Copeland, and colleagues[42] found that having a psychiatric disorder in childhood was a "potent risk factor" for psychiatric problems later in development, with heterotypic and homotypic transitions noted in all disorder categories. Longitudinal studies in a variety of populations suggest that abnormalities in childhood may be precursors of schizophrenia, even if not all children with these early precursors manifest schizophrenia later.[43] Recent research suggests that heavy cannabis use in adolescents, particularly those with these precursors or prodromal symptoms of schizophrenia, may be more at risk for developing a thought disorder.[43] This complex interaction of early biological risk with compounding factors during transitional stages are important areas to study and may help us understand the continuity or discontinuity in the expression of psychiatric disorders.

Also, studying public policy issues which impact on TAY access to appropriate, available, and affordable psychiatric treatment is crucial. Copeland and colleagues,[44] in a study of changes of rates of service use and untreated psychiatric disorders during the transition from adolescence to adulthood, found that young adults often have much less psychiatric treatment (28.9%) compared with adolescents (50.9%), though issues of insurance and poverty were unrelated to use of psychiatric services.

Developmental psychopathology is particularly interested in continuity and discontinuity in development and the impact that transitions in development may have on the next stage of growth and the emergence of or improvement of psychiatric disorders. For example, why do some teens with successful and productive adolescent years become handicapped with debilitating substance abuse disorders and tumultuous interpersonal relationships following the transition to college? Likewise, why do some troubled high schoolers manage to turn their lives around and become functioning and often successful adults? Schulenberg and colleagues[5] point out that there is much to learn from these discontinuities in development. Discontinuities may be related to early childhood factors that could be predicted and could be lessened or magnified to affect an adult outcome. Alternatively, changes in functioning may be related to the stress or nature of the transition itself and exposures that may be common during the transition but not in earlier stages of development. Finally, the change seen during this developmental transition should be considered as a turning point leading to a different developmental course (positive or negative).[5]

Continuities and discontinuities become particularly important concerning children and adolescents with current or potentially emerging mental illnesses and the impact that these illnesses may have on educational and occupational attainment.[42,44] For example, a 30-year, 3-generation, longitudinal study of mental health demonstrated that mental health in adolescence was an important predictor of educational and occupational outcomes 12 years later, even more than IQ scores and family socioeconomic status.[6]

SUMMARY

The transition to adulthood is an important stage of life that connects childhood and adolescence to adulthood. Given the complex nature of development, multiple factors in the individual and in the environment interact over a lifespan to create a unique life. Developmental transitions can help consolidate new behaviors for the next stage of life, can provide opportunities to change pathways, or can be fraught with risk and danger for the fragile or unprepared individual. Understanding these continuities and discontinuities in a life requires an intimate appreciation of the individual. As Rutter[45] notes, "Transitions need to be considered in personal terms."

TAY have unique vulnerabilities that may make their pathway to adulthood particularly challenging. Given the plasticity of brain development, which continues well into the twenties, as well as neuroscience research, which continues to identify allelic variants that might confer protection against environmental insults,[3,38] the period of development of TAY deserves increased scientific scrutiny, as well as financial support for effective policy and therapeutic interventions to assist TAY with mental illness with a successful navigation to adulthood. Future research can help focus on identifying mediating processes (eg, biological, environmental, epigenetic, educational, therapeutic) that might improve the long-term trajectory of at-risk youth.[43]

Also, it is crucial for child and adolescent psychiatrists, and others who work with this age group, to:

- Understand the distinct characteristics of this period of development[31]
- Recognize signs and symptoms of emerging psychiatric disorders[3]
- Know risk and resilience factors that may prevent or promote successful transitions to adulthood[33,35,38]
- Be aware of changes in the world today that place greater demands on young adults[20,30]
- Be able to implement effective therapeutic interventions to lessen the impact of mental illnesses in this age group.[3]

Having an understanding of an individual's developmental challenges and opportunities will help set the stage for a successful path to adulthood.

Likewise, it is imperative for fiscal and social policy makers, medical and mental health providers, and parents to realize the impact of the changing trends of transition to adulthood so they can support young adults with appropriate medical, mental health, and social services that focus on their special needs. Specialized college programs can help the transition to higher education of TAY with special needs.[46,47] Because college students with psychiatric illness drop out of college at twice the rate of the general population, some TAY will benefit from programs such as supported education, which have focused on the factors that influence risk (eg, cognitive impairment, social stigma) and resilience (peer relationships, coping skills) to promote retention at the college level.[48] For young adults with autism, VanBergeijk and colleagues[49] have suggested using the transition plan component of the individualized education program in high school to make a detailed plan for transition to college, creating an individualized college plan that would "outline academic modifications, independent living skills, socialization skills and goals, vocational goals, and mental health supports."

Other potential solutions are financial assistance or loan forgiveness programs for those with large educational debts and affordable child care for working parents.

Additionally, viable occupational options are needed for immigrant youth (documented and undocumented), for those emerging from incarceration, for those in highly structured special education programs, and for those leaving the military, or foster care, to promote a variety of successful pathways to independence. International studies suggest the following to improve transitions to adulthood for all youths: (1) more vocational or educational programs for young people who choose not to attend college, (2) more vocational guidance for all adolescents, and (3) more connections between educational programs and employment through internships or apprenticeships.[32]

Research, programs, and financial investment are all needed to help improve the chances of all youths to succeed in adulthood. Most importantly, as Luthar and Prince[34] remind us, "resilience rests, fundamentally, on relationships." Being a parent, teacher, tutor, mentor, therapist, psychiatrist, coach provide opportunities to connect with children and families to help build competences, confidences, and community.

We are social beings, with a need for connection to the "magnetic chain of humanity."

—*Nathaniel Hawthorne, Ethan Brand, 1850*

REFERENCES

1. Maslow AH, Stephens DC. The Maslow business reader. New York: John Wiley & Sons; 2000.
2. Transition (n.d.). Available at: https://www.google.com/#q=transition. Accessed October 08, 2016.
3. Wilens TE, Rosenbaum JF. Transitional aged youth: a new frontier in child and adolescent psychiatry. J Am Acad Child Adolesc Psychiatry 2013;52:887–90.
4. Lebowitz ER. Failure to launch: shaping intervention for highly dependent adult children. J Am Acad Child Adolesc Psychiatry 2016;55:89–90.
5. Schulenberg JE, Sameroff AJ, Cicchetti D. The transition to adulthood as a critical juncture in the course of psychopathology and mental health. Dev Psychopathol 2004;16:799–806.
6. Slominski L, Sameroff A, Rosenblum K, et al. Longitudinal predictors of adult socioeconomic attainment: the roles of socioeconomic status, academic competence, and mental health. Dev Psychopathol 2011;23:315–24.
7. U.S. Census Bureau, Current population Survey, Annual Social and Economic Supplement, 2012.
8. U.S. Census Bureau; Annual Estimates of the Resident Population by Sex, Age, Race, and Hispanic Origin for the United States and States: April 1, 2010 to July 1, 2015; generated by Edwin Williamson; using American FactFinder. 2016. Available at: http://factfinder2.census.gov. Accessed September 18, 2016.
9. U.S. Census Bureau projections show a slower growing, older, more diverse nation a half century from now. Newsroom Archive. Washington, DC: US Census Bureau; 2012. Web September 20, 2016.
10. Fast Facts. Fast Facts. Washington, DC: National Center for Education Statistics; 2016. Web September 18, 2016.
11. U.S. Bureau of Labor Statistics. College enrollment and work activity of 2015 high school graduates. Washington, DC: U.S. Bureau of Labor Statistics; 2016. Web September 05, 2016.
12. Norris F. Fewer U.S. Graduates Opt for College After High School. New York Times 2016.

13. U.S. Bureau of Labor Statistics. A-10. Unemployment rates by age, sex, and marital status, seasonally adjusted. Washington, DC: U.S. Bureau of Labor Statistics; 2016. Web September 20, 2016.
14. United States Bureau of Labor Statistics. Highlights of women's earnings in 2014. Washington, DC: US Department of Defense; 2015. Print. Report 1058.
15. Source, Military One. Demographics Profile of the military community. Washington, DC: US Department of Defense; 2014. p. 35.
16. Powers R. What are the Iraq and Afghanistan casualty statistics? The Balance; 2016. Web September 20, 2016.
17. Travis J, Redburn S, Western B. Rising incarceration rates. The growth of incarceration in the United States: exploring causes and consequences. Chapter 2. Washington, DC: National Academies; 2014. p. 33.
18. Child Trends Databank. Young adults in jail or prison. 2012. Available at: http://www. childtrends.org/?indicators=young-adults-in-jail-or-prison. Accessed September 18, 2016.
19. US Department of Justice. Bureau of Justice Statistics. Probation and Parole in the United States, 2014. By Danielle Kaeble. 2015.
20. Investing in the health and well-being of young adults. In: Institute of Medicine of the National Academies, October, 2014. Available at: www.nationalacademies.org/ hmd/~/media/Files/Report Files/2014/YAYAreportbrief.pdf. Accessed September 6, 2016.
21. Brault MW. Americans with disabilities 2010. Washington, DC: U.S. Dept. of Commerce, Economics and Statistics Administration, U.S. Census Bureau; 2012. Available at: http://www.census.gov/prod/2012pubs/p70-131.pdf. Accessed September 11, 2016.
22. Gallup, Inc. Special report: 3.4% of U.S. adults identify as LGBT. Gallup.com 2012. Web September 24, 2016.
23. Sanlo R. Lesbian, gay, and bisexual college students: risk, resiliency, and retention. J Coll Stud Ret 2004;6(1):97–110, p98.
24. Alexander T, Genadek K, Goeken R, et al. Children in U.S. Immigrant families. Migrationpolicy.org; 2016. Web October 18, 2016.
25. Alexander T, Genadek K, Goeken R, et al. Age-sex pyramids of U.S. immigrant and native-born populations, 1970-present. Migrationpolicy.org; 2016. Web October 18, 2016.
26. The AFCARS report, vol. 22. Household economic studies, administration for children and families. Washington, DC: U.S. Department of Health and Human Services, Administration for Children and Families, Administration on Children, Youth and Families, Children's Bureau; 2010.
27. Courtney M, Dworsky A, Brown A, et al. Midwest evaluation of the adult functioning of former foster youth: outcomes at age 26. Chicago: Chapin Hall at the University of Chicago; 2011.
28. Stroud C, Mainero T, Olson S, editors. Improving the health, safety, and well-being of young adults: workshop summary. Washington, DC: National Academies Press; 2013.
29. Anderson SL. Trajectories of brain development: point of vulnerability or window of opportunity? Neurosci Biobehav Rev 2003;27:3–18.
30. Waters MC, Carr PJ, Kefalas MJ, et al. Coming of age in America: the transition to adulthood in the twenty-first century. Berkeley (CA): University of California Press; 2011. p. 1–19, 191–204.
31. Cohen P, Kasen S, Chen H, et al. Variations in patterns of developmental transitions in the emerging adulthood period. Dev Psychol 2003;39(4):657–69.

32. Shanahan MJ. Pathways to adulthood in changing societies: variability and mechanisms in life course perspective. Annu Rev Sociol 2000;26:667–92.
33. Masten AS. Global perspectives on resilience in children and youth. Child Dev 2014;85(1):6–20.
34. Luthar SS, Prince RP. Developmental psychopathology. In: Martin A, Volkmar FR, editors. Lewis's child and adolescent psychiatry: a comprehensive textbook. 4th edition. Philadelphia: Lippincott Williams; 2007. p. 291–9.
35. Kim-Cohen J. Resilience and developmental psychopathology. Child Adolesc Psychiatr Clin N Am 2007;16:271–83.
36. Kandel ER. A new intellectual framework for psychiatry. Am J Psychiatry 1998; 155(4):457–69.
37. Felitti VJ, Anda RF, Nordenberg D, et al. Relationship of childhood abuse and household dysfunction to many of the leading causes of death in adults: the Adverse Childhood Experiences (ACE) Study. Am J Prev Med 1998;14(4):245–58.
38. Kim-Cohen J, Turkewitz R. Resilience and measured gene–environment interactions. Dev Psychopathol 2012;24(04):1297–306.
39. Masten AS, Hubbard JJ, Gest SD, et al. Competence in the context of adversity: pathways to resilience and maladaptation from childhood to late adolescence. Dev Psychopathol 1999;11(01):143–69.
40. Masten AS. Ordinary magic: resilience in development. New York: Guilford Publications; 2015.
41. Costello EJ, Copeland W, Angold A. The Great Smoky Mountains study: developmental epidemiology in the southeastern United States. Soc Psychiatry Psychiatr Epidemiol 2016;51(5):639–46.
42. Copeland WE, Adair CE, Smetanin P, et al. Diagnostic transitions from childhood to adolescence to early adulthood. J Child Psychol Psychiatry 2013;54(7):791–9.
43. Rutter M, Kim-Cohen J, Maughan B. Continuities and discontinuities in psychopathology between childhood and adult life. J Child Psychol Psychiatry 2006; 47(3–4):276–95.
44. Copeland WE, Shanahan L, Davis M, et al. Increase in untreated cases of psychiatric disorders during the transition to adulthood. Psychiatr Serv 2015;66: 397–403.
45. Rutter M. Pathways from childhood to adult life. J Child Psychol Psychiatry 1989; 30(1):23–51.
46. Hong D. Adolescence to adulthood: are some children falling into the gap? J Am Acad Child Adolesc Psychiatry 2013;52:885–6.
47. Chan V. Special needs: scholastic disability accommodations from K-12 and transitions to higher education. Curr Psychiatry Rep 2016;18(21):1–7.
48. Hartley MT. Increasing resilience: strategies for reducing dropout rates for college students with psychiatric disabilities. Am J Psychiatr Rehabil 2010;13(4): 295–315.
49. VanBergeijk E, Klin A, Volkmar F. Supporting more able students on the autism spectrum: college and beyond. J Autism Dev Disord 2008;38(7):1359–70.
50. Oesterle S. Background paper: pathways to young adulthood and preventive interventions targeting young adults. Institute of Medicine and National Research Council, improving the health, safety, and well-being of young adults: workshop summary. Washington, DC: National Academies of Sciences, Engineering, and Medicine; 2013. p. 147–76.

The Transitional Age Brain
"The Best of Times and the Worst of Times"

Winston W. Chung, MD[a], James J. Hudziak, MD[b],*

KEYWORDS

- Transitional age youth • Brain development • Transitional age brain • Behavior
- Neuroscience

KEY POINTS

- Over the past 2 decades, there have been substantial developments in the understanding of brain development.
- Progress in neuroimaging has allowed us to better understand the nuances of the development of cortical, subcortical, and white matter structures.
- Modern neuroscience, genomics, and epigenomic studies allow us a lens through which to develop an understanding of transitional age youth (TAY) behavior from a neurodevelopmental perspective.
- Developing brain building health promotion and illness prevention approaches for TAY will likely yield reductions in morbidity and mortality, enhance individual life trajectories, and have a life-long impact.

INTRODUCTION

A great deal of attention has been paid to the so-called zero to 3 period of brain development. Although clearly an important focus of neuroscience and public health, there is emerging evidence that a second critical period of neurodevelopment exists, bracketed by the onset of the peripubertal process to the completion of cortical organization (roughly ages 13–25). This 'transitional age brain' (TAB) epoch is marked by an increase in risk for morbidity, mortality, drug and alcohol use/misuse, and the onset of persistent psychiatric and nonpsychiatric medical conditions.

The central hypothesis is that the TAB has fully matured risk-taking hardware because of early maturation of subcortical brain regions (amygdala, nucleus

Disclosure Statement: The authors have nothing to disclose.
[a] Vermont Center for Children, Youth, and Family, University of Vermont Medical Center, 1 South Prospect Street, Arnold 3, Burlington, Vermont 05401, USA; [b] University of Vermont College of Medicine and Medical Center, 1 South Prospect Street, Arnold 3, Burlington, Vermont 05401, USA
* Corresponding author.
E-mail address: James.Huziak@med.uvm.edu

accumbens, etc) but does not yet have matured regulatory hardware (fully pruned pre-frontal and related cortical regions). We maintain that adolescents (13–17 of age) and their TABs benefit from imposed external regulatory systems in the form of parents, family members, teachers, and coaches. Even with external control and expectations, transitional age youth (TAY) remain at very high risk for morbidity and mortality associated with suicide, substance use and misuse, psychiatric illness, and accidents. At the same time that TAY and their maturing brains need more external regulatory support and lower risk environments, they instead have easier access to alcohol and drugs, high-risk social activities, and loss of close parenting and supervision. In other words, these negative environmental factors are in play at a very vulnerable time of brain development, in which the regulatory regions of the brain are undergoing the critical process of maturation.

Herein, we discuss the neurodevelopmental processes (with a special emphasis on pruning) that place TAY at high risk to make impulsive, poorly regulated decisions. We present a description of the symphony of brain development (neurogenesis, synaptogenesis, myelination, and pruning) from fertilization to the end of the TAB period to set the stage for just why the TAB epoch is a critical period. Although we emphasize the potential negative consequences of the TAB epoch, we also want to acknowledge that the same features of adolescent and young adult brain development may be a strength that allows TAY and TAB to respond to psychosocial interventions or to changes in environmental context with improved trajectories into adulthood.

EARLY BRAIN DEVELOPMENT

With advances in both structural (MRI) and functional (fMRI) imaging techniques, along with creative experimental designs using fMRI, information about the development of the human brain has been rapidly expanding. Still, research in the field continues to rely on studies the using other mammalian species with the extrapolation of data to humans.[1]

Human brain development begins during the third week of gestation and continues to about the middle of the second decade, when the components involved in executive function become fully formed. It is a process that is intricate and tightly controlled, yet allows for some flexibility to adapt to the idiosyncrasies of the environment. One theme that emerges is that the brain matures by becoming more interconnected and each region becoming more specialized. Another theme that emerges is the process of overproduction before the elimination of excessive cells and connections based on experience, ultimately resulting in an efficient and unique processor.

The process begins with gastrulation, with differentiation of neural progenitor cells, followed by formation of the neural tube, then the neocortex and synaptic pathways. Around gestational week 28, the number of neurons in the human brain is at its peak, a level 40% greater than in adults. Dendritic growth, arborization, and synaptogenesis begin to accelerate rapidly.[2–9] The rate of synaptogenesis reaches its peak around gestational week 34, but the net decrease of synapses does not begin to decrease until the onset of puberty.[2,7–10] At the same time, up to 50% of the neurons undergo cell death to begin the process of establishing definitive connections.[11]

After birth, neurogenesis is largely complete, and a dynamic process of synaptogenesis, myelination, programmed cell death, and pruning ensues as intrinsic and extrinsic signals interact. In the initial critical period up to age 3, development is dominated by synaptogenesis and by age 2 to 3, a toddler has more synapses than an adult and peaks at a level nearly twice that of adults.[12,13] Some networks connections are exuberant, and entire networks are sometimes formed that are not found in adults.[14–16] This process is regulated by neurotrophic factors such as brain-derived neurotrophic factor (BDNF), which blocks apoptosis.[17,18]

Gray and white matter develop in concert with sensorimotor areas developing first, and then progressing to spatial orientation and language, before concluding with association regions (frontal lobe). There is a profound temporal mismatch between early subcortical development (limbic areas including the nucleus accumbens, amygdala, and others) and cortical regulatory regions. This period of cortical organization or pruning takes place during this second critical period during the transitional age (13–25 years), when the final pruning and myelination takes place. This leads to improved executive function such as attention, concentration, impulse control, reasoning, planning, problem solving, and mood regulation.

BRAIN PATTERNING AND PLASTICITY

During the prenatal period, a basic structure of brain organization is developed. The core structures from the spinal cord to the neocortex and the major compartments within these structures are formed, and there is an initial partitioning of the neocortex into well-defined functional areas.[19–23] This initial patterning is underdefined, malleable, and based largely on intrinsic signaling.[24] Beginning in the late prenatal period, brain development is exquisitely responsive to extrinsic signaling or experience. Significant alterations to the brain structure can occur depending on whether the environment is enriched or deprived. This plasticity allows the mammalian brain to adapt to its environment.

The early patterning of the brain is well illustrated through the development of the neocortex. Emx2 and Pax6 are 2 signaling molecules produced in opposite gradients along the anterior–posterior axis in the neocortical proliferative zone.[25] The concentration of Pax6 is greatest in the anterior and lateral regions, whereas the highest concentration of Emx2 is in the posterior and medial regions. It is the relative concentration of each of these signaling molecules that contribute to the early patterning.[19,25,26] High concentration of Pax6 and low concentration of Emx2 leads to the development of motor cortex (M1). However, a low concentration of Pax6 and a high concentration of Emx2 toward the caudal end lead to the development of the visual cortex (v1). The somatosensory cortex emerges in between, where the concentrations of Pax6 and Emx2 are intermediate; knockout mouse models of Pax6 and Emx2 confirm that it is indeed the concentration of 1 signaling molecule in conjunction with the other that produces the specific patterning. When Pax6 expression is blocked, visual areas enlarge and somatosensory and motor areas shrink. When Emx2 expression is blocked, the opposite is true.

Despite this early patterning, the structure and function of these areas remain highly malleable and subject to experience. Greenough and coworkers have coined the term "experience expectant processes" to explain the phenomenon of synaptic and neuronal exuberance and subsequent pruning. This process allows for adaptation to ubiquitous environmental conditions that are common to all species.[27] However, it also suggests that the environment is a necessary condition for the normal development of certain neurobehavioral functions. An example of this would be the seminal study conducted by Hubel and Weisel on the early postnatal development of the visual cortex.[28,29] By limiting the visual input of 1 eye on a primate, the bands of the active eye in the ocular dominance column expanded into the area of the deprived eye. Similarly, in Bachevalier and Mishkin's study, infant monkeys who sustained early lesions to the inferior temporal cortex were able to regain most of their function with only minimal deficits compared with adults who were not able to regain their function.[30] It is also noteworthy that infant monkeys that sustained medial temporal lobe lesions were not able to regain their function, suggesting that neural plasticity also has its limits.

Studies of human brain development also highlight the importance of experience and the environment. For example, poverty has been shown to be associated with significant impacts on brain development. Hanson and colleagues[31] have shown lower total gray matter volumes, frontal and parietal volumes, and decreased total gray matter trajectory in children from lower income families. Additionally, early life stressors, which include low socioeconomic status, but also neglect and abuse, led to smaller amygdala and hippocampal volumes.[32] Decreases in cortical gray matter thickness, right hemispheric volume, and left and right anterior insula volume[33,34] are associated with early childhood depression. Interestingly, a variation of parent–child interaction therapy developed by Luby and associates,[35] named parent–child interaction therapy—emotion development, seems to be helpful for early childhood depression. Connectivity among regions important for emotional regulation is also similarly affected. Increased early life stressors was associated with decreased and atypical connectivity between the amygdala and the prefrontal cortex.[36–39] And, Luby reported that lower income-to-need ratio was associated with reduced negative connectivity between left hippocampus and amygdala and the right superior frontal gyrus in addition to connectivity of both the amygdala and hippocampus bilaterally.[40]

Although depravation can lead to thinning, atypicality, and loss of function, an enriched environment can have the opposite effect. Early on, Hebb noted rats reared in a "home" environment outperformed rats reared in a laboratory environment.[41] Later, Rosenzweig and his colleagues also noted difference in brain weight, and other physical and histologic differences between rats reared in enriched versus impoverished environments.[42–50] More recently, Greenough and coworkers showed that rats reared in a complex environment (large groups and objects in a cage that was frequently cleaned) had 20% to 25% more dendrites per neuron, and in those animals that were fitted with a monocular occluders, the exuberance was noted only unilaterally.[51–55] Moreover, the glial cells were also affected, with greater numbers and complexity, as well as an enhanced capillary system.[51,56] Similar effects have been observed in adult rats reared in complex environments.[57,58] In human studies, practice of specific skills such as juggling or playing a musical instrument has led to structural and white matter changes.[59–69]

GRAY AND WHITE MATTER MATURATION

Early MRI morphometry studies compared children and adults. In Jernigan and Tallal's seminal study, gray matter volumes were shown to be considerably larger in school-aged children than in young adults.[70,71] And in Giedd's landmark study, he showed that the volume of the cortical gray matter follow an inverted U shape, with peaks in late childhood and a surge just before puberty and occurring about 1 to 2 years earlier in girls.[72,73] In subsequent studies, Shaw and Raznahan have also reported a curvilinear growth pattern of cortical thickness, a component underlying cortical volume along with cortical surface area.[74,75] However, other studies have not identified the "inverted U" shape but rather monotonic linear decreases in cortical thickness. Sowell, Muftuler, Koolschijn, Mutlu, and Ducharme and their colleagues all primarily found first-order linear declines with the youngest children in this study being around 5 years old.[76–80] More important, Ducharme and associates[78] found postprocessing quality control procedures significantly impacted the complexity of the growth trajectories.

When no quality control procedures were implemented, there were more areas with quadratic and cubic trajectories. The biological underpinnings of the volumetric and cortical thickness changes are owing to arborization as well as continued glial cell maturation opposed by pruning of neuronal processes.[11] Changes in neuronal size, glial cell density, and vasculature could also contribute to cortical thickness changes.[81]

More recent structural MRIs allowed for more precise measurements of cortical thickness.[82,83] These more detailed studies were able to show a modal pattern of cortical development, suggesting regional specificity in cortical thickness.[81] Gogtay and coworkers[84] reported that phylogenetically older regions matured (thinned) earlier than newer regions. They also observed that the maturation process starts with lower order somatosensory and visual cortices before proceeding to multimodal and supramodal cortices.[84] The lateral prefrontal cortex and the temporal poles, regions processing motivation, goal-setting, and integration of emotion, are the last regions to mature.[84–87] The maturation of various cortical regions has been correlated with performance measures. Maturation of the prefrontal cortex is related to cognitive intelligence, the anterior cingulate cortex is related to impulse control, the motor cortex is related to fine motor skills, and the left hemisphere area is related to increased language processing skills.[88–91] Our group has shown that, in typically developing children followed across development, it is possible to relate specific cortical thickness regions in whole brain analyses that correlate with quantitatively different expressions of common traits such as aggression, anxiety, attention, emotional regulation, and externalizing problems.[92–96]

The subcortical gray matter also undergoes significant changes, although to a lesser degree compared with the neocortex.[79,97–100] The caudate, which has traditionally been implicated in control of movement and muscle tone, and more recently in mediating higher order cognitive functions, had previously been shown in some but not all studies to also have a curvilinear developmental trajectory with peaks during the preadolescent to adolescent years.[101,102] However, in a more recent study, Ostby and associates[100] analyzed multiple structures in the basal ganglia (caudate, putamen, and pallidum), and nucleus accumbens, and found a linear decrease over time. The hippocampus and the amygdala on the other hand, showed an increase in size with age.[97–99,103,104]

Unlike gray matter, white matter volume begins to increase in the postnatal period and continues into middle adulthood.[105–107] The development of diffusion tensor imaging has allowed the visualization of white matter by measuring proton diffusivity. As fiber tracts mature and myelination proceeds, diffusion or fractional anisotropy increases.[108] Although many studies found that white matter volume linearly increases over time, some studies have suggested it may have a curvilinear inverted U function, reaching its peak during the second decade.[71,72,109,110] Also like gray matter, different tracts mature at different times. Tracts such as the corticospinal tract and corona radiata are mature by adolescence, but tracts responsible for executive function and emotional and behavioral control such as the internal capsule are still maturing in the adolescent. The continued maturation of these tracts likely is a major contributor to the improvements in modulation of adolescent behavior.[111–113] The maturation of the white matter tracts has implications for other cognitive functions, such as intelligence, visuospatial skills, response inhibition, memory, reading skills, and language.[114]

The nuances in the development of various cortical and subcortical regions are noteworthy, but further investigations with a longitudinal design are needed to confirm the results.

TRANSITIONAL AGE BRAIN MISMATCH HYPOTHESIS

In almost every measurable domain, adolescence is a developmental period of strength and resilience. Compared with young children, adolescents are stronger, bigger, and faster, and are achieving maturational improvements in reaction time, reasoning abilities, immune function, and capacity to withstand cold, heat, injury, and physical stress. Yet, despite these robust maturational improvements in many domains, overall morbidity and mortality rates increase by 200% over the same interval of time.[115] This doubling in rates of death and disability from the period of early school age into late adolescence/early adulthood is likely owing to difficulties in the control of behavior and emotion. This period is, therefore, marked for the high rates of accident suicide, violence, and health problems related to risky sexual behaviors.[115] In addition, adolescence is the peak time of emergence for several types of mental illnesses, including anxiety disorders, bipolar disorder, depression, eating disorders, psychosis, and substance abuse. In the National Comorbidity Survey Replication Study, Kessler and colleagues[116] found that 50% of most mental illnesses people experience emerge by age 14 and 75% start by age 24.

A simplistic explanation of the developmental mismatch can be understood through the emerging understanding of the development of 3 key regions of the brain: the nucleus accumbens, amygdala, and prefrontal cortices.

The nucleus accumbens is the home of motivation, passion and pleasure. Afferents from the ventral tegmental area, specifically the A9 and A10 nuclei travel over the mesolimbic dopamine pathway to stimulate the nucleus accumbens via dopaminergic neurons. Activity in the nucleus accumbens influences how much effort an individual will expend in pleasure and reward-seeking behavior. A developing nucleus accumbens is believed to contribute to the often observed tendency that some TAY prefer activities that require low effort yet produce high excitement. When mature, the mesolimbic dopaminergic pathway terminates in prefrontal and frontal cortical regions and is responsible for attentional control, concentration, and mood regulation. However, those frontal regions are not yet organized and the mismatch of drive without control is the essence of the TAB and central to the developmental mismatch theory.

The amygdala plays a key role in both emotional recognition and regulation. It increases in volume from late childhood until late adolescence, with a decelerating rate of growth after the age 16.[117] Pathways into and out of the amygdala are responsible for integrating emotional reactions to both pleasurable and aversive experiences. It is hypothesized that, during the developmental mismatch epoch, the amygdala contributes to 2 behavioral effects: the tendency for adolescents to react to situations with "hot" emotions rather than more controlled and "cool" emotions and the propensity for youth to misread neutral or inquisitive facial expressions from other individuals as a sign of anger.[74] As the TAB matures, the functional connectivity of the amygdala changes dramatically and amygdala activity becomes more closely linked to activity in those prefrontal cortex regions involved in emotional regulation. This signals an end to the TAB period and the beginning of a more neurologically regulated period referred to as adulthood.[118]

Last, the prefrontal cortex is the key area of the brain involved in attention, emotional regulation, impulse control, cognitive flexibility, planning, and judgment. To do this, it processes complex information, requiring inputs from many brain regions. It allows a person to make decisions and select a course of action based on impulse inhibition, foreseeable consequences, and personal goals. It also happens to develop much later than the nucleus accumbens or the amygdala because cortical thinning or gray matter volume loss (maturation) occurs from the back of the brain to the front. In fact, the prefrontal cortex is the last brain region to complete development. As a consequence, TAY rely much more on the emotional regions of their brain, such as the amygdala and other limbic regions, to guide their behavior compared with adults.[74,119] In other words, TAY do not yet have the brain structures in place that allow the consistent use of the prefrontal cortex for its primary responsibilities of planning, judgment, cognitive flexibility, and impulse control. This mismatch in maturational timing is most exaggerated during the adolescent period, when the subcortical structures including the hormone fueled limbic system is already developed while the prefrontal cortex and the white matter tracts connecting to the prefrontal cortex continue to mature.[120] Most recent studies seem to bear this out, indicating that risk-taking behaviors, sensation seeking, and heightened emotional reactivity are linked to the developmental mismatch in maturation of cortical and subcortical structures.[121] The fact that puberty seems to be starting earlier means that the "mismatch years" are being extended.

As a result of this mismatch, TAY at times use poor judgment and take excessive risks. The relative delay in the maturation of frontal cortical areas as well as those networks connecting to them leaves adolescents vulnerable to performance impairments of higher order cognitive functions, such as cognitive control and response inhibition when stressed.[122–125] TAY have increased activation of the ventral striatum to rewards and decreased activation during reward anticipation, which leaves them vulnerable to risk taking.[126–130] Further, their amygdala are less activated in response to aversive outcomes while exhibiting social emotional bias, resulting in more risky behavior in the presence of others.[131–135] As such, they more frequently make poor decisions and take excessive risk.[84]

Similarly, the protracted development of the uncinated fasciculus provides insight into the difficulty TAY have in emotional regulation. The uncinated fasiculus is a fiber pathway composed of frontotemporal connections that include projections from orbitofrontal cortex to the anterior temporal cortex, as well as the amygdala.[136,137] It has been shown to display age-related increases in microstructural integrity well into adulthood.[138] Although the amygdala has been implicated in mediating negative affective states such as fear and anxiety, hemodynamic activity within aspects of the orbitofrontal cortex has been associated with emotion regulatory processes.[139] The continued development of the orbitofrontal cortex and this pathway that links it to the amygdala is what allows for improved affective regulation as TAY grow into adulthood.

EMOTION REGULATION AND THE BRAIN

The neuropsychological processes important for emotion perception, allowing the generation of contextually appropriate, complex affective states, emotional experiences (feelings), and behaviors, include the identification of the emotional significance of an environmental stimulus, the production of an affective state and emotional behavior, and the regulation of the affective state and emotional behavior. Findings of neuroimaging studies indicate that specific neural regions may be important for more than one of these processes. The processes may be depend on the functioning of 2 main neural systems: a ventral system and a dorsal system. The ventral system, including the amygdala, insula, ventral striatum, and ventral regions of the anterior cingulate gyrus and prefrontal cortex, is important for the identification of the emotional significance of environmental stimuli and the production of affective states. It is additionally important for automatic regulation and mediation of autonomic responses to emotive stimuli and contexts accompanying the production of affective states. The dorsal system, including the hippocampus and dorsal regions of the anterior cingulate gyrus and prefrontal cortex, regions where cognitive processes are integrated, is important for the performance of executive functions, including selective attention, planning, and effortful rather than automatic regulation of affective states.[140]

The emotional circuitry of the brain is being shaped continuously by experiences that impinge on the nervous system during prenatal development and throughout life. This experience-induced plasticity has been documented in the brain in a variety of animal models and there is now substantial evidence on the effect of stressful and stimulating environments on the developing human brain and associated behavior. Most evidence is obtained by structural MRI studies of children that experienced adversity. Abused children are shown to have smaller orbitofrontal volumes and, the smaller the orbitofrontal volume in the abused sample, the more severe the social stress was reported.[141] In another study, higher parental ratings of internalizing behavior and anxiety were correlated with a larger amygdala volume. Furthermore, children continuously exposed to maternal depressive symptoms from birth had significantly larger left and right amygdala than children with no such exposure.[142] Such a developmental pattern in the amygdala has been suggested to occur in the autistic brain.[143,144] Research suggests that some of these alterations in brain structure are caused by epigenetic regulations. For example, child abuse is associated with alterations in the epigenetic regulation of the glucocorticoid receptor extracted from the hippocampus of suicide victims with a history of child abuse compared with those with no abuse history along with controls. In the hippocampus, decreased levels of glucocorticoid receptor messenger RNA were observed.[145] Several pathologic conditions (eg, major depression, posttraumatic stress disorder) are associated with decreased density or volume of the hippocampus.[146,147]

EPIGENETICS, GENE EXPRESSION, AND A PERIOD OF VULNERABILITY AND OPPORTUNITY

As discussed, epigenetic regulations can have powerful effects on the brain. The main factors that contribute to epigenetic changes in the adolescent brain are DNA methylation, histone modification, and microRNAs or noncoding RNAs. DNA methylation is generally associated with gene silencing as a methyl group binds to CpG islands blocking RNA polymerase, although recent evidence suggests that the effects of methylation could be more complicated.[148–150] Histone modifications alter the accessibility of the transcription machinery to the DNA and include methylation, acetylation phosphorylation, and ubiquitination.[151] And last, microRNAs are small noncoding RNAs that regulate posttranscriptional gene expression by affecting the translational efficiency of specific messenger RNA targets.[152–154] Noncoding RNAs regulate many levels of transcriptional process such as modulating chromatin structure by recruiting coregulators to the transcriptional unit.[153,154]

During normal mammalian brain development, adolescence seems to be a time of great epigenetic shift. Somel and associates[155] showed that there was heightened level of epigenetic modulation during adolescence, which the authors believed extended neuronal plasticity. Similarly, Lister and colleagues[156] also identified large-scale reconfiguration of the epigenome during periods of heightened synaptogenesis such as during adolescence. These changes in the epigenome likely help to regulate sex differences in the brain. The preoptic area is an area important for sexual, parenting, and thermoregulating behaviors. In this area, the expression of the ERα is modulated by estradiol resulting in 30% greater methylation in females compared with males.[149] In males, higher levels of histone deacetylases play a key role in programming male sexual behavior.[157] And last, Zinc Fingers, which represses transcription by binding to regulatory regions of DNA, plays a role in modulating pubertal onset in both males and females.[158,159]

With the elevated level of epigenetic modulation and increased brain flexibility, adolescents are at increased risk of detriment and long-term impairment. In fact, studies were able to show the differential effects of substances on the adolescent brain compared with the adult brain. With repeated exposure to ethanol, adolescent rats showed reduced expression of dopamine receptor D_2, and glutamate ionotropic receptor NMDA type subunit 2 in the prefrontal cortex and altered acetylation levels of histones H3 and H4, which was mediated by elevated histone acetyltransferase (histone deacetylase), in the frontal cortex, striatum, and nucleus accumbens.[160] The same exposure to adult rats showed no changes in the measures as listed. Other studies have shown similar long-term changes to the organization of the reward and emotional circuitry.[161–164] Nicotine studies showed the greatest gene alterations occurred during the mid-to-late adolescent periods, corresponding with the age of greatest dependence.[165] Similarly, psychostimulant studies showed more pronounced effects in the adolescents compared with adults. Amphetamine and methylphenidate both showed decreased messenger RNA levels of BDNF in the prefrontal cortex and hippocampus but actually increased BDNF levels in adult prefrontal cortex.[166] The attenuation of a factor involved in neuronal growth and plasticity in adolescents is certainly concerning.

But, just as the heightened brain plasticity could result in detrimental effects, an enriched environment could produce benefits. A single week of voluntary exercise in adolescent rats led to significant increases in BDNF, and epigenetic regulators such as histone deacetylase and DNA methyltransferase decreased.[167] With 4 weeks of exercise, the adolescent rats demonstrated improved memory that was sustained into adulthood.[168] Adults who exercised showed immediate benefits in memory enhancement and elevation of BDNF but no long-term benefits. Interestingly, low-to-moderate intensity exercise was sufficient for increased neurogenesis and increased level of BDNF, whereas high-intensity exercise may have triggered a stress response that offset the benefits of exercise.[169] Even more impressive, social enrichment was able to mitigate impact of prenatal alcohol exposure in a rat model of fetal alcohol spectrum disorder.[170]

Evolutionarily speaking, adolescence is a time of transition where independent skills are acquired to facilitate the transition into adulthood. Brain plasticity provides opportunity for the developmental changes in TAY, creating a physiologic environment that intersects with the environmental and emotional changes that contribute to independent skill development. Increases in peer-directed social interactions, and intensification of risk taking and novelty seeking behaviors mediated by increases in dopamine levels and enervation may contribute to more successful mating and independence.[1,171,172] To balance this increase in risk, the increased emotional reactivity may contribute to heightened vigilance of risks and threats thereby increasing opportunity for survival.[122] Increased epigenetic modulation and brain plasticity may contribute during this time of great change by mediating learning of new information. It was possibly a survival advantage at some point in human evolution, especially when one considers the differences in life expectancy and social pace across the history of human development. However, given the statistics on morbidity and mortality, it is important to consider both the advantages and the potential risks that result from this mismatch in modern TAY. The question as to whether this elevated plasticity is a unique adolescent risk factor or a transition to a more stable brain remains.[173]

SUMMARY

Over the past 2 decades, there have been substantial developments in the understanding of brain development. Progress in neuroimaging has allowed us to better understand the nuances of the development of cortical, subcortical, and white matter structures. Modern neuroscience, genomics, and epigenomic studies allow us a lens through which to develop an understanding of TAY behavior from a neurodevelopmental perspective. We now understand, to a greater degree, why adolescents have difficulty with impulse control, risky behavior, and are disproportionately influenced by their peers. Although our current science has not provided us with all the answers, we can now state confidently that negative environmental influences impact the structure and function of the human brain and the thoughts, actions, and behaviors that result. Armed with emerging evidence that positive environmental influences can influence positively the structure and function of the brain and foment improved academic, memory, mood, and emotional regulatory outcomes,[174] it is now time for child and adolescent psychiatry to design brain-building health promotion and illness prevention approaches for all children, but particularly those in the TAB risk epoch. Developing brain-building health promotion and illness prevention approaches for TAB individuals will likely yield reductions in morbidity and mortality in this high-risk period, enhance individual life trajectories, and possibly have life-long impact on friends and families of TAY.

REFERENCES

1. Spear LP. The adolescent brain and age-related behavioral manifestations. Neurosci Biobehav Rev 2000;24(4):417–63.
2. Huttenlocher PR, de Courten C, Garey LJ, et al. Synaptogenesis in human visual cortex–evidence for synapse elimination during normal development. Neurosci Lett 1982;33(3):247–52.
3. Becker LE, Armstrong DL, Chan F, et al. Dendritic development in human occipital cortical neurons. Brain Res 1984;315(1):117–24.
4. Mrzljak L, Uylings HB, Kostovic I, et al. Prenatal development of neurons in the human prefrontal cortex: I. A qualitative Golgi study. J Comp Neurol 1988; 271(3):355–86.
5. Mrzljak L, Uylings HB, Kostovic I, et al. Prenatal development of neurons in the human prefrontal cortex. II. A quantitative Golgi study. J Comp Neurol 1992; 316(4):485–96.
6. Mrzljak L, Uylings HB, Van Eden CG, et al. Neuronal development in human prefrontal cortex in prenatal and postnatal stages. Prog Brain Res 1990;85: 185–222.
7. Bourgeois JP, Goldman-Rakic PS, Rakic P. Synaptogenesis in the prefrontal cortex of rhesus monkeys. Cereb Cortex 1994;4(1):78–96.
8. Bourgeois JP. Synaptogenesis, heterochrony and epigenesis in the mammalian neocortex. Acta Paediatr Suppl 1997;422:27–33.
9. Rakic P, Bourgeois JP, Eckenhoff MF, et al. Concurrent overproduction of synapses in diverse regions of the primate cerebral cortex. Science 1986;232(4747): 232–5.
10. Levitt P. Structural and functional maturation of the developing primate brain. J Pediatr 2003;143(4 Suppl):S35–45.
11. Stiles J, Jernigan TL. The basics of brain development. Neuropsychol Rev 2010; 20(4):327–48.

12. Bourgeois JP, Rakic P. Changes of synaptic density in the primary visual cortex of the macaque monkey from fetal to adult stage. J Neurosci 1993;13(7): 2801–20.

13. Huttenlocher PR, Dabholkar AS. Regional differences in synaptogenesis in human cerebral cortex. J Comp Neurol 1997;387(2):167–78.

14. Stanfield BB, O'Leary DD. The transient corticospinal projection from the occipital cortex during the postnatal development of the rat. J Comp Neurol 1985; 238(2):236–48.

15. Stanfield BB, O'Leary DD, Fricks C. Selective collateral elimination in early postnatal development restricts cortical distribution of rat pyramidal tract neurones. Nature 1982;298(5872):371–3.

16. Innocenti GM, Price DJ. Exuberance in the development of cortical networks. Nat Rev Neurosci 2005;6(12):955–65.

17. Isackson PJ, Huntsman MM, Murray KD, et al. BDNF mRNA expression is increased in adult rat forebrain after limbic seizures: temporal patterns of induction distinct from NGF. Neuron 1991;6(6):937–48.

18. Huang EJ, Reichardt LF. Neurotrophins: roles in neuronal development and function. Annu Rev Neurosci 2001;24:677–736.

19. Bishop KM, Rubenstein JL, O'Leary DD. Distinct actions of Emx1, Emx2, and Pax6 in regulating the specification of areas in the developing neocortex. J Neurosci 2002;22(17):7627–38.

20. Nakamura H, Katahira T, Matsunaga E, et al. Isthmus organizer for midbrain and hindbrain development. Brain Res Brain Res Rev 2005;49(2):120–6.

21. Kiecker C, Lumsden A. Hedgehog signaling from the ZLI regulates diencephalic regional identity. Nat Neurosci 2004;7(11):1242–9.

22. Lumsden A, Keynes R. Segmental patterns of neuronal development in the chick hindbrain. Nature 1989;337(6206):424–8.

23. Gavalas A, Ruhrberg C, Livet J, et al. Neuronal defects in the hindbrain of Hoxa1, Hoxb1 and Hoxb2 mutants reflect regulatory interactions among these Hox genes. Development 2003;130(23):5663–79.

24. Stiles J. The fundamentals of brain development: integrating nature and nurture. Cambridge (MA): Harvard University Press; 2008.

25. Bishop KM, Goudreau G, O'Leary DD. Regulation of area identity in the mammalian neocortex by Emx2 and Pax6. Science 2000;288(5464):344–9.

26. Hamasaki T, Leingärtner A, Ringstedt T, et al. EMX2 regulates sizes and positioning of the primary sensory and motor areas in neocortex by direct specification of cortical progenitors. Neuron 2004;43:359–72.

27. Greenough WT, Black JE, Wallace CS. Experience and brain development. Child Dev 1987;58(3):539–59.

28. Hubel DH, Wiesel TN. Ferrier lecture. Functional architecture of macaque monkey visual cortex. Proc R Soc Lond B Biol Sci 1977;198(1130):1–59.

29. Hubel DH, Wiesel TN, LeVay S. Plasticity of ocular dominance columns in monkey striate cortex. Philos Trans R Soc Lond B Biol Sci 1977;278(961):377–409.

30. Bachevalier J, Mishkin M. Effects of selective neonatal temporal lobe lesions on visual recognition memory in rhesus monkeys. J Neurosci 1994;14(4):2128–39.

31. Hanson JL, Hair N, Shen DG, et al. Family poverty affects the rate of human infant brain growth. PLoS ONE 2013;8(12):e80954.

32. Hanson JL, Nacewicz BM, Sutterer MJ, et al. Behavioral problems after early life stress: contributions of the hippocampus and amygdala. Biol Psychiatry 2015; 77(4):314–23.

33. Luby JL, Belden AC, Jackson JJ, et al. Early childhood depression and alterations in the trajectory of gray matter maturation in middle childhood and early adolescence. JAMA Psychiatry 2016;73(1):31–8.

34. Belden AC, Barch DM, Oakberg TJ, et al. Anterior insula volume and guilt: neurobehavioral markers of recurrence after early childhood major depressive disorder. JAMA Psychiatry 2015;72(1):40–8.

35. Luby J, Lenze S, Tillman R. A novel early intervention for preschool depression: findings from a pilot randomized controlled trial. J Child Psychol Psychiatry 2012;53(3):313–22.

36. Burghy CA, Stodola DE, Ruttle PL, et al. Developmental pathways to amygdala-prefrontal function and internalizing symptoms in adolescence. Nat Neurosci 2012;15(12):1736–41.

37. Fan Y, Herrera-Melendez AL, Pestke K, et al. Early life stress modulates amygdala-prefrontal functional connectivity: implications for oxytocin effects. Hum Brain Mapp 2014;35(10):5328–39.

38. Gee DG, Gabard-Durnam I J, Flannery J, et al. Early developmental emergence of human amygdala-prefrontal connectivity after maternal deprivation. Proc Natl Acad Sci USA 2013;110(39):15638–43.

39. Grant MM, Wood K, Sreenivasan K, et al. Influence of early life stress on intra- and extra-amygdaloid causal connectivity. Neuropsychopharmacology 2015; 40(7):1782–93.

40. Barch D, Pagliaccio D, Belden A, et al. Effect of hippocampal and amygdala connectivity on the relationship between preschool poverty and school-age depression. Am J Psychiatry 2016;173(6):625–34.

41. Hebb DO. The organization of behavior. New York: Wiley; 1949.

42. Diamond MC, Krech D, Rosenzweig MR. The effects of an enriched environment on the histology of the rat cerebral cortex. J Comp Neurol 1964;123:111–20.

43. Rosenzweig MR, Bennett EL, Diamond MC. Brain changes in response to experience. Scientific American. 1972. Available at: http://psycnet.apa.org/psycinfo/1972-22480-001. Accessed October 4, 2016.

44. Bennett EL, Rosenzweig MR. Difference in occipital cortical synapses from environmentally enriched, impoverished, and standard colony rats. J Neurosci Res 1975;1(2):109–19.

45. Bennett EL, Rosenzweig MR. Quantitative synaptic changes with differential experience in rat brain. Int J Neurosci 1971;2(3):113–27.

46. Bennett EL, Rosenzweig MR, Diamond MC. Rat brain: effects of environmental enrichment on wet and dry weights. Science 1969;163(3869):825–6. Available at: http://science.sciencemag.org/content/163/3869/825.short.

47. Rosenzweig MR, Bennett EL, Diamond MC. Effects of differential environments on brain anatomy and brain chemistry. Proc Annu Meet Am Psychopathol Assoc 1967;56:45–56.

48. Diamond MC, Rosenzweig MR, Bennett EL, et al. Effects of environmental enrichment and impoverishment on rat cerebral cortex. J Neurobiol 1972;3(1): 47–64.

49. Diamond MC, Law F, Rhodes H, et al. Increases in cortical depth and glia numbers in rats subjected to enriched environment. J Comp Neurol 1966; 128(1):117–26.

50. Rosenzweig MR, Bennett EL, Diamond MC, et al. Influences of environmental complexity and visual stimulation on development of occipital cortex in rat. Brain Res 1969;14(2):427–45.

51. Black JE, Sirevaag AM, Greenough WT. Complex experience promotes capillary formation in young rat visual cortex. Neurosci Lett 1987;83(3):351–5.

52. Greenough WT, Chang FL. Dendritic pattern formation involves both oriented regression and oriented growth in the barrels of mouse somatosensory cortex. Brain Res 1988;471(1):148–52.

53. Jones TA, Greenough WT. Ultrastructural evidence for increased contact between astrocytes and synapses in rats reared in a complex environment. Neurobiol Learn Mem 1996;65(1):48–56.

54. Markham JA, Greenough WT. Experience-driven brain plasticity: beyond the synapse. Neuron Glia Biol 2004;1(4):351–63.

55. Chang FL, Greenough WT. Lateralized effects of monocular training on dendritic branching in adult split-brain rats. Brain Res 1982;232(2):283–92.

56. Sirevaag AM, Greenough WT. Differential rearing effects on rat visual cortex synapses. III. Neuronal and glial nuclei, boutons, dendrites, and capillaries. Brain Res 1987;424(2):320–32.

57. Uylings HB, Kuypers K, Veltman WA. Environmental influences on the neocortex in later life. Prog Brain Res 1978;48:261–74.

58. Uylings HB, Kuypers K, Diamond MC, et al. Effects of differential environments on plasticity of dendrites of cortical pyramidal neurons in adult rats. Exp Neurol 1978;62(3):658–77.

59. Boyke J, Driemeyer J, Gaser C, et al. Training-induced brain structure changes in the elderly. J Neurosci 2008;28(28):7031–5.

60. Driemeyer J, Boyke J, Gaser C, et al. Changes in gray matter induced by learning–revisited. PLoS ONE 2008;3(7):e2669.

61. Draganski B, Gaser C, Busch V, et al. Neuroplasticity: changes in grey matter induced by training. Nature 2004;427(6972):311–2.

62. Pantev C, Okamoto H, Teismann H. Music-induced cortical plasticity and lateral inhibition in the human auditory cortex as foundations for tonal tinnitus treatment. Front Syst Neurosci 2012;6:50.

63. Pantev C, Roberts LE, Schulz M, et al. Timbre-specific enhancement of auditory cortical representations in musicians. Neuroreport 2001;12(1):169–74.

64. Pantev C, Oostenveld R, Engelien A, et al. Increased auditory cortical representation in musicians. Nature 1998;392(6678):811–4.

65. Hudziak JJ, Albaugh MD, Ducharme S, et al. Cortical thickness maturation and duration of music training: health-promoting activities shape brain development. J Am Acad Child Adolesc Psychiatry 2014;53(11):1153–61, 1161.e1–2.

66. Bengtsson SL, Nagy Z, Skare S, et al. Extensive piano practicing has regionally specific effects on white matter development. Nat Neurosci 2005;8(9):1148–50.

67. Scholz J, Klein MC, Behrens TE, et al. Training induces changes in white-matter architecture. Nat Neurosci 2009;12(11):1370–1.

68. Takeuchi H, Taki Y, Nouchi R, et al. Working memory training impacts the mean diffusivity in the dopaminergic system. Brain Struct Funct 2015;220(6):3101–11.

69. Takeuchi H, Sekiguchi A, Taki Y, et al. Training of working memory impacts structural connectivity. J Neurosci 2010;30(9):3297–303.

70. Jernigan TL, Tallal P. Late childhood changes in brain morphology observable with MRI. Dev Med Child Neurol 1990;32(5):379–85.

71. Jernigan TL, Trauner DA, Hesselink JR, et al. Maturation of human cerebrum observed in vivo during adolescence. Brain 1991;114(Pt 5):2037–49.

72. Giedd JN, Blumenthal J, Jeffries NO, et al. Brain development during childhood and adolescence: a longitudinal MRI study. Nat Neurosci 1999;2(10):861–3.

73. Giedd JN, Snell JW, Lange N, et al. Quantitative magnetic resonance imaging of human brain development: ages 4-18. Cereb Cortex 1996;6(4):551–60.

74. Shaw P, Kabani NJ, Lerch JP, et al. Neurodevelopmental trajectories of the human cerebral cortex. J Neurosci 2008;28(14):3586–94.

75. Raznahan A, Shaw P, Lalonde F, et al. How does your cortex grow? J Neurosci 2011;31(19):7174–7.

76. Sowell ER, Thompson PM, Leonard CM, et al. Longitudinal mapping of cortical thickness and brain growth in normal children. J Neurosci 2004;24(38):8223–31.

77. Muftuler LT, Davis EP, Buss C, et al. Cortical and subcortical changes in typically developing preadolescent children. Brain Res 2011;1399:15–24.

78. Ducharme S, Albaugh MD, Nguyen T-VV, et al. Trajectories of cortical thickness maturation in normal brain development–The importance of quality control procedures. Neuroimage 2016;125:267–79.

79. Koolschijn PC, Crone EA. Sex differences and structural brain maturation from childhood to early adulthood. Dev Cogn Neurosci 2013;5:106–18.

80. Mutlu AK, Schneider M, Debbané M, et al. Sex differences in thickness, and folding developments throughout the cortex. Neuroimage 2013;82:200–7.

81. Zatorre RJ, Fields RD, Johansen-Berg H. Plasticity in gray and white: neuroimaging changes in brain structure during learning. Nat Neurosci 2012;15(4): 528–36.

82. Fischl B, Dale AM. Measuring the thickness of the human cerebral cortex from magnetic resonance images. Proc Natl Acad Sci USA 2000;97(20):11050–5.

83. Kabani N, Goualher Le G, MacDonald D, et al. Measurement of cortical thickness using an automated 3-D algorithm: a validation study. Neuroimage 2001; 13(2):375–80.

84. Gogtay N, Giedd JN, Lusk L, et al. Dynamic mapping of human cortical development during childhood through early adulthood. Proc Natl Acad Sci USA 2004;101(21):8174–9.

85. Sowell ER, Thompson PM, Holmes CJ, et al. In vivo evidence for post-adolescent brain maturation in frontal and striatal regions. Nat Neurosci 1999; 2(10):859–61.

86. Giedd JN, Rapoport JL. Structural MRI of pediatric brain development: what have we learned and where are we going? Neuron 2010;67(5):728–34.

87. Olson IR, Plotzker A, Ezzyat Y. The Enigmatic temporal pole: a review of findings on social and emotional processing. Brain 2007;130(Pt 7):1718–31.

88. Shaw P, Greenstein D, Lerch J, et al. Intellectual ability and cortical development in children and adolescents. Nature 2006;440(7084):676–9.

89. Casey BJ, Trainor R, Giedd J, et al. The role of the anterior cingulate in automatic and controlled processes: a developmental neuroanatomical study. Dev Psychobiol 1997;30(1):61–9.

90. Lu L, Leonard C, Thompson P, et al. Normal developmental changes in inferior frontal gray matter are associated with improvement in phonological processing: a longitudinal MRI analysis. Cereb Cortex 2007;17(5):1092–9.

91. Sowell ER, Thompson PM, Toga AW. Mapping changes in the human cortex throughout the span of life. Neuroscientist 2004;10(4):372–92.

92. Nguyen T-VV, McCracken JT, Albaugh MD, et al. A testosterone-related structural brain phenotype predicts aggressive behavior from childhood to adulthood. Psychoneuroendocrinology 2016;63:109–18.

93. Ducharme S, Albaugh MD, Hudziak JJ, et al. Anxious/depressed symptoms are linked to right ventromedial prefrontal cortical thickness maturation in healthy children and young adults. Cereb Cortex 2014;24(11):2941–50.

94. Albaugh MD, Ducharme S, Collins DL, et al. Evidence for a cerebral cortical thickness network anti-correlated with amygdalar volume in healthy youths: implications for the neural substrates of emotion regulation. Neuroimage 2013; 71:42–9.

95. Ducharme S, Hudziak JJ, Botteron KN, et al. Decreased regional cortical thickness and thinning rate are associated with inattention symptoms in healthy children. J Am Acad Child Adolesc Psychiatry 2012;51(1):18–27.e2.

96. Ameis SH, Ducharme S, Albaugh MD, et al. Cortical thickness, cortico-amygdalar networks, and externalizing behaviors in healthy children. Biol Psychiatry 2014;75(1):65–72.

97. Giedd JN, Vaituzis AC, Hamburger SD, et al. Quantitative MRI of the temporal lobe, amygdala, and hippocampus in normal human development: ages 4-18 years. J Comp Neurol 1996;366(2):223–30.

98. Toga AW, Thompson PM, Sowell ER. Mapping brain maturation. Trends Neurosci 2006;29(3):148–59.

99. Sowell ER, Trauner DA, Gamst A, et al. Development of cortical and subcortical brain structures in childhood and adolescence: a structural MRI study. Dev Med Child Neurol 2002;44(1):4–16.

100. Ostby Y, Tamnes CK, Fjell AM, et al. Heterogeneity in subcortical brain development: a structural magnetic resonance imaging study of brain maturation from 8 to 30 years. J Neurosci 2009;29(38):11772–82.

101. Giedd JN, Clasen LS, Lenroot R, et al. Puberty-related influences on brain development. Mol Cell Endocrinol 2006;254-255:154–62.

102. Lenroot RK, Giedd JN. Brain development in children and adolescents: insights from anatomical magnetic resonance imaging. Neurosci Biobehav Rev 2006; 30(6):718–29.

103. Guo X, Chen C, Chen K, et al. Brain development in Chinese children and adolescents: a structural MRI study. Neuroreport 2007;18(9):875–80.

104. Gogtay N, Nugent TF, Herman DH, et al. Dynamic mapping of normal human hippocampal development. Hippocampus 2006;16(8):664–72.

105. Benes FM, Turtle M, Khan Y, et al. Myelination of a key relay zone in the hippocampal formation occurs in the human brain during childhood, adolescence, and adulthood. Arch Gen Psychiatry 1994;51(6):477–84.

106. Paus T, Collins DL, Evans AC, et al. Maturation of white matter in the human brain: a review of magnetic resonance studies. Brain Res Bull 2001;54(3): 255–66.

107. Walhovd KB, Fjell AM, Reinvang I, et al. Effects of age on volumes of cortex, white matter and subcortical structures. Neurobiol Aging 2005;26(9):1261–70 [discussion: 1275–8].

108. Hermoye L, Saint-Martin C, Cosnard G, et al. Pediatric diffusion tensor imaging: normal database and observation of the white matter maturation in early childhood. Neuroimage 2006;29(2):493–504.

109. Li TQ, Noseworthy MD. Mapping the development of white matter tracts with diffusion tensor imaging. Developmental Science 2002;5:293–300.

110. Imperati D, Colcombe S, Kelly C, et al. Differential development of human brain white matter tracts. PLoS ONE 2011;6(8):e23437.

111. Luna B, Garver KE, Urban TA, et al. Maturation of cognitive processes from late childhood to adulthood. Child Dev 2004;75(5):1357–72.

112. Luna T, Munoz M. Maturation of widely distributed brain function subserves cognitive development. Neuroimage 2001;13(5):786–93.

113. Zald I. The development of spatial working memory abilities. Dev Neuropsychol 2004;26(1):487–512.
114. Dahl RE. Adolescent brain development: a period of vulnerabilities and opportunities. Keynote address. Ann N Y Acad Sci 2004;1021:1–22.
115. Dahl RE, Gunnar MR. Heightened stress responsiveness and emotional reactivity during pubertal maturation: implications for psychopathology. Dev Psychopathol 2009;21(1):1–6.
116. Kessler BP, Berglund P, Demler O, et al. Lifetime prevalence and age-of-onset distribution of DSM-IV disorders in the National Comorbidity Survey Replication. Arch Gen Psychiatry 2005;62:593–603. Available at: https://www.ncbi.nlm.nih.gov/pubmed/?term=Demler%20O%5BAuthor%5D&cauthor=true&cauthor_uid=159 39837.
117. Giedd JN. The amazing teen brain. Sci Am 2015;312(6):32–7.
118. Gabard-Durnam LJ, Flannery J, Goff B, et al. The development of human amygdala functional connectivity at rest from 4 to 23 years: a cross-sectional study. Neuroimage 2014;95:193–207.
119. Yurgelun-Todd D. Emotional and cognitive changes during adolescence. Curr Opin Neurobiol 2007;17(2):251–7.
120. Dahl RE. Biological, developmental, and neurobehavioral factors relevant to adolescent driving risks. Am J Prev Med 2008;35(3 Suppl):S278–84.
121. Mills KL, Goddings A-LL, Clasen LS, et al. The developmental mismatch in structural brain maturation during adolescence. Dev Neurosci 2014;36(3–4): 147–60.
122. Casey BJ, Jones RM, Hare TA. The adolescent brain. Ann N Y Acad Sci 2008; 1124:111–26.
123. Liston C, McEwen BS, Casey BJ. Psychosocial stress reversibly disrupts prefrontal processing and attentional control. Proc Natl Acad Sci USA 2009; 106(3):912–7.
124. Rubia K, Halari R, Smith AB, et al. Dissociated functional brain abnormalities of inhibition in boys with pure conduct disorder and in boys with pure attention deficit hyperactivity disorder. Am J Psychiatry 2008;165(7):889–97.
125. Stevens MC, Kiehl KA, Pearlson GD, et al. Functional neural networks underlying response inhibition in adolescents and adults. Behav Brain Res 2007;181(1): 12–22.
126. Andersen SL. Changes in the second messenger cyclic AMP during development may underlie motoric symptoms in attention deficit/hyperactivity disorder (ADHD). Behav Brain Res 2002;130(1–2):197–201.
127. Galvan A, Hare TA, Parra CE, et al. Earlier development of the accumbens relative to orbitofrontal cortex might underlie risk-taking behavior in adolescents. J Neurosci 2006;26(25):6885–92.
128. Cohen JR, Asarnow RF, Sabb FW, et al. A unique adolescent response to reward prediction errors. Nat Neurosci 2010;13(6):669–71.
129. Van Leijenhorst L, Gunther Moor B, Op de Macks ZA, et al. Adolescent risky decision-making: neurocognitive development of reward and control regions. Neuroimage 2010;51(1):345–55.
130. Schneider S, Peters J, Bromberg U, et al. Risk taking and the adolescent reward system: a potential common link to substance abuse. Am J Psychiatry 2012; 169(1):39–46.
131. Ernst M, Nelson EE, Jazbec S, et al. Amygdala and nucleus accumbens in responses to receipt and omission of gains in adults and adolescents. Neuroimage 2005;25(4):1279–91.

132. Bjork JM, Smith AR, Danube CL, et al. Developmental differences in posterior mesofrontal cortex recruitment by risky rewards. J Neurosci 2007;27(18): 4839–49.
133. Steinberg LA. Social neuroscience perspective on adolescent risk-taking. Dev Rev 2008;28(1):78–106.
134. Steinberg L, Graham S, O'Brien L, et al. Age differences in future orientation and delay discounting. Child Dev 2009;80(1):28–44.
135. Hare TA, Tottenham N, Galvan A, et al. Biological substrates of emotional reactivity and regulation in adolescence during an emotional go-nogo task. Biol Psychiatry 2008;63(10):927–34.
136. Klingler J, Gloor P. The connections of the amygdala and of the anterior temporal cortex in the human brain. J Comp Neurol 1960;115:333–69.
137. Ebeling U, von Cramon D. Topography of the uncinate fascicle and adjacent temporal fiber tracts. Acta Neurochir (Wien) 1992;115(3–4):143–8.
138. Lebel C, Walker L, Leemans A, et al. Microstructural maturation of the human brain from childhood to adulthood. Neuroimage 2008;40(3):1044–55.
139. Banks SJ, Eddy KT, Angstadt M, et al. Amygdala-frontal connectivity during emotion regulation. Soc Cogn Affect Neurosci 2007;2(4):303–12.
140. Phillips ML, Drevets WC, Rauch SL, et al. Neurobiology of emotion perception I: the neural basis of normal emotion perception. Biol Psychiatry 2003;54(5): 504–14.
141. Hanson JL, Chung MK, Avants BB, et al. Early stress is associated with alterations in the orbitofrontal cortex: a tensor-based morphometry investigation of brain structure and behavioral risk. J Neurosci 2010;30:7466–72.
142. Lupien SJ, Parent S, Evans AC, et al. Larger amygdala but no change in hippocampal volume in 10-year-old children exposed to maternal depressive symptomatology since birth. Proc Natl Acad Sci U S A 2011;108:14324–9.
143. Nacewicz BM, Dalton KM, Johnstone T, et al. Amygdala volume and nonverbal social impairment in adolescent and adult males with autism. Arch Gen Psychiatry 2006;63:1417–28.
144. Mosconi MW, Cody-Hazlett H, Poe MD, et al. Longitudinal study of amygdala volume and joint attention in 2- to 4-year-old children with autism. Arch Gen Psychiatry 2009;66:509–16.
145. Davidson RJ, McEwen BS. Social influences on neuroplasticity: stress and interventions to promote well-being. Nat Neurosci 2012;15(5):689–95.
146. Sheline YI. 3D MRI studies of neuroanatomic changes in unipolar major depression: the role of stress and medical comorbidity. Biol Psychiatry 2000;48(8): 791–800.
147. Kasai K, Yamasue H, Gilbertson MW, et al. Evidence for acquired pregenual anterior cingulate gray matter loss from a twin study of combat-related posttraumatic stress disorder. Biol Psychiatry 2008;63(6):550–6.
148. Champagne FA. Epigenetic influence of social experiences across the lifespan. Dev Psychobiol 2010;52(4):299–311.
149. McCarthy MM, Nugent BM. Epigenetic contributions to hormonally-mediated sexual differentiation of the brain. J Neuroendocrinol 2013;25(11):1133–40.
150. Chahrour M, Jung SY, Shaw C, et al. MeCP2, a key contributor to neurological disease, activates and represses transcription. Science 2008;320(5880): 1224–9.
151. Fagiolini M, Jensen CL, Champagne FA. Epigenetic influences on brain development and plasticity. Curr Opin Neurobiol 2009;19(2):207–12.

152. Bartel DP. MicroRNAs: genomics, biogenesis, mechanism, and function. Cell 2004;116(2):281–97.
153. Mattick JS, Amaral PP, Dinger ME, et al. RNA regulation of epigenetic processes. Bioessays 2009;31(1):51–9.
154. Mehler MF. Epigenetic principles and mechanisms underlying nervous system functions in health and disease. Prog Neurobiol 2008;86(4):305–41.
155. Somel M, Franz H, Yan Z, et al. Transcriptional neoteny in the human brain. Proc Natl Acad Sci USA 2009;106(14):5743–8.
156. Lister R, Mukamel EA, Nery JR, et al. Global epigenomic reconfiguration during mammalian brain development. Science 2013;341(6146):1237905.
157. Matsuda KI, Mori H, Nugent BM, et al. Histone deacetylation during brain development is essential for permanent masculinization of sexual behavior. Endocrinology 2011;152(7):2760–7.
158. Lomniczi A, Wright H, Castellano JM, et al. Epigenetic regulation of puberty via Zinc finger protein-mediated transcriptional repression. Nat Commun 2015;6: 10195.
159. Lomniczi A, Loche A, Castellano JM, et al. Epigenetic control of female puberty. Nat Neurosci 2013;16(3):281–9.
160. Pascual M, Boix J, Felipo V, et al. Repeated alcohol administration during adolescence causes changes in the mesolimbic dopaminergic and glutamatergic systems and promotes alcohol intake in the adult rat. J Neurochem 2009; 108(4):920–31.
161. Coleman LG, He J, Lee J, et al. Adolescent binge drinking alters adult brain neurotransmitter gene expression, behavior, brain regional volumes, and neurochemistry in mice. Alcohol Clin Exp Res 2011;35(4):671–88.
162. Pandey SC, Sakharkar AJ, Tang L, et al. Potential role of adolescent alcohol exposure-induced amygdaloid histone modifications in anxiety and alcohol intake during adulthood. Neurobiol Dis 2015;82:607–19.
163. Kyzar EJ, Zhang H, Sakharkar AJ, et al. Adolescent alcohol exposure alters lysine demethylase 1 (LSD1) expression and histone methylation in the amygdala during adulthood. Addict Biol 2016. [Epub ahead of print].
164. Sakharkar AJ, Tang L, Zhang H, et al. Effects of acute ethanol exposure on anxiety measures and epigenetic modifiers in the extended amygdala of adolescent rats. Int J Neuropsychopharmacol 2014;17(12):2057–67.
165. Polesskaya OO, Fryxell KJ, Merchant AD, et al. Nicotine causes age-dependent changes in gene expression in the adolescent female rat brain. Neurotoxicol Teratol 2007;29(1):126–40.
166. Banerjee PS, Aston J, Khundakar AA, et al. Differential regulation of psychostimulant-induced gene expression of brain derived neurotrophic factor and the immediate-early gene Arc in the juvenile and adult brain. Eur J Neurosci 2009;29(3):465–76.
167. Abel JL, Rissman EF. Running-induced epigenetic and gene expression changes in the adolescent brain. Int J Dev Neurosci 2013;31(6):382–90.
168. Hopkins ME, Nitecki R, Bucci DJ. Physical exercise during adolescence versus adulthood: differential effects on object recognition memory and brain-derived neurotrophic factor levels. Neuroscience 2011;194:84–94.
169. Lou SJ, Liu JY, Chang H, et al. Hippocampal neurogenesis and gene expression depend on exercise intensity in juvenile rats. Brain Res 2008;1210:48–55.
170. Ignacio C, Mooney SM, Middleton FA. Effects of acute prenatal exposure to ethanol on microRNA expression are ameliorated by social enrichment. Front Pediatr 2014;2:103.

171. Rosenberg DR, Lewis DA. Postnatal maturation of the dopaminergic innervation of monkey prefrontal and motor cortices: a tyrosine hydroxylase immunohisto-chemical analysis. J Comp Neurol 1995;358(3):383–400.
172. Laviola G, Adriani W, Terranova ML, et al. Psychobiological risk factors for vulnerability to psychostimulants in human adolescents and animal models. Neurosci Biobehav Rev 1999;23(7):993–1010.
173. Spear LP. Adolescent neurodevelopment. J Adolesc Health 2013;52(2 Suppl 2): S7–13.
174. O'Loughlin K, Hudziak JJ. Health promotion and prevention in child and adoles-cent mental health. In: Rey JM, editor. IACAPAP Textbook of Child and Adoles-cent Mental Health. Geneva (Switzerland): International Association for Child and Adolescent Psychiatry and Allied Professions; 2017. p. 1–23.

Aligning Mental Health Treatments with the Developmental Stage and Needs of Late Adolescents and Young Adults

Brian Skehan, MD, PhD*, Maryann Davis, PhD

KEYWORDS

- Transitional age youth • Emerging adult • Engagement

KEY POINTS

- Transitional age youth (TAY) with serious mental health conditions require a variety of developmentally appropriate options for care to achieve autonomy in mature adulthood.
- Treatment options for TAY need to incorporate educational, vocational, mental health, and medical care to facilitate transition to mature adulthood.
- Further evidence is needed to operationalize the current theories regarding best practices for engagement and treatment of TAY with serious mental health conditions.

INTRODUCTION

Navigating the pathway to adulthood for late adolescents and young adults is a complicated journey that consists of self-discovery and learning through multiple stages of developmental growth. Despite legal definitions, sociocultural norms, and historical precedence, the definition of mature adulthood is less defined by chronologic age and more appropriately defined by developmental milestones. Thus, transitional age youth (TAY) are perhaps best described as individuals in the developmental period between adolescence and mature adulthood. Acceleration in the transition to mature adulthood begins as early as 14 and can extend through age 25 or 30.[1,2] Psychologically, during the early ages of transition, youth continue to progress through cognitive, social, moral, and social-sexual development that began earlier in childhood, with a particular focus on identity formation, typically under the supervision of

The authors have nothing to disclose.
Department of Psychiatry, University of Massachusetts Medical School, 55 Lake Avenue North, Worcester, MA 01655, USA
* Corresponding author.
E-mail address: Brian.Skehan@umassmemorial.org

Abbreviations

SMHC   Serious mental health condition
TAY   Transitional age youth

parents or parental figures, and social institutions, such as schools. This psychosocial development continues into young adulthood, and underlies their abilities to achieve adult goals such as long-term employment, financial independence, stable romantic relationships, and raising children.[1] The transition years are also a time that coincides with the onset of many mental health conditions.[3] Among those who develop psychiatric disorders, their onset occurs before age 25 in approximately 75%, and the typical age of onset of the most serious mental health conditions occurs during the transition years.[4,5] Results from the National Comorbidity Survey–Replication, an epidemiologic study of psychiatric disorders in the United States, found that 1 in every 4 to 5 youth will have a serious mental illness with severe impairment during adolescence.[6] We refer to TAY with either serious emotional disturbance or serious mental illness as having a serious mental health condition (SMHC).[7] Youth with SMHC have significant delays in their psychosocial development that can impair their functional capacities as they enter adulthood.[8] The combination of critical developmental milestones and risk of mental health conditions makes the transition years particularly important for intervening quickly when mental health needs arise.

TYPICAL PSYCHOSOCIAL DEVELOPMENT

Typically developing TAY develop increasing cognitive abilities related to abstract thinking, including anticipating the consequences of their choices and actions, engaging in complex strategic planning, and gaining increasing insight. They also develop better behavior and cognitive control toward emotional or distracting stimuli.[9–11] Social development during this stage comprises complex friendships involving intimacy and loyalty, a peak then reduction in the influence of peer networks on decision making,[12] and subsequent development of smaller, more intimate social networks. Concurrently, psychosexual development involves new forms of emotional intimacy, negotiation of sexual relationships, and resolution of sexual orientation and gender identity. Identity formation and moral development at this stage lead to increased empathic responses, the ability to sacrifice for the greater good, and exploration of boundaries to seek answers about their own identity.

Numerous studies have shown that brain development during the early transition age stage is not yet complete. In fact, it is unclear at what point during the 20s that brain development appears as in fully mature adults.[13] The prefrontal cortex, which is responsible for executive functioning and cognitive control, is the last region to develop fully.[14,15] Impaired judgment and executive functioning during this period are particularly challenging for youth who have increasing reliance on peers and rejection of authority to guide their decision making. Studies have shown that youth are more willing to accept risk than older adults and that the presence of peers during the decision making process can lead to a greater emphasis on the potential benefits and increased acceptance of risk than if they were confronted with a similar decision alone.[16] Further complicating matters is the high prevalence of substance abuse in this age range. Emerging adulthood is the peak age for developing a substance use disorder and approximately 36% of young adults with mental health conditions have comorbid substance abuse.[17] TAY also have a unique role within families. Typically, they use family resources for financial and emotional support, particularly during the early years of the transition stage, while at the same time attempting to achieve greater self-determination.[18] Family systems see distinct changes as young adults mature along developmental lines to accommodate autonomy and independence of the youth with decreased parental roles in decision making.[19,20] The degree of independence from family varies cross-culturally, reflecting diverse emphases on ways of being both independent and interdependent,[21] thus also reflecting cultural differences in parental involvement in the decision making of their young adult children.[22]

PSYCHOSOCIAL DEVELOPMENT IN TRANSITIONAL AGE YOUTH WITH SERIOUS MENTAL HEALTH CONDITIONS

There are an estimated 1.9 million 15- to 25-year-olds with SMHCs in the United States.[23,24] As a group, adolescents with SMHCs have significant delays in their psychosocial development, which may impair their functional capacities as they enter adulthood.[8] Given their psychosocial delays, and other factors, such as trauma, associated with the development of SMHCs, it is not surprising, that these adolescents struggle to complete their high school education,[25–27] enroll in and complete college,[28–30] and establish adult work lives.[31] They are also at high risk for homelessness,[32,33] justice system involvement,[34] and cooccurring substance use disorders.[17]

Delays in psychosocial development can impede a youth's ability to develop and execute plans, demonstrate judgment based on their own principles rather than peer-influenced ideas, and change behaviors based on self-reflection and awareness.[35] Delays in social development at this age may lead to poor quality and quantity of friendships, compromised family relations, and compromised success in school, college, or the workplace. Although sexual maturity is not delayed in TAY with SMHCs, healthy negotiations around sexual relationships call for social skills and self-confidence that is often reduced in this group. Young women with SMHCs are more likely than their peers to have become pregnant.[25]

Other Important Characteristics of Youth with Serious Mental Health Conditions

Many TAY with SMHCs who have received services enter the transition age with complex family relationships. Many have families living in poverty, single heads of households,[36] and may have more strained relationships with parents than typical of this age.[37] This can make the challenging balance of parental supervision and guidance while fostering healthy adolescent self-determination even more complicated.

Particularly for youth with SMHCs who have received public services, such as foster care, juvenile justice, or public mental health, the abrupt end of services, which may include residential services, upon reaching the upper age limit of these services, can pose severe additional barriers to the successful transition into adulthood.[2]

BARRIERS AND FACILITATORS TO HELP-SEEKING IN TRANSITION AGE YOUTH

We have not done a good job engaging and retaining TAY in mental health treatment; they have higher rates of attrition than more mature adults.[38–40] Despite the persistence of many mental health conditions into adulthood, TAY with mental health issues also have decreased rates of accessing services compared with more mature adults.[41] There are a number of barriers to TAY seeking care. Health care providers, insurers, and system constraints can all contribute to difficulties engaging these youth in care. For example, although the Affordable Care Act has provided much greater continuity of health care coverage for young adults who can now remain on parental private insurance until the age of 26, finding providers who accept that particular insurance, who have openings, and who work well with the TAY can require extreme persistence in effort. This persistence may be compromised by both their youthfulness and the impact of their mental health condition. Furthermore, youth may not recognize their symptoms of mental ill health, may have stigmatizing views of mental illness owing to cultural differences or parent perspective, and have ambivalence about seeking help or treatment. Addressing these barriers to connecting TAY with good mental health care requires a multifaceted approach. The complexity of this issue is in part the reason for the largest federal program to facilitate TAY connection to mental health treatment, namely, Now Is the Time—Healthy Transitions.[42]

ROLE OF THE MENTAL HEALTH PROVIDER

Mental health providers play a critical role in the treatment of TAY with SMHCs, but can also inadvertently create barriers in their ability to access care. Youth rejection of treatment from mental health providers can be explained partly by the ongoing development of identity formation, which includes the rejection of authority figures to develop autonomy. Real or perceived recommendations and endorsements of ongoing treatment by providers can result in youth viewing the provider as an authority figure, particularly if they disagree with the recommendation, resulting in early termination of treatment.[43] TAY may have misperceptions about the duration and efficacy of treatment[38,44] and terminate helpful treatments as part of their rejection of authority. Shared decision making is critical at this stage, although many youth engaged in treatment have little or no experience in making complex decisions regarding their own treatment. The ability and mandate to make these decisions often arrives suddenly at the legal age of 18 with little preparation for participation in the process. Some youth may even be unaware that they have a right to participate in these discussions and may not be able to formulate questions regarding medications or treatment plans to obtain the information that they deem necessary to make an informed decision. Others may be hypervigilant when it comes to side effects of psychotropic medications, particularly those that result in weight gain or dermatologic concerns, in part owing to their developmental life stage and desire for romantic relationships. In light of these issues, the ability of the provider to address these concerns adequately in the context of high-volume clinical practice is critical to the youth's understanding of recommendations. Paternalism of providers or limited discussion about shared decision making and youth preferences can limit the engagement of youth in the process and result in treatment attrition or limited engagement.[43] Providers may be unprepared to work with emerging adults in a developmentally appropriate fashion[13,45–47] or fail to recognize the need for increased time and attention to collaborative treatment plans, shared decision making, and psychoeducation, leading to poor engagement or treatment attrition.

SYSTEMIC BARRIERS TO CARE

Youth and providers face numerous systemic challenges when developing treatment plans for TAY. Many TAY view youth and adult services unfavorably, resulting in low use of services despite persistence of mental illness through this developmental period.[48,49] In fact, although office-based treatment is accessed by more than 750,000 emerging adults each year, there is limited impact because they are almost 8 times more likely to terminate treatment when compared with more mature adults.[38,39,50] Although there are many options for adult services once youth reach 18 years of age, the adult service system has its own set of complexities that make it difficult for youth to navigate, especially for those who have not been provided adequate preparation while still receiving adolescent services. The confusion of navigating adult services independently, including insurance eligibility, vocational opportunities, limiting housing options, and eligibility for additional services, can add to their emotional distress as they try to maintain the increasing demands of adulthood with less preparation than their age-matched peers owing to psychosocial delays.[51] Knowledge about the services and available funding is often limited to those who are familiar with the supporting agencies and change rapidly based on available state and federal funding. This can lead to discontinuities in care when a youth no longer meets criteria and decreases collaboration between providers.[2]

TAY with SMHCs often interact with multiple systems and agencies. Many have been in child welfare, special education, or the juvenile justice system, in addition to the child mental health system. Many will come into contact with the criminal justice system,[34] or will need vocational rehabilitation services, housing, or substance use services, in addition to mental health services as an adult. Service coordination models to help bridge the complex crossroads of child and adult services for this population are just beginning to be developed, specified, and tested.[52–54] In most locations in the United States, care coordination models reside within either the child system (eg, wraparound) or the adult system (eg, assertive community treatment) but do not bridge the two. Furthermore, some services do not have similar counterparts between adult and child services. Special education and child welfare services do not continue in the adult system beyond age 21, and substance abuse treatment is often very limited in the child system or supported through different agencies with different eligibility requirements in each service silo.[2] Standard adult services that are typical for adults age 30 to 60 who undergo minimal developmental change are often inappropriate for TAY who encompass numerous stages of psychosocial development and brain maturation.[13] Young adults are also unlikely to be eligible for any child and adolescent services that may be helpful once they reach the age of 18 or are no longer on an individualized educational plan.

INDIVIDUAL BARRIERS

Some youth may view the need to seek help from others as a failure to achieve a successful transition to adulthood. Predictors of dropout from mental health care in TAY include barriers to access, perceived relevance of treatment, and quality of the therapeutic relationship.[41] Engagement in treatment, identifying goals, and developing a future vision can be intimidating during this developmental stage for a multitude of reasons.

Many emerging adults enter this developmental period with excitement about their increasing autonomy and fewer restrictions from parents or other custodial systems. Those with SMHCs may struggle with their increased autonomy owing to their symptoms, psychosocial delay, or inexperience in navigating and practicing typical social interactions in the adult world. Youth often eagerly anticipate increased independence, but the prospect of increasing responsibility and consequences with less support from parents or authority figures can be terrifying.[55] Those who have spent time in institutions such as the foster care system, correctional facilities, group homes, or recurrent hospitalizations may be at increased risk owing to the long separations from their families and supports. These prolonged absences also decrease their exposure to adult modeling of careers and families. Of course, some youth have limited exposure to positive adult modeling and may not have been involved in any of these systems. These youth may benefit tremendously from having peer supports with lived experiences or from connections with other sources of positive modeling, such as vocational mentors, mentorship in higher education, or spiritual counselors based on the youth's strengths and preferences.

Obtaining a higher education or engagement in vocation can be critical to developing autonomy and role identity during the transition years. Youth with serious mental illness have lower rates of education and higher school dropout rates than others their age without mental illness.[8,25,47,56] Leaving school may require youth to enter the workforce to develop financial independence. Major economic changes have resulted in a workforce that has shifted away from trade and manufacturing toward service and information. This shift demands higher levels of education to obtain better paying jobs, which can be difficult to achieve for youth struggling with mental illness.[51] Jobs that have lower education requirements have relatively lower wages than in the past, especially when inflation is taken into account,[57] and unemployment is a serious risk.[58] Furthermore, youth with serious mental health issues have an increased risk of arrest by age 25, many of them multiple times,[34] and they are at high risk for other poor outcomes including homelessness[59] and unwanted pregnancy.[25] One study showed that 65% to 70% of youth involved in the juvenile justice system have mental health disorders with 80% meeting criteria for more than 1 disorder and 61% having comorbid substance use disorders.[60] Criminal charges, especially more serious offences, can restrict access to housing, college loans, Medicaid, or employment, further limiting financial means or access to care. These limitations can be prohibitive in youth who are seeking recovery and can have long-lasting implications on their development, far beyond the intended sentence.[2] These barriers create obstacles in accessing care either owing to incarceration, lack of insurance, poor financial means, or transportation limitations to get youth to appointments with providers.

FACILITATORS OF TREATMENT FOR TRANSITIONAL AGE YOUTH

The mental health care system could become an important resource for TAY by rethinking the delivery of services to this discrete population and using existing frameworks that are already accessed by other age groups. Psychiatrists and other providers treating this age group should have familiarity with the systems of care model[61] and would benefit from taking a developmental process approach to engaging with young adults and consider highly individualized treatment plans that pay attention to youth's strengths and preferences.[40,52,62,63] Training current and future providers to think of TAY as a discrete developmental stage that is distinctly different from both younger adolescents and more mature adults can help to facilitate treatment engagement. More research needs to be done in this area to understand how to support and engage youth because most of the evidence base on therapeutic interventions focuses on children or adults and misses this age group.[64,65]

Accessible services for TAY should comprise multidimensional supports that include psychiatric, vocational, and transitional services and development of these types of services may increase use.[52,56,66] Although adult mental health services often include vocational and housing supports, they are rarely tailored to the specific needs of young adults, and do not include transition supports that help build the skills for adult functioning.[67] The Transitions to Independence model is used in several states and in Canada to address this person-centered approach.[52] High-fidelity wraparound services may also serve this age group well.[68] The "systems of care" model, commonly practiced in child and adolescent psychiatry, uses youth- and family-guided treatment plans. These plans may include integrated care coordination, therapeutic mentors, and family partners (parents of children with serious emotional disturbances with lived experience within the system). The Transitions to Independence system and other person-centered planning approaches for TAY are extensions of this system of care framework. One common approach to making services more age appropriate for TAY is to add peer mentors or coaches[69,70] to person-centered planning processes. Youth voice is critical in developing programs and formulating a treatment plan, even before the age of 18, to maintain engagement after a youth can decline services. Implicit in this principle is that there needs to be a variety of services for youth to have a choice in the process. The Substance Abuse and Mental Health Services Administration has provided 3 national programs to improve services for TAY, Partnerships for Youth Transitions, the Healthy Transitions Initiative, and Now is the Time—Healthy Transitions,[42] each of which requires grantees to use strengths-based treatments to provide services that incorporate multiple life domains in a person-centered approach.[52]

Effective engagement can also be achieved by providing young-adult friendly information. Using social media to engage youth and provide nonjudgmental information about services is a way to introduce service options in an appealing way. Current technology can also allow youth to maintain relationships that they have created in residential programs that can potentially have positive long-term effects in helping to create their own peer support network.[55]

Treatment focused on transitioning to adulthood rather than a transition to adult services can be helpful in keeping youth engaged in treatment. Services for emerging adults need to be both appealing and developmentally appropriate to engage youth once they are at a legal age where they can decline services. In recognition of this, the Institute of Medicine recommended that developmentally appropriate treatments for young adults be a focus of research, and not be assumed to be the case for existing evidence-based treatments for adults.[13] Existing programs with expanding evidence base have been successful in treating other developmental age groups and could be expanded or redesigned to care for emerging adults. For example, coordination between adult services that are largely unfamiliar with a system of care approach and are further limited by the Federal Educational Records Privacy Act of 1974, Health Insurance Portability and Accountability Act of 1996, and other privacy barriers will be necessary to incorporate the increased vocational supports and substance abuse treatments required to care for emerging adults with SMHCs.[2,67] Educational supports that can facilitate additional training in community colleges, universities, or trades will help young people to be more productive members of their community and mitigate the risk of poor outcomes if these developmental milestones are unmet.

EVIDENCE-BASED TREATMENTS AND STRATEGIES FOR THIS POPULATION

In a recent review of the literature on evidence-based treatments, the Academy of Science's Institute of Medicine recommended a research priority to develop or discover evidence-based behavioral health interventions specifically for young adults, based on the paucity of such treatments to date.[13] Others have similarly concluded that there is a significant dearth of evidence-based treatments for the entire age range of TAY.[52,65,66,71] Traditional study design and funding parameters that focused on gathering data for either adults or children and adolescents both fragment this age group (ie, some data in adolescent research, other data in adult research) and fail to obtain specific data on this age group (ie, data on young adults lumped in with data on all adults). This greatly limits the evidence base needed to provide effective treatment for this population.[2,65] The Institute of Medicine recommendations are as follows13p.329:

- Identify those EBPs [evidence-based practices] that hold promise for being effective in this age group and test them for efficacy;

- Identify EBPs that are likely to be effective with modification for this age group and test the efficacy of the modified versions; and
- Identify behavioral and medical health care needs that are unlikely to be addressed by existing or modified EBPs and conduct research to develop and establish new EBPs for young adults in these areas.

Fortunately, the knowledge gap has been identified and there is growing interest in identifying effective treatments for this population to decrease morbidity, disability, and mortality and the cost of increased social services that become necessary in part owing to ineffective mental health treatment through this developmental stage. Services and treatments need to be both attractive and culturally sensitive to those they serve and reflect the diverse backgrounds, languages, and cultures of the populations involved.

There is no research to date that assesses the pharmacologic effectiveness of Food and Drug Administration-approved treatments specifically in TAY. Inferences can be made from the associated literature about adolescents and mature adults. The complicating factor for treating these youth involves shared decision making. If the youth is below the age of 18, a parent or guardian needs to consent to the treatment, but assent from the youth should be obtained as well. Similarly, youth older than 18 may continue to lean heavily on parental guidance. Involving additional family members in the informed consent process may be beneficial in these cases to increase adherence to the regimen. Knowledge of the family dynamics and support system in place for each individual and consent from youth greater than 18 years of age should dictate involvement of both youth and family in the shared decision making process. There are no known long-term studies looking at the impact of psychotropic medication use over the typical lifespan when these medications were initiated during adolescence and there are many barriers to designing such studies.[72] Furthermore, there is little evidence base to inform practitioners when medications may be tapered and removed, if at all, after transition through this developmental stage, an important implication and safety concern when one considers the risk of the metabolic syndrome and other long-term effects of some psychotropic medications. Moreover, given this unique developmental stage, being able to discuss the benefits and risks of medication with young people in a manner that is developmentally appropriate, nonjudgmental, and engaging, and that includes parental figures as appropriate, is critical to successful pharmacologic treatment.[73] Generally, young adults prefer more active health care decision making than adults who are older.[74,75] Although a recent systematic review of shared decision making in health care settings concluded that it was beneficial for adults, particularly those with anxiety or affective disorders, there were no findings specific to TAY.[76] There is, unfortunately, a paucity of specific guidelines for shared decision making with individuals in this age group. Given the many developmental differences between younger and older adults, and the changing role of families in TAYs' lives, a specific set of guidelines is needed. Although several approaches have been described for use with adolescents with other health conditions,[77] or with mental health conditions,[78] none have examined the impact on clinical outcomes. A small qualitative study looking at TAY who were seeing a psychiatrist found that short visits were a barrier to treatment engagement and youth looked for increased amounts of time in session to participate in shared decision making. Psychiatrists who were able to engage in respectful and caring communications, encourage collaboration from the patient, and reduce professional boundaries were found to be more effective from the youth's perspective.[43]

Generally, any cognitive–behavioral or behavioral therapy that has efficacy in both adolescents and adults is likely to have efficacy in young adults because they are between these 2 groups in cognitive maturity. However, the ability to help this age group stay in treatment long enough to benefit is more challenging than in other age groups. Thus, the challenge to implementing likely effective interventions may be finding strategies to help young adults and older adolescents remain in treatment long enough to benefit. Motivational interviewing-based strategies have been shown to be effective in this age group, not only for reducing behavioral health symptoms, but for increasing session attendance.[79,80] Mistler and colleagues[40] developed a motivational enhancement therapy for treatment attrition, a brief pretherapy intervention that can be administered before a typical course of recommended treatment or revisited during times of resistance or prolonged absence from therapy to increase engagement in treatment. Motivational enhancement therapy for treatment attrition has good feasibility findings, although outcomes have not been evaluated yet.

Some other treatments that have developed evidence of efficacy in this age group include individual placement and support[81] and the NAVIGATE program, a comprehensive, multidisciplinary, team-based treatment approach for first episode psychosis.[82] A variety of other models and interventions are currently under development as evidence based practices. These include Just Do You, a service engagement intervention[83]; Achieve My Plan,[68,84] a person-centered care planning model; Multisystemic Therapy for Emerging Adults,[54,85] a comprehensive intervention to reduce recidivism and treat mental illness in justice-system involved emerging adults with mental illness; and Better Futures,[70] an intervention to enhance the success of postsecondary school engagement in former foster care youth with mental health conditions.

SUMMARY AND DISCUSSION

Providers and systems must be able to recognize the need for continuity of care between the ages of 16 and 30 for TAY with mental health conditions. Care needs to be continuous and coordinated across services in both the adult and youth systems of care to be effective. Furthermore, the services need to provide adequate variety, as well as options that are both appealing and developmentally appropriate, to increase access to services and prevent treatment attrition. Families and peers, as defined by the youth, should be encouraged to be involved in developmentally appropriate ways because these youth have not yet acquired the skills and knowledge required to navigate the existing complex systems in adult services and may lack the vocational and financial means to do so during this developmental stage. To achieve this goal, treating providers must have training and expertise in caring for this discrete developmental cohort that includes familiarity with the systems of care model and the ability to speak to the emerging adult in a developmentally appropriate way. They should use evolving technology to engage youth in care and disseminate information about services. To achieve these goals, further research must be done focusing on treatment engagement in this population as well as federal and state policies and funding streams that inadvertently create barriers and discontinuities at the same time that SMHCs is most likely to emerge and evolve.

REFERENCES

1. Arnett JJ. Emerging adulthood. A theory of development from the late teens through the twenties. Am Psychol 2000;55(5):469–80.

2. Davis M, Green M, Hoffman C. The service system obstacle course for transition-age youth and young adults. 2009. Available at: https://works.bepress.com/maryann_davis/8/. Accessed September 30, 2016.

3. Kessler RC, Berglund P, Demler O, et al. Lifetime prevalence and age-of-onset distributions of DSM-IV disorders in the national comorbidity survey replication. Arch Gen Psychiatry 2005;62(6):593–602.

4. de Girolamo G, Dagani J, Purcell R, et al. Age of onset of mental disorders and use of mental health services: needs, opportunities and obstacles. Epidemiol Psychiatr Sci 2012;21(1):47–57.

5. Kessler RC, Angermeyer M, Anthony JC, et al. Lifetime prevalence and age-of-onset distributions of mental disorders in the world health organization's world mental health survey initiative. World Psychiatry 2007;6(3):168–76.

6. Merikangas KR, He JP, Burstein M, et al. Lifetime prevalence of mental disorders in U.S. adolescents: results from the national comorbidity survey replication–adolescent supplement (NCS-A). J Am Acad Child Adolesc Psychiatry 2010; 49(10):980–9.

7. Clark HB, Unger KV, Stewart ES. Transition of youth and young adults with emotional/behavioral disorders into employment, education and independent living. Community Alternatives: International Journal of Family Care; 1993.

8. Davis M, Vander Stoep A. The transition to adulthood for youth who have serious emotional disturbance: developmental transition and young adult outcomes. J Ment Health Adm 1997;24(4):400–27.

9. Hare RD, Neumann CS. Psychopathy: assessment and forensic implications. Can J Psychiatry 2009;54(12):791–802.

10. Liston C, Watts R, Tottenham N, et al. Frontostriatal microstructure modulates efficient recruitment of cognitive control. Cereb Cortex 2006;16(4):553–60.

11. Christakou A, Halari R, Smith AB, et al. Sex-dependent age modulation of frontostriatal and temporo-parietal activation during cognitive control. Neuroimage 2009; 48(1):223–36.

12. Steinberg L. Cognitive and affective development in adolescence. Trends Cogn Sci 2005;9(2):69–74.

13. Stroud C, Walker LR, Davis M, et al. Investing in the health and well-being of young adults. Journal of Adolescent Health 2015;56(2):127–9.

14. Gogtay N, Giedd JN, Lusk L, et al. Dynamic mapping of human cortical development during childhood through early adulthood. Proc Natl Acad Sci U S A 2004; 101(21):8174–9.

15. Cohen AO, Breiner K, Steinberg L, et al. When is an adolescent an adult? assessing cognitive control in emotional and nonemotional contexts. Psychol Sci 2016; 27(4):549–62.

16. Gardner M, Steinberg L. Peer influence on risk taking, risk preference, and risky decision making in adolescence and adulthood: an experimental study. Dev Psychol 2005;41(4):625–35.

17. Sheidow AJ, McCart M, Zajac K, et al. Prevalence and impact of substance use among emerging adults with serious mental health conditions. Psychiatr Rehabil J 2012;35(3):235–43.

18. Malian I, Nevin A. A review of self-determination literature: implications for practitioners. Remedial Spec Edu 2002;23(2):68–74.

19. Carter BE, McGoldrick ME. The changing family life cycle: a framework for family therapy. New York: Gardner Press; 1988.

20. Settersten RA Jr, Ray B. What's going on with young people today? The long and twisting path to adulthood. Future Child 2010;20(1):19–41.

21. Vignoles VL, Owe E, Becker M, et al. Beyond the 'East–West' dichotomy: global variation in cultural models of selfhood. J Exp Psychol Gen 2016;145:966–1000.

22. Supple AJ, Ghazarian SR, Peterson GW, et al. Assessing the cross-cultural validity of a parental autonomy granting measure comparing adolescents in the United States, China, Mexico, and India. J Cross Cult Psychol 2009;40(5):816–33.

23. Lipari RN, Hedden SL. Serious mental health challenges among older adolescents and young adults. The CBHSQ Report. Rockville (MD): Substance Abuse and Mental Health Services Administration (US); 2013.

24. U.S. Census Bureau. Annual estimates of the resident population by single year of age and sex for the united states: April 1, 2010 to July 1, 2014 (NC-EST2014-AGE-SEX-RES). 2014. Available at: https://www.census.gov/popest/data/datasets.html.

25. Vander Stoep A, Beresford SA, Weiss NS, et al. Community-based study of the transition to adulthood for adolescents with psychiatric disorder. Am J Epidemiol 2000;152(4):352–62.

26. Armstrong KH, Dedrick RF, Greenbaum PE. Factors associated with community adjustment of young adults with serious emotional disturbance: a longitudinal analysis. J Emot Behav Disord 2003;11(2):66–76.

27. Wagner M, Newman L, Cameto R, et al. Changes over time in the early post-school outcomes of youth with disabilities. A report of findings from the national longitudinal transition study (NLTS) and the national longitudinal transition study-2 (NLTS2). Menlo Park (CA): SRI International; 2005.

28. Wagner M, Newman L. Longitudinal transition outcomes of youth with emotional disturbances. Psychiatr Rehabil J 2012;35(3):199–208.

29. Hartley MT. Increasing resilience. Am J Psychiatr Rehabil 2010;13(4):295–315. Available at: https://arizona.pure.elsevier.com/en/publications/increasing-resilience-strategies-for-reducing-dropout-rates-for-c. Accessed September 28, 2016.

30. Kessler RC, Sonnega A, Bromet E, et al. Posttraumatic stress disorder in the national comorbidity survey. Arch Gen Psychiatry 1995;52(12):1048–60.

31. Davis M, Delman J, Duperoy T. Employment and careers in young adults with psychiatric disabilities. Worcester (MA): University of Massachusetts Medical School, Department of Psychiatry, Center for Mental Health Services Research, Transitions RTC; 2013.

32. Fernandes-Alcantara A. Runaway and homeless youth: demographics and programs. Washington, DC: Congressional Research Service; 2013.

33. Cauce AM, Paradise M, Ginzler JA, et al. The characteristics and mental health of homeless adolescents: age and gender differences. J Emotional Behav Disord 2000;8(4):230–9.

34. Davis M, Banks SM, Fisher WH, et al. Arrests of adolescent clients of a public mental health system during adolescence and young adulthood. Psychiatr Serv 2007;58(11):1454–60.

35. Chung HL, Little M, Steinberg L. The transition to adulthood for adolescents in the juvenile justice system: a developmental perspective. Chicago (IL): University of Chicago Press; 2005. p. 68–91.

36. Wagner MM, Wei X, Thornton SP, et al. Accessing services for youth with emotional disturbances in and after high school. Career Dev Transit Except Individ 2015;39(3):164–74.

37. Prange ME, Greenbaum PE, Silver SE, et al. Family functioning and psychopathology among adolescents with severe emotional disturbances. J Abnorm Child Psychol 1992;20(1):83–102.

38. Edlund MJ, Wang PS, Berglund PA, et al. Dropping out of mental health treatment: patterns and predictors among epidemiological survey respondents in the United States and Ontario. Am J Psychiatry 2002;159(5):845–51.

39. Olfson M, Marcus SC, Druss B, et al. National trends in the use of outpatient psychotherapy. Am J Psychiatry 2002;159(11):1914–20.

40. Mistler L, Sheidow AJ, Davis M. Trans-diagnostic motivational enhancement therapy to reduce treatment attrition: use in emerging adults. Cogn Behav Pract 2016;23(3):368–84.

41. Copeland WE, Shanahan L, Davis M, et al. Increase in untreated cases of psychiatric disorders during the transition to adulthood. Psychiatr Serv 2015;66(4):397–403.

42. Substance Abuse and Mental Health Services Administration (SAMHSA). Now is the time. Web site. Available at: http://www.samhsa.gov/priorities/now-is-the-time. Accessed October 14, 2016.

43. Delman J, Clark JA, Eisen SV, et al. Facilitators and barriers to the active participation of clients with serious mental illnesses in medication decision making: the perceptions of young adult clients. J Behav Health Serv Res 2015;42(2):238–53.

44. Pulford J, Adams P, Sheridan J. Therapist attitudes and beliefs relevant to client dropout revisited. Community Ment Health J 2008;44(3):181–6.

45. United States Government Accountability Office. Young adults with serious mental illness: some states and federal agencies are taking steps to address their transition challenges. Washington, DC: United States Government Accountability Office; 2008.

46. Pottick KJ, Bilder S, Stoep AV, et al. US patterns of mental health service utilization for transition-age youth and young adults. J Behav Health Serv Res 2007;35(4):373–89. Available at: http://link.springer.com/article/10.1007/s11414-007-9080-4. Accessed September 29, 2016.

47. Davis M, Banks S, Fisher W, et al. Longitudinal patterns of offending during the transition to adulthood in youth from the mental health system. J Behav Health Serv Res 2004;31(4):351–66.

48. Delman J, Jones A. Voices of youth in transition: the experience of aging out of the adolescent public mental health service system in Massachusetts: policy implications and recommendations. 2002. Available at: http://works.bepress.com/jonathan_delman/12/. Accessed January 17, 2017.

49. Jivanjee P, Kruzich J, Gordon LJ. Community integration of transition-age individuals: views of young with mental health disorders. J Behav Health Serv Res 2008;35(4):402–18.

50. Wang J, Patten SB, Williams JV, et al. Help-seeking behaviours of individuals with mood disorders. Can J Psychiatry 2005;50(10):652–9.

51. Hoffman C, Heflinger CA, Athay M, et al. Policy, funding, and sustainability: issues and recommendations for promoting effective transition systems. 2009. Available at: http://works.bepress.com/maryann_davis/2/. Accessed January 17, 2017.

52. Walker JS. A theory of change for positive developmental approaches to improving outcomes among emerging adults with serious mental health conditions. J Behav Health Serv Res 2015;42(2):131–49. Available at: http://link.springer.com/article/10.1007/s11414-015-9455-x. Accessed September 29, 2016.

53. Walker JS, Flower KM. Provider perspectives on principle-adherent practice in empirically supported interventions for emerging adults with serious mental health conditions. J Behav Health Serv Res 2015;43(4):525–41.

54. Sheidow AJ, McCart MR, Davis M. Multisystemic therapy for emerging adults with serious mental illness and justice involvement. Cogn Behav Pract 2016;23(3):356–67.

55. Fagan M, Davis M, Denietolis BM, et al. Innovative residential interventions for young adults in transition. Residential interventions for children, adolescents, and families: a best practice guide. East Sussex (UK): Taylor & Francis; 2014. p. 126.

56. Gilmer TP, Ojeda VD, Leich J, et al. Assessing needs for mental health and other services among transition-age youths, parents, and providers. Psychiatr Serv 2012;63(4):338–42.

57. Settersten RA. Linking the two ends of life: what gerontology can learn from childhood studies. J Gerontol B Psychol Sci Soc Sci 2005;60(4):173.

58. Haber MG, Karpur A, Deschenes N, et al. Predicting improvement of transitioning young people in the partnerships for youth transition initiative: findings from a multisite demonstration. J Behav Health Serv Res 2008;35(4):488–513.

59. Embry LE, Vander Stoep AV, Evens C, et al. Risk factors for homelessness in adolescents released from psychiatric residential treatment. J Am Acad Child Adolesc Psychiatry 2000;39(10):1293–9.

60. Callahan L, Cocozza J, Steadman HJ, et al. A national survey of US juvenile mental health courts. Psychiatr Serv 2012;63(2):130–4.

61. Stroul B, Blau G, Friedman R. Updating the system of care concept and philosophy. Washington, DC: Georgetown University Center for Child and Human Development; National Technical Assistance Center for Children's Mental Health; 2010.

62. Clark DM, Layard R, Smithies R, et al. Improving access to psychological therapy: initial evaluation of two UK demonstration sites. Behav Res Ther 2009; 47(11):910–20.

63. Wagner KD, Martinez M, Joiner T. Youths' and their parents' attitudes and experiences about participation in psychopharmacology treatment research. J Child Adolesc Psychopharmacol 2006;16(3):298–307.

64. Block AM, Greeno CG. Examining outpatient treatment dropout in adolescents: a literature review. Child Adolesc Social Work J 2011;28(5):393–420.

65. Davis M, Koroloff N, Ellison ML. Between adolescence and adulthood: rehabilitation research to improve services for youth and young adults. Psychiatric Rehabilitation Journal 2012;35(3):167–70.

66. Marsenich L, Kelch LD. A roadmap to mental health services for transition age young women: a research review. Sacramento (CA): California Institute for Mental Health; 2005.

67. Davis M, Hunt B. State efforts to expand transition supports for young adults receiving adult public mental health services. Systems and Psychosocial Advances Research Center Publications and Presentations. 436; 2005. Available at: http://escholarship.umassmed.edu/psych_cmhsr/436. Accessed January 17, 2017.

68. Walker JS, Pullmann MD, Moser CL, et al. Does team-based planning" work" for adolescents? findings from studies of wraparound. Psychiatr Rehabil J 2012; 35(3):189.

69. Klodnick VV, Davis KE, Fagan MA, et al. Launching into adulthood from institutional care with a serious mental health condition. Community Ment Health J 2014;50(2):209–15.

70. Geenen S, Powers LE, Phillips LA, et al. Better futures: a randomized field test of a model for supporting young people in foster care with mental health challenges to participate in higher education. J Behav Health Serv Res 2015;42(2):150–71.

71. Lane KL, Carter EW. Supporting transition-age youth with and at risk for emotional and behavioral disorders at the secondary level: a need for further inquiry. J Emotional Behav Disord 2006;14(2):66–70.

72. Gupta S, Cahill JD. A prescription for "Deprescribing" in psychiatry. Psychiatr Serv 2016;67(8):904–7.

73. Hetrick S, Simmons M, Merry S. SSRIs and depression in children and adolescents: the imperative for shared decision-making. Australas Psychiatry 2008; 16(5):354–8.

74. Arora NK, McHorney CA. Patient preferences for medical decision making: who really wants to participate? Med Care 2000;38(3):335–41.

75. Catalan J, Brener N, Andrews H, et al. Whose health is it? Views about decision-making and information-seeking from people with HIV infection and their professional carers. AIDS Care 1994;6(3):349–56.

76. Shay LA, Lafata JE. Where is the evidence? A systematic review of shared decision making and patient outcomes. Med Decis Making 2015;35(1):114–31.

77. Herlitz A, Munthe C, Torner M, et al. The counseling, self-care, adherence approach to person-centered care and shared decision making: moral psychology, executive autonomy, and ethics in multi-dimensional care decisions. Health Commun 2016;31(8):964–73.

78. Metz MJ, Franx GC, Veerbeek MA, et al. Shared decision making in mental health care using routine outcome monitoring as a source of information: a cluster randomised controlled trial. BMC Psychiatry 2015;15(1):1.

79. Grote NK, Swartz HA, Geibel SL, et al. A randomized controlled trial of culturally relevant, brief interpersonal psychotherapy for perinatal depression. Psychiatr Serv 2009;60(3):313–21.

80. Buckner JD, Schmidt NB. A randomized pilot study of motivation enhancement therapy to increase utilization of cognitive–behavioral therapy for social anxiety. Behav Res Ther 2009;47(8):710–5.

81. Bond GR, Drake RE, Campbell K. Effectiveness of individual placement and support supported employment for young adults. Early Interv Psychiatry 2014;10(4): 300–7.

82. Kane JM, Robinson DG, Schooler NR, et al. Comprehensive versus usual community care for first-episode psychosis: 2-year outcomes from the NIMH RAISE early treatment program. Am J Psychiatry 2015;173(4):362–72.

83. Munson MR, Cole A, Jaccard J, et al. An engagement intervention for young adults with serious mental health conditions. J Behav Health Serv Res 2014; 43(4):542–63.

84. Moser C, Walker J, Allen J, et al. No title. Achieve My Plan (AMP!): youth participation in planning teams. Webinar Research & Training Center for Pathways to Positive Futures. Portland (OR): Portland State University.

85. Davis M, Sheidow AJ, McCart MR. Reducing recidivism and symptoms in emerging adults with serious mental health conditions and justice system involvement. J Behav Health Serv Res 2015;42(2):172–90.

Conceptualization of Success in Young Adulthood

Maryland Pao, MD

KEYWORDS

- Successful transition • Mental health • Mental illness • Physical illness • Treatment

KEY POINTS

- Successful transition from childhood to adolescence and into adulthood is context and culture dependent.
- There may be a few universal concepts of what is thought to be fundamental to being a successful adult.
- Parents, educators, mental health professionals, and policymakers need to be cognizant of their assumptions about what successful adult is and understand they play essential roles in developing policies and practices to promote this.
- It is important to discuss what "success" looks like with transitional age youth and their family members because treatment approaches may adapt accordingly.

INTRODUCTION

Success, like beauty, is in the eye of the beholder. As such, there are many forms that success can take at the individual, familial, and societal levels. The concept of a successful transition to adulthood is, therefore, completely context (including geographic and historical moment) and culture dependent. However, from Marcus Aurelius, a Roman Emperor in 170 AD, who told us centuries ago in his collection of *Meditations*, "When you arise in the morning, think of what a precious privilege it is to be alive - to breathe, to think, to enjoy, to love"[1] to Martin Luther King, Jr., who last century told us, "If you can't fly then run, if you can't run then walk, if you can't walk then crawl, but whatever you do you have to keep moving forward,"[2] we can see there may be a few universal concepts of what is thought to be fundamental to being a successful adult as we help transitional age youth (TAY) reach for realization and try to thrive in adulthood.

The author has nothing to disclose.
Office of the Clinical Director, NIMH, NIH, 10 Center Drive, Bethesda 20817, MD, USA
E-mail address: paom@mail.nih.gov

Child Adolesc Psychiatric Clin N Am 26 (2017) 191–198
http://dx.doi.org/10.1016/j.chc.2016.12.002
1056-4993/17/Published by Elsevier Inc.

This article first presents definitions of mental health and mental illness that have evolved in the field of psychiatry. Applying a developmental lens, the author then reviews several dimensions of successful young adult development that have been described in the literature. It is important to note that the assumptions articulated by these definitions and ideals represent a Western value system, often based on self-determination theory,[3] which postulates that 3 innate psychological needs—competence, autonomy, and relatedness—underlie mental health. Because there is not one specific pathway to successful adulthood, and there will be tensions between personal, familial, and community ambitions, it is essential that TAY, parents or guardians, clinicians, educators, and policymakers recognize, clearly articulate and evaluate their vision together and clarify common goals of "success," because this will lead us to specific treatment interventions and particular governmental and educational policies.

HISTORICAL DEFINITION OF MENTAL HEALTH

Historically, mental illness was described by ancient civilizations including the Egyptians and Greeks, who recognized and named hysteria and melancholy.[4] Because the flagrant symptoms of mental illness are readily apparent to others, individuals with these symptoms were often seen by society in medieval times as criminals, insane, or morally corrupt. As the field of psychiatry began to develop in the late 1800s, it became more humane, but was still primarily focused on understanding and treating psychopathology and deviant behavior.[4] In the early 20th century, the fields of mental hygiene and psychology began to evolve and the concept of mental health started to be studied, although Freud is reported to have dismissed mental health as "an ideal fiction."[5] Until after World War II, mental health had eluded definition in the literature, although it was clearly more than the absence of mental illness, but little research had been done on to how to measure positive mental health.

WORLD HEALTH ORGANIZATION DEFINITIONS OF HEALTH, MENTAL HEALTH, AND QUALITY OF LIFE

First defined in 1946 and last modified in 1948, the World Health Organization (WHO) defined health as, "Health is a state of complete physical, mental and social well-being and not merely the absence of disease or infirmity."[6] As of 2014, the WHO states the following, "Mental health is defined as a state of well-being in which every individual realizes his or her own potential, can cope with the normal stresses of life, can work productively and fruitfully, and is able to make a contribution to her or his community."[7] To measure well-being, the WHO developed a cross-cultural tool to measure the improvement in quality of life related to health care through monitoring changes in the frequency and severity of diseases. Encompassing multiple factors including positive mental and physical health, WHO defines quality of life as "an individual's perception of their position in life in the context of the culture and value systems in which they live and in relation to their goals, expectations, standards and concerns."[8]

In the past decade, the WHO has recognized that, internationally, people are reporting as much disability from disabling mental conditions as from physical conditions and that mental disorders are affecting their activities of daily living, ability to communicate, personal relationships and occupational functioning. Mental disorders rank among the most disabling conditions in terms of total disability-adjusted life years, a WHO metric developed in 1990 to estimate the global burden of disease; disability-adjusted life years are an estimate of how many years of life are lost owing to premature death or to being in a state of poor health and disability.[9] The WHO has issued the Mental Health Action Plan 2013 to 2020 to encourage world leaders to provide more comprehensive plans and services to promote mental health as well as to prevent mental disorders.[10]

MENNINGER DEFINITION OF MENTAL HEALTH

At about the same time as the introduction of the WHO definition of health, a prominent US psychiatrist, Karl Menninger, defined mental health as "an adjustment of human beings to the world and to each other with a maximum of effectiveness and happiness."[11] The Menninger research group, led by psychologist Lester Luborsky, developed the Health-Sickness Rating Scale,[12] a precursor to the *Diagnostic and Statistical Manual of Mental Disorders,* 4th edition, Global Assessment of Functioning scale.[13] On Luborsky's scale, a score of 80 or above reflected positive mental health, which has been subsequently supported in cross-cultural settings as well.[14] Of note, the Global Assessment of Functioning scale has been dropped recently, in the *Diagnostic and Statistical Manual of Mental Disorders, 5th edition,*[15] and the WHO Disability Assessment Schedule 2.0 (WHODAS 2.0) is proposed as an option for measuring disability.[8]

MODELS OF MENTAL HEALTH

George Vaillant,[5] a researcher who has studied a longitudinal cohort of Harvard graduates for more than 50 years, described in a review of models of mental health the following conceptualizations of mental health as:

- Above normal, a mental state that is objectively desirable—as in the capacity to work and to love;
- Positive psychology, an early example of which was Maslow's "self-actualizing" individual[16];
- Maturity;
- Emotional or social intelligence;
- Subjective well-being—a mental state that is subjectively experienced as happy, contented, and desired; and
- Resilience, as in successful adaptation and homeostasis.

Most likely, it is some combination of all of these factors. Vaillant[5] described, "Of course, healthy adult development does not follow rigid rules, nor are butterflies healthier than caterpillars. Some individuals, often because of great stress, tackle developmental tasks out of order or all at once." He recognizes that attributes or skills may have different developmental trajectories and that is certainly what TAY, particularly with mental and physical problems, may experience in even more exaggerated and disparate ways that can make transition to young adulthood and mental health treatment challenging.

One personal quality that has gained significant prominence in our society in the past couple of decades is the importance of high social–emotional intelligence. Gardner[17] described emotional intelligence as the capacity to "discern and respond appropriately to the moods, temperaments, motivations and desires of other people." Goleman[18] more explicitly defined emotional intelligence with the following criteria:

- Accurate conscious perception and monitoring of one's own emotions;
- Modification of one's emotions so that their expression is appropriate, including the capacity to self-soothe anxiety, sadness, and anger;
- Accurate recognition of and response to emotions in others;
- Skill in negotiating close relationships with others; and
- Capacity for focusing emotions (motivation) on a desired goal (delayed gratification).[5]

MODELS OF POSITIVE YOUTH DEVELOPMENT

Erikson[19] described the developmental tasks of young adulthood of becoming independent from family and known supports (psychologically as well as physically), of developing one's identity and role in society, and of developing intimacy or relationships with others, including romantic ones. These complex tasks, concretely denoted as leaving the parental home to establish one's own residence, establishing financial independence (eg, paying one's bills), completing high school or college, moving into full-time employment, getting married, and becoming a parent, are often considered by society as key markers of adulthood but clearly vary by culture and opportunity.[20] These tasks that, over time, expand an individual's social circle and impact,[5] must also be accomplished against a tumultuous backdrop of rapid hormonal and brain changes in a constantly changing external environment.

In an extensive review of the developmental literature, from a strength-based approach, Scales and colleagues[20] distilled research findings from the Search Institute and the Social Development Research Group to identify 8 consensus core dimensions of successful young adult development. These include:

- Physical health,
- Psychological and emotional well-being,
- Life skills,
- Ethical behavior,
- Healthy family and social relationships,
- Educational attainment,
- Constructive educational and occupational engagement, and
- Civic engagement.

Scales and colleagues[20] acknowledge that, "No set of dimensions of developmental success, for any life stage, possibly can be entirely valid for all imaginable variations of class, gender, sexual orientation, racial-ethnic, and religious, diversities, among others." In a separate study, the Pathways Mapping Initiative at Harvard University, also found as desired outcomes young adults who were effectively educated; embarked on or prepared for a productive career; physically, mentally, and emotionally healthy; active participants in civic life; and prepared for parenting.[21]

For each of the core dimensions identified by Scales and colleagues,[20] assumptions were made; for example, a healthy physical or emotional state will not be free of risk or experimentation or without the normal developmental feelings of anxiety, sadness, or self-doubt. Also, successful young adults develop skills to diminish risks and handle challenges typical of this life stage, such as use of alcohol and other drugs and relationship disappointments. The review also describes the social development model,[22] which presupposes that, to stay on a positive developmental trajectory, TAY need to establish bonds with family, partners, and peers at developmentally appropriate ages and be given prosocial opportunities to build competencies and skills in school, work, and community settings over time.[20] The social development model has been researched extensively and found to predict health-related outcomes, including sub-stance use and misuse, depression, violence, school misbehavior, and other problem behaviors.[20] Evolving models of the social development model that focus on develop-mental relationships suggest a framework of more bidirectional interactions[23] that "rather than being seen as a lock-step progression of invariant stages of development neatly correlated with specific chronologic ages, development [is] seen more as an evolving person-context double helix structure."[20] This highlights that the process of forming developmental relationships is iterative and there are potentially multiple opportunities and timepoints to intervene to try to change a youth's trajectory in pos-itive directions.

One purpose of identifying the core dimensions for successful young adulthood is to be able to measure and track the dimensions if educators, policymakers, and govern-ment leaders establish programs for youth and positive development in the commu-nity at large. Scales and colleagues[20] conclude, "This suggests that far greater *intentionality* in helping young people and their socializing systems deal with that shift in relationships, contexts, demands, and opportunities is vital for a successful transi-tion to young adulthood." Similarly, Nagaoka and colleagues,[24] from the University of Chicago Consortium on Chicago School Research led a group of educators and pol-icymakers on a report entitled: *Foundations for Young Adult Success: A Develop-mental Framework.* They define success in young adulthood as well as underscore the developmental experiences that are necessary to build a strong foundation to navigate the transition throughout a youth's school and community experiences. Organized around the 3 key factors of (1) agency, (2) an integrated identity, and (3) competencies, they found that self-regulation, awareness, reflection on or making meaning out of experiences, and critical thinking skills were important foundations for success.[24] The report describes agency as one's ability to make active choices while developing competencies such as responsible decision making and being able to collaborate with others, which eventually becomes incorporated into an inte-grated identity, or a consistent internal framework across time.[24] This model, although proposed to address bridging the opportunity gap for youth living in impoverished ur-ban areas, can also inform program and policy development for other vulnerable youth populations, such as those with mental illness.

IMPLICATIONS OF THE MODELS

Vaillant[25] posed the fundamental question: "What facets of mental health are fixed and which are susceptible to change?" These definitions and models seem to converge on the idea that self-determination, skills to adapt to the vagaries of life, and the skills to relate to others lead to a sense of well-being and the concept of quality of life as described. Further, the various models lead clinicians to ponder the modifiable factors for advocacy and treatment of TAY at the individual, familial, educational and societal levels. They also point out the need for identifying specific goals, harmonization, and persistent planning. Nagaoka and colleagues[24] instruct in their concept paper, "Pre-paring all youth for meaningful, productive futures requires coordinated efforts and intentional practices by adults across all the settings youth inhabit on a daily basis." Young people's opportunities will vary significantly by race and socioeconomic class, but also by experiences such as hospitalizations for mental and physical illnesses and other events such as war or natural disaster. At an educational level, Nagaoka and col-leagues[24] suggest different institutional emphases will be needed at different develop-mental stages that, although obvious to child mental health workers, may not be foremost on the minds of policymakers and city, state, and national leaders.

HOW DOES THE DEFINITION OF SUCCESS INFLUENCE OUR TREATMENT APPROACH?

As medical professionals, along with parents and educators, we may consider our task as the following, "To maximize children's functional abilities and sense of well-being, their health-related quality of life, and their development into healthy and productive adults."[26] So, why is it important to articulate our vision of successful transition to adulthood for TAY? Because our vision influences our treatment goals and strategies and methods used. In helping families, we need to take a self-assessment of what our own expectations are in addition to those of the TAY patient and the TAY's family. Clinicians often help TAY to take stock of their strengths and difficulties, assess where and why they may have fallen off their trajectory, and reevaluate whether their goals need adjustment. Facilitating creativity, such as writing music, painting, or taking photographs, or technical proficiency in an area, such as cooking, electrical wiring, or car engine repair, may be more helpful for a particular TAY than attending college, as an example. Families play a critical role in helping TAY meet or accept altered expectations, such as living in a supervised home with case managers or participating in supported employment. Clinicians will need to be able to work with a full spectrum of parenting styles, from authoritarian or over-involved parents to laissez-faire or free-range parents. As clinicians, we may hope to strike a balance, but must do so with intentionality and flexibility to adapt to whatever events or crises arise and to whatever the TAY brings to the table with regard to abilities and temperament. It is crucial for all involved to have expectations for the next achievement. Without expectations and goals, failure can be a self-fulfilling prophecy for the TAY, but sometimes goals do need to be adjusted. Although the early development of a mental illness may disrupt developmental trajectories and certainly alters the timelines of achieving different developmental milestones, we should not believe that youth with serious mental illnesses should expect any less quality of life. It is important, however, to discuss what "success" looks and feels like with TAY and their family members, because treatment approaches may need to adapt accordingly.

TRANSITION AGE YOUTH, ADULTHOOD, AND BEYOND

Research shows that in the absence of disease, the brain continues to work well until at least age 80.[27] Current neuroscience research increasingly indicates that, even in adulthood, the brain is plastic and that learning and memory are lifelong adaptive brain processes. In their book about aging, Holland and Greenstein[28] share, "research has shown that among people between the ages of 18 and 85, the age group that feels the greatest sense of well-being is 82 to 85." This serves to remind us that developmental trajectories may be altered as we continue to grow, learn and mature and we can continue to strive for well-being well into old age.

SUMMARY

Successful transition for TAY is context and culture dependent. It can be defined not only as preventing problems, but as positive functioning in several domains including autonomy, competence, and relationships. Many of the goals to be achieved are fundamental and universal for us as humans, regardless of physical or mental illnesses that may develop as we age. The successful development of youth into young adulthood includes positive psychological self-perceptions and skills building with the hopes of achieving some universal societal markers. Conscious understanding and discussion of what "success" looks like with TAY and their family members as well as among educators, clinicians, and policy leaders can lead to the creation of intentional programs and appropriate innovative treatment approaches.

REFERENCES

1. Aurelis M. Meditations. New York: Penguin Books; 2005.
2. King ML. Available at: https://www.goodreads.com/author/quotes/23924.Martin_Luther_King_Jr_. Accessed November 13, 2016.
3. Ryan RM, Deci EL. Self-determination theory and the facilitation of intrinsic motivation, social development, and well-being. Am Psychol 2000;55:68–78.
4. Alexander FG, Sheldon TS. The history of psychiatry: an evaluation of psychiatric thought and practice from prehistoric times to the present. New York: Harper and Row, Publishers; 1966.
5. Vaillant GE. Mental health. Am J Psychiatry 2003;160:1373–84.
6. Preamble to the Constitution of the World Health Organization as adopted by the International Health Conference, New York, 19-22 June, 1946; signed on 22 July 1946 by the representatives of 61 States (Official Records of the World Health Organization, no. 2, p. 100) and entered into force on 7 April 1948. Available at: http://www.who.int/about/definition/en/print.html. Accessed November 13, 2016.
7. World Health Organization. Mental health: a state of well-being. Available at: http://www.who.int/features/factfiles/mental_health/en/. Accessed November 13, 2016.
8. World Health Organization. WHOQOL: measuring quality of life. Available at: http://www.who.int/mental_health/media/68.pdf. Accessed November 13, 2016.
9. World Health Organization. Metrics: disability-adjusted life year (DALY). Quantifying the burden of disease from mortality and morbidity. Available at: http://www.who.int/healthinfo/global_burden_disease/metrics_daly/en/. Accessed November 13, 2016.
10. World Health Organization. Comprehensive mental health action plan 2013–2020. Available at: http://www.who.int/mental_health/action_plan_2013/en/. Accessed November 13, 2016.
11. Menninger WC. A psychiatrist for a troubled world. In: Hall BH, editor. Selected papers of William C. Menninger. New York: The Viking Press; 1967. p. 607.
12. Luborsky L. Clinicians' judgments of mental health: a proposed scale. Arch Gen Psychiatry 1962;7:407–17.
13. Endicott J, Spitzer RL, Fleiss JL, et al. The Global Assessment Scale: a procedure for measuring overall severity of psychiatric disturbance. Arch Gen Psychiatry 1976;33:766–71.
14. Armelius BA, Gerin P, Luborsky L, et al. Clinician's judgment of mental health: an international validation of HSRS. Psychother Res 1991;1:31–8.
15. American Psychiatric Association. Diagnostic and statistical manual of mental disorders: DSM-5. Washington, DC: American Psychiatric Association; 2013.
16. Maslow AH. Motivation and personality. 2nd edition. New York: Harper & Row; 1970.
17. Gardner H. Frames of mind. New York: Basic Books; 1983.
18. Goleman D. Emotional intelligence. New York: Bantam Books; 1995.
19. Erikson E. Childhood and society. New York: Norton; 1950.
20. Scales PC, Benson PL, Oesterle S, et al. The dimensions of successful young adult development: a conceptual and measurement framework. Appl Dev Sci 2016;20:150–74.

21. Schorr LB, Marchand V. Pathway to the prevention of childhood abuse and neglect. Project on Effective Interventions & Pathways Mapping Initiative 2007. Available at: http://www.dss.cahwnet.gov/CDSSWEB/entres/pdf/Pathway.pdf. Accessed November 13, 2016.

22. Catalano RF, Hawkins JD. The social development model: a theory of antisocial behavior. In: Hawkins JD, editor. Delinquency and crime: current theories. New York: Cambridge University Press; 1996.

23. Pekel K, Roehlkepartain EC, Syvertsen AK, et al. Don't forget the families: the missing piece in America's effort to help all children succeed. Minneapolis (MN): Search Institute; 2015.

24. Nagaoka J, Farrington CA, Ehrlich SB, et al. Foundations for young adult success: a developmental framework. Chicago (IL): The University of Chicago Consortium on Chicago School Research; 2015. Available at: https://consortium.uchicago.edu/publications/foundations-young-adult-success-developmental-framework. Accessed November 13, 2016.

25. Vaillant GE. Positive mental health: is there a cross-cultural definition? World Psychiatry 2012;11:93–9.

26. American Academy of Pediatrics, Committee on Children with Disabilities and Committee on Psychosocial Aspects of Child and Family Health. Psychosocial risks of chronic health conditions in childhood and adolescence. Pediatrics 1993;92:876–8.

27. Schaie KW. The Seattle Longitudinal Study: a 21-year exploration of psychometric intelligence in adulthood. In: Schaie KW, editor. Longitudinal studies of adult psychological development. New York: Guilford; 1983. p. 64–135.

28. Holland J, Greenstein M. Lighter as we go: virtues, character strengths and aging. New York: Oxford University Press; 2015. p. 10.

Common Challenges

Involving Parents/Family in Treatment during the Transition from Late Adolescence to Young Adulthood

Rationale, Strategies, Ethics, and Legal Issues

Cecilia M.W. Livesey, MD[a], Anthony L. Rostain, MD, MA[b],*

KEYWORDS

- Emerging adulthood • Young adults • Family therapy • Mental health

KEY POINTS

- Transition to adulthood is a time of great change in youths' relational patterns with parents, family, and peers.
- Familial factors and relational dynamics significantly contribute to the ability of transitional age youth (TAY) to successfully evolve into adulthood, with its hallmarks of autonomy, stable sense of self, personal responsibility, and financial independence.
- Parenting styles, family stresses, and cultural considerations have an impact on this process of separation-individuation-differentiation.
- Clinical assessment of family structure, patterns of interaction, and underlying values should be understood and incorporated into the treatment planning for TAY.
- Family involvement in the treatment of TAY with mental health concerns has been demonstrated to have a significant impact on treatment outcomes.

INTRODUCTION

The period of transition from adolescence to adulthood is a time of tremendous change characterized by identity formation, independence, and shifting relationship dynamics among peers and parents. The family is embedded in all aspects of this transition and serves as both a protective support and a limiting factor, a complicated duality that raises psychological, practical, ethical, and legal issues. This article discusses the influence of familial factors and provides assessment strategies for evaluating the family in relation to mental health treatment of TAY. Although the family of

Disclosure Statement: The authors have nothing to disclose.
[a] Department of Psychiatry, The University of Pennsylvania Health System, 3535 Market Street, Room 4039, Philadelphia, PA 19104, USA; [b] Department of Psychiatry, Perelman School of Medicine, University of Pennsylvania, 3535 Market Street, Room 2007, Philadelphia, PA 19104, USA
* Corresponding author.
E-mail address: rostain@mail.med.upenn.edu

origin is always relevant, it is important to neither pathologize nor romanticize the family; rather, the integral role of the family should be appreciated and assessed with respect to a youth's mental health, global functioning, and trajectory into adulthood.

FAMILY RELATIONSHIPS IN THE TRANSITION TO ADULTHOOD
The Evolving Definition of Family

In recent decades, the concept of family has expanded to include strongly supportive, long-term relationships between people who may not be related by blood or marriage. Young adults may assign familial roles to friends or mentors, belong to unconventional or blended families, or have their own committed partners and children. The demographic shift toward a protracted period of group socialization and a sharp decline in durable romantic partnerships underscore the importance of extrafamilial entities on TAY trajectories.[1] The proliferation of social media and collapse of traditional communication barriers allow for uninterrupted identification with like-minded peer groups (although not without well-documented risks). As supportive members of TAY's physical and virtual communities, peers serve an integral role in the transition to adulthood: assisting in identity formation, clarifying values, and normalizing changes. For lesbian, gay, bisexual, transgender, and questioning (LGBTQ) youth, peers may be incorporated into their chosen expanded family, especially if parents are not accepting of their gender or sexuality. And, for non–European American youth, family norms of intergenerational interdependence may clash with peer group ideals of autonomy.

It is critical to ask youth whom they identify as family and their preferences for involvement of their defined family in treatment.

Cultural Differences

Conflict between ancestral kin and self-defined support networks occurs more readily in cultural groups that prioritize family obligation and self-sacrifice in opposition to youth's struggle for self-determination.[2–4] Non-European immigrant families may grapple with reconciling their collectivist cultural orientation with the individualistic values of American society. For example, although in both native and immigrant families the degree of psychological autonomy afforded to adolescents is positively correlated with enhanced self-worth, Mexican American youth do not perceive parental psychological control as negatively as their European American counterparts. This indicates integration of the Mexican emphasis on family involvement with the American ideal of independence.[5] Youth who are able to establish this type of bicultural identity have better adaptational outcomes than those who embrace full assimilation, marginalization, or cultural separation.[6]

TAY with 2 or more ethnic or racial backgrounds face an even more complex set of identity issues. They must explore both their racial identity, frequently associated with their appearance, and their ethnic background, which has an impact on their sense of group belonging. Multiracial young adults who have attained many indicators of adulthood, such as financial independence and an established career, may still be dealing with fundamental identity questions and conflicts with older family members.

Clinicians should identify cultural components of barriers to treatment; expand their cultural knowledge base; address acculturation stress and incorporate cultural strengths in treatment; maintain a culturally curious and sensitive stance; and be cognizant of cultural biases.[6,7]

Generational Issues

Generational differences (gaps) relating to social norms, knowledge, and values also contribute to the complexities encountered in the transition to adulthood, as each generation has its own investment in the family structure. Adolescents have a stake in believing their parents are limited and old-fashioned, but this divergence helps propel youth to separate and individuate from their parents. More research is needed to explore the challenges and effects of multigenerational households and intergenerational conflict on TAY.

Trauma

In addition, clinicians must evaluate for transgenerational transmission of the effects of trauma on TAY, even in the absence of direct child trauma. Parent trauma can affect youth outcomes through influences on parenting behavior and through vicarious trauma. Significant associations have been found between a parent's history of childhood sexual abuse and higher rates of permissive parenting, boundary distortions, and use of physical discipline.[8] These parenting behaviors may increase anxiety in the family system and have a direct impact on TAY's mental health. It is crucial to engage these parents in treatment, to frame their experience, and to promote their ability to serve a protective function for their own children.[9]

Changes in Family Relationships

The period of emerging adulthood in contemporary US society is marked by efforts to become a more self-sufficient person, as evidenced by self-responsibility, autonomous decision making, and financial independence.[10] There are numerous protective and risk factors when considering mental health in TAY, which can be classified as biological, psychological, or social and cultural (**Table 1**). Understanding the discrete influences and superposition of these components can inform clinicians about youth's potential resources and vulnerabilities.

Although it is normative to cultivate autonomy and set boundaries with family during emerging adulthood,[11] youth often require parental assistance in managing conflicts and demands.[12] Clinicians should address these contradictory realities because they may create ambivalence and turbulence within the family system. If youth's efforts for independence are insufficiently respected and encouraged by parents, navigating developmental tasks may prove challenging.[13] Equally important for continued growth, however, may be the parents' and siblings' ability to provide emotional connectedness and instrumental support.

During childhood, sibling relationships (as experienced by 76% of Americans)[14] are frequently marked by power inequality and periods of intense conflict,[15] whereas, young adult sibling affiliation is more voluntary in nature,[16] with a demonstrated reduction in intimacy[17] and contact.[11] Continued strong attachment to siblings, often the norm in cultures that emphasize interdependence and familistic values,[18] is positively correlated with socioemotional well-being and perceived support.[19] In the clinical context, it is essential to explore the quality of sibling relationships, particularly in cases of friction in the family system.

Although siblings typically form enduring relationships, romantic attachments during the transition to adulthood are often unstable, consuming, and impermanent. The achievement of interpersonal intimacy is one of the central developmental tasks of emerging adulthood, but volatility in these relationships can be extremely distressing for TAY and may require extensive focus in the treatment context.

Conceptualizing how relationship dynamics, communication patterns, parental background, cultural factors, and family structure affect youth functioning and development is essential to interpreting their impact on the treatment of mental health in TAY (**Fig. 1**).

Table 1
Protective and risk factors for mental health disorders in youth

	Protective Factors	Risk Factors
Biological	Good physical health Robust intellectual functioning Age-appropriate physical development	In utero exposure to toxins (eg, alcohol) Family (genetic) psychiatric history Head trauma Malnutrition Other illness
Psychological	Self-esteem; self-worth Social skills Coping and problem-solving skills Emotional self-regulation	Learning disorders Maladaptive personality traits Challenging temperament Sexual, physical, emotional abuse; neglect Substance abuse
Social and Cultural		
Family	Family attachment Supportive relationships Extended family support Adequate socioeconomic status Acculturation	Single parent Family conflict; parental strain Death of a family member Poverty Acculturation gap
School	School engagement Positive reinforcement for academic achievement Peer social support Presence of mentors	Academic failure Unsafe, unsupportive school environment Bullying Isolation from peer social groups
Community	Community connectedness Positive role models Positive cultural experiences Opportunities for leisure	Community disorganization Exposure to violence Discrimination; marginalization

Adapted from World Health Organization. Mental health policy and service guidance package: child and adolescent mental health policies and plans. Available at: http://www.who.int/mental_health/policy/Childado_mh_module.pdf; and Wille N, Bettge S, Ravens-Sieberer U, et al. Risk and protective factors for children's and adolescents' mental health: results of the BELLA study. Eur Child Adolesc Psychiatry 2008;17 Suppl 1:133–47

Parenting Styles

In addition to known biological risk factors, parenting styles[20,21] have a significant impact on TAY's developmental progression as paradigms of family communication and conflict resolution are internalized by children and replicated in their adult relationships.[22] Clinicians should always consider the attachment expectations of TAY; they are a crucial dimension of the familial construct and may inform the degree of parental involvement that the youth is willing to tolerate. For European Americans, the effect of the generational shift away from a less accessible, authoritarian style of parenting toward a more joining, permissive stance has been widely debated. Reviewing recent changes in parenting terminology is a useful way to conceptualize current parent-TAY dynamics. Although these terms are most often used in European American cultures, there are cross-cultural variations on these themes that should also be considered.

Helicopter parenting

Helicopter parenting, a term that connotes overly intrusive hyperhovering parents,[23] is associated with several dimensions of parenting, including parental involvement and information seeking, behavioral and psychological control, and reinforced dependence.[24,25] Helicopter parenting, as distinct from other parental styles,[25] may constrict

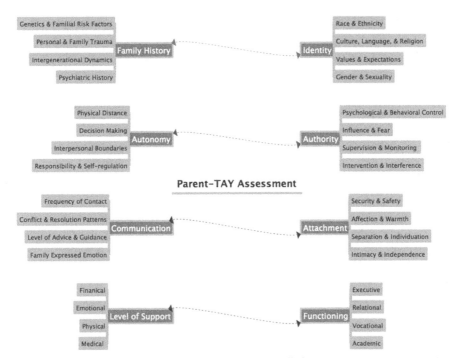

Fig. 1. Domains of parental and TAY assessment potentially having an impact on transition to adulthood.

autonomy, decrease engagement in school, affect perception of competence, and raise the risk of depression and anxiety.[26]

Causality, however, is unclear; parents of anxious children may be overprotective, and parents of highly dependent young adults may be more involved in their children's decisions. Early adulthood is a period of time when parents act as scaffolding or safety nets,[27] and this support confers an emotional and economic advantage to youth.[28,29] Surprisingly, intense parental involvement, as measured by frequency of involvement rather than quantity or quality of time spent, is positively correlated with young adults' sense of life satisfaction and well-being.[29] Extrapolating these findings to all emerging adults, however, may not be valid because employment or educational difficulties, traumatic life events, and chronic illness may be independently associated with increased parental involvement.[27,28]

In addition, cultural and generational norms vary widely. The American lens on helicopter parenting may exaggerate the negative impact of the behaviors and thus serve to increase resentment in a youth who does not want to be viewed as dependent.[30]

Clinicians should consider the extent to which helicopter parents overfunction for TAY, thereby inhibiting the development of autonomy and self-regulation.

Failure-to-launch and boomerang families

Leaving the family home is a central marker of the transition to adulthood. The average age of home-leaving has increased dramatically over the past century and ranges from late teens to early 30s,[31] depending on country, ethnicity, gender, religion, and socioeconomic status. A 2016 Pew Research Center analysis highlights recent demographic shifts that explain this trend; today's emerging adults delay partnerships and employment,[32] have lower earning potential, enroll in further schooling, receive more support from parents, and coreside with parents more than any other type of living arrangement.[33]

Failure-to-launch families include children who continue to live at home and are unable to move toward self-sufficiency, whereas boomerang families include children returning home, often due to financial concerns related to the new economic climate.[34] These paradigms, however, can undermine autonomy, self-esteem, and decision making.[35] A negative correlation between young adults coresiding with parents and those young adults' life satisfaction has been identified,[36] although the perception of choice weakens this correlation.[37]

In addition, parents often feel the strain of the emotional and economic needs of their adult children[35]; nonetheless, if TAY are focused on achieving developmentally appropriate tasks, parents are more supportive of youth living at home.[38] The public perception of these young adults as spoiled or disabled, along with the increased shame and alienation from peer groups, results in a pattern of avoidant or provocative behaviors. Lebowitz[39] discusses decreasing family accommodation as an effective strategy for moving these youth into more normative and independent familial roles.

Clinicians should consider the extent to which family members are in agreement with the living arrangement, the implicit and explicit expectations regarding coresidency, and stated plans for the future.

Letting go

The concept of letting go has changed dramatically over several generations. Frontier-style autonomy and independence have given way to managed childhood[40] with bidirectional resistance to individuation and independence. Within certain demographics, such as the 10% of adolescents with a chronic illness, the struggle to separate from overprotective parents is complicated by physical or behavioral difficulties and requires all parties to find a compromise solution of quasi-independence.[41] For a majority of parents, their willingness to let go is based on their perception of TAY's achievements, maturity, and degree of acceptance for TAY's lifestyle choices.[42] Although they acknowledge the importance of the separation-individuation process, parents often have ambivalence toward home-leaving and independent decision making, at times erecting conscious and unconscious obstacles or engaging in power struggles.[42]

Clinicians should consider the extent to which parental expectations and attitudes are based on a realistic appraisal of the youth's capabilities for autonomy and self-regulation, the youth's judgment, the ability of the family to discuss issues of separation-individuation, and the impact of cultural norms and values (**Table 2**).

MENTAL HEALTH DISORDERS IN TRANSITIONAL AGE YOUTH

During the transition to adulthood, demands on youth can overwhelm their ability to cope. This period is marked by changes in perspective, emotional regulation, identity, independence, and relations with others.[43] Along with the important influences of genetic and epigenetic factors, mental health is also the successful psychosocial adaptation to changing life situations,[44] with psychopathology reflecting maladaptive behavior or distress that interferes with adaptation.[45] For youth trying to emerge from the strain and stigma of adolescent mental health disorders, identity formation, social functioning, and familial attachment can be compromised. This vulnerable TAY population along with youth aging out of institutional settings, such as foster care and the criminal justice system, face greater challenges during this stage of maturation.

Family Assessment

Clinical assessment of family functioning and periodic inclusion of the family in care is not the same as family therapy. It is a way of establishing trust, opening channels of communication, and engaging all significant parties in treatment planning. Beyond

Table 2
Questions to consider during clinical assessment of transitional age youth who are not fully individuated from parents or family

Helicopter parenting	• What is the difference between perceived and actual received support? • Is it the youth or the parent who is prompting the increase in support? • Are parent and youth expectations and cultural norms congruent? • Are there opportunities for discussion about these expectations, especially when disagreements emerge?
Residing with parents	• Are economic or developmental issues impeding the youth's ability to live outside the home? • What developmentally inappropriate tasks are parents continuing to do for the youth (eg, all cooking, laundry, and social planning)? • Is the family accommodating avoidant or acting out behaviors? • Is the youth able to articulate the need for autonomy and balance this against the parents' expectations for accountability and respect for family needs? • What are the key areas of concern and conflict that seem to be hampering family functioning? How might these best be addressed clinically?
Financially supported by parents	• How is the economic and emotional burden of support affecting the dynamics of family relationships? For example, are parents using money to influence the youth's activities or to induce guilt? • Is financial support a positive motivator, allowing the youth to reach goals (eg, education), or a negative motivator, preventing the youth from pursuing goals (eg, employment)? • What practical steps can the youth take to seek employment and contribute to family finances?
Difficulty letting go	• What role does parental separation anxiety play in the difficulty of letting go? • How do parents view the youth's abilities to manage affairs, engage in independent decision making, and handle the predictable stresses of daily life? To what extent are parents in agreement? What happens when there is disagreement? • When there are major disagreements, how do these get raised and discussed? Are the conflicts overt or covert? Do they exert a negative impact on the parent-child relationship (eg, lack of trust, resentment, or secrecy)? • How does the youth view readiness for autonomy vs need for parental contact and involvement? • What is the impact of parents' difficulties with letting go on the youth's sense of competence and confidence?

these basic objectives, it is appropriate and advisable to establish a therapeutic framework that includes family sessions, especially in cases of youth seriously impaired by their symptoms.

The steps of conducting a family assessment include joining with family members and validating their importance in the care of the TAY, exploring obstacles to family involvement, identifying additional supports, and obtaining detailed family medical and psychiatric histories.[46] Assessment should identify strengths and vulnerabilities, TAY's fears and perceptions about their situation, and prior efforts to achieve developmental milestones.

Multisystemic, language, logistical, ethnopharmacologic, and financial barriers prevent cultural parity in mental health treatment, with minority families half as likely to seek mental health treatment of their children.[6] And, depending on background, minority families may conceptualize time, boundaries, self-disclosure, and familial interdependence differently. Whenever cultural barriers arise, such as stigma regarding psychiatric care, it may be necessary to extend the assessment process to ensure trust and reduce misconceptions about diagnosis and treatment.

A key determination to make is the degree to which TAY can accept and understand their mental health issues and advocate for support, as these practices predict better adjustment over time.[47] TAY may minimize their suffering or exaggerate the extent to which they can handle developmental challenges, life demands, and the treatment proposed. There is an inevitable tension experienced by most parents between the desire to protect their children from harm and permitting them to face the consequences of their decision making. It is virtually universal for parents to feel responsible for their child's psychiatric problems and, by acknowledging this emotional burden and avoiding parent blaming, family members can be supported in identifying and processing their own conflicted emotions.

Given the variety of developmental tasks of emerging adulthood, the extent to which youth's psychiatric difficulties are interfering with their progress toward self-responsibility and autonomy needs to be assessed. **Fig. 2** provides a framework for grasping the interaction of complex factors affecting youth with a chronic developmental and/or psychiatric disorder. Along with assessing adjustment along a variety of dimensions, the neuropsychological capacities of youth must be considered as these play a key role in preparedness and maturity.

Family assessment is an iterative process that generates possibilities for treatment planning and encourages family members to consider their respective roles. In cases of individual treatment as the chosen modality, a clear set of expectations for keeping the family engaged should be discussed. TAY may need to be educated about the benefits of some level of family input and involvement. If the youth and clinician agree,[48] periodic family meetings can be arranged, and these may evolve, if indicated, into family therapy.

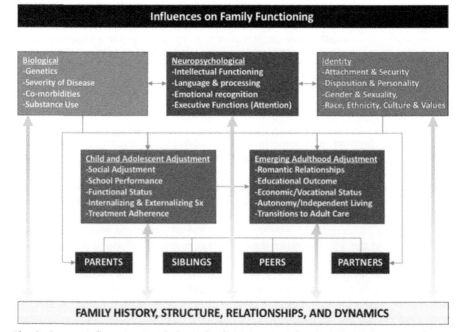

Fig. 2. Factors influencing psychological adjustment and family functioning in youth and emerging adults. Sx, symptoms. (*Adapted from* Holmbeck GN, Devine KA. Psychosocial and family functioning in spina bifida. Dev Disabil Res Rev 2010;16(1):41.)

Situations in which the family should be kept out of treatment include the need to preserve autonomy and the therapeutic alliance[10] and the unwillingness of the family to engage in the work of therapy. *Boundary violations, attempts to undermine or terminate treatment, physical or sexual abuse, and concerns about intrafamilial violence are all contraindications for regular family sessions.* It is almost inevitable, due to the developmental challenges of this phase of life, that the clinician is drawn into conflicts between TAY and family. It is best to adopt an open, flexible approach by taking a reasonable middle ground, whereby a variety of options are offered, such as separate parent and child meetings, sessions with subsystems of the family, and, when appropriate, referring to a family therapist to directly address family issues.[49]

Clinical questions, included in **Table 3**, may provide clinicians with a clearer picture of repetitive and reinforcing family interactional patterns. The concept of executive functioning[55] should be introduced to analyze how the family sees the youth's capacity for self-regulation. Another critical dimension to address is expressed emotion,

Table 3	
Clinical questions to consider during the family assessment of transitional age youth	
General assessment	• How much is the youth engaged with other family members on a day-to-day basis, and how do people feel about daily family interactions? • What aspects of family life are mutually satisfying and which are unfulfilling or stressful? • What does each family member see as the family's core values and greatest assets or strengths? • How are conflicts handled? What issues are most difficult for family members to resolve? • What explanations do family members have for why things are not going well? Is there agreement or disagreement about this? • What are the individual's and family's hopes and dreams for the future?
Executive functioning	• To what extent is the young person able to manage his/her own life? • How much assistance does the youth need to carry out activities of daily living, engage in age-appropriate activities, make reasonable decisions, exercise good judgment, manage time and organize a daily schedule, and regulate negative emotions? • What supports and scaffolding do family members provide in order for the youth to develop these skills? • Are these helping the youth make progress toward self-responsibility and autonomy, or do these efforts seem ineffective? • What explanations do people offer for why progress doesn't seem to be occurring? Clinical assessment tools: Behavior Rating Inventory of Executive Function[50] and the Barkley Deficits of Executive Functioning Scale[51]
Expressed emotion	• What is the level of tension and conflict in the household? • Is criticism, hostility, intrusiveness, warmth, or positive remarks evident in family communication patterns? • Does the youth perceive family members to be emotionally overinvolved? • The clinician should provide family education that high parental expressed emotion predicts worse outcomes in a variety of mental health conditions in pediatric and adult populations (psychosis, depression, anxiety, and bipolar disorder)[52] and is associated with temperament problems, externalizing disorders, and self-injurious behavior.[53] • Expressed emotion can be assessed through direct observation of family interactions, especially when discussing emotionally charged topics. Clinical assessment tools: Level of Expressed Emotion Scale, Perceived Criticism Scale, Family Emotional Involvement and Criticism Scale, Family Attitude Scale[54]

among the most salient and robust predictors of long-term functioning in studies of psychopathology.[56]

Transdiagnostic Family Systems Intervention

Although evidence-based family systems approaches have been developed and studied for specific conditions, there are shared therapeutic strategies that can be applied to most clinical situations.[57] Once the youth and family have agreed to participate in family-based treatment, the clinician should explain the principles, enlist active participation of family members, discuss parameters, and clarify questions the family has about the treatment process (**Table 4**).

Table 4
General structure and clinical questions for family systems intervention

Initial phase	• Establish ground rules for the sessions; create safe space for dialogue. • Discuss goals (self-regulation and autonomy), objectives, and key problems. • Identify cultural values, strengths, and barriers. • Address concerns and fears about the treatment. • Acknowledge that the family might be in or have a history of crisis.
Example questions	• What are the most stressful familial conflictual interactions that arise within the family setting? How do arguments unfold? • What patterns of thinking, feeling, and behaving does each family member experience during these negative interactions? • What are the beliefs that family members hold that may be distorting their views of the situation or contributing to symptoms?
Intermediate phase	• Explore problematic family dynamics that arise in day-to-day life. • Determine which factors are perpetuating these difficulties, and which prior approaches the family has taken to address them. • Examine the ways in which each family member contributes to the situation. • Assess if family dynamics may be causing discord between the parents. • Facilitate family members in renegotiating their expectations. • Devise new approaches to communication and problem solving. • Between sessions, it is important for TAY and family to try new strategies.
Final phase	• This phase is signaled by a shift in the family's dynamics toward greater harmony, better communication, and improved problem solving skills. • Decrease the frequency of sessions and monitor how the family tackles remaining challenges. • Family determines when goals of treatment have been achieved and develops plan for maintaining gains.

As with all interventions, treatment unfolds in phases.[58] During the early phase, the family is encouraged to communicate and clarify issues, to embrace collaboration, and to respect each member in the process. Throughout the middle phase, the family is guided to become more effective in exploring conflicts, to support the youth's efforts in assuming greater responsibility, and to give parents opportunities to change their behaviors, such as becoming less reactive or directive. When successful, the final phase of treatment is signaled by a shift in the family's dynamics away from focusing on crises and disabling symptoms and toward improved communication and enhanced confidence in the family's ability to solve problems on its own. Termination involves decreasing the frequency of sessions, monitoring the family's capacity to tackle remaining challenges, and ensuring the family develops a plan for maintaining gains.

Evidence for Family Involvement in Improving Treatment Outcomes

A rapidly expanding body of literature supports family involvement in the treatment of young adults with specific mental health diagnoses, although data on the implications of the diversity of this demographic are limited. **Table 5** reviews studies on family therapies for youth and adolescents (subset of TAY ages 16–19), and, for the latter, caution should be used in extrapolating the results. For example, increased conflict with parents at age 18 is associated with worsening depressed mood, but by age 25 the negative correlation is

Table 5
Evidence for the efficacy of family-based treatment strategies for mental health disorders in youth

Disorder	Therapy Modality	Efficacy of Treatment
Bipolar disorder	FFT	8 RCTs (adults and adolescents) showed faster recovery from mood episodes, reduction in recurrence, reduced symptom severity (greater effect with families with high EE).[59]
Suicidality and self-harm	Home-based family intervention; multisystemic therapy; ABFT; family intervention for suicide prevention	Meta-analysis of 19 RCTs (adolescents) showed treatment interventions with strong family component (>50% of sessions attended by family) had risk reduction of 0.14 but no specific type of family intervention was significantly superior.[60]
Psychotic disorders	FFT; family intervention; psychoeducation; crisis-oriented family therapy; behavioral family therapy	RCT showed increase in active listening, calm communication, and decrease in irritability, anger, and criticism.[61] Meta-analyses of 25 studies[62] and 1 of 8 RCTs[63] showed family intervention alone reduced relapse and hospital admission rates. Review of 27 studies of first episode psychosis in young adults shows need to intervene with high EE families.[64]
Obsessional disorders	FBCBT; including family in behavioral treatments; reducing family accommodation; family psychoeducation; multifamily behavioral treatment	Meta-analysis of 10 studies of FBCBT for adolescents showed large effect size, but FBCBT was not significantly superior to individual CBT.[65] Intensive and weekly FBCBT have same results.[66] Review indicating advantages to parental involvement in treatment of young adults.[67]
Feeding and eating disorders	FBT; SFT; MFT	Single content analysis[68] on FBT with TAYs showed FBT with adaptations (more individual sessions, focus on therapeutic alliance, and engaging TAY in treatment) is a successful treatment of AN. Pilot study[69] showed no difference in efficacy between SFT and MFT in treatment of adult AN.

(continued on next page)

Table 5
(continued)

Disorder	Therapy Modality	Efficacy of Treatment
Substance use disorders	Functional family therapy; multisystemic therapy; multidimensional family therapy; brief strategic family therapy; family behavior therapy; ecologically based family therapy; culturally informed and flexible family treatment of adolescents; strengths-oriented family therapy; AIM program	Meta-analysis shows family involvement in adolescent substance abuse is more effective than behavioral therapy, CBT, motivational interviewing, motivational enhancement therapy, group counseling, and TAU.[70] Meta-analysis (adolescent) of 24 studies was statistically significant for increased efficacy over TAU for 4 different models of family therapy; no model had superior effectiveness.[71] Review (adolescent) of efficacy of 7 models of family therapy showed increased abstinence, recovery, parental involvement and family functioning, and decreased substance use, relapse, criminal behavior, family conflict, and externalizing/internalizing behaviors.[72] RCT of AIM program for African American TAY showed decrease in substance use disorders.[73]
Depression	ABFT; family psychoeducation	RCT (adolescents) engaged in ABFT resulted in 81% no longer meeting criteria for MDD.[74]
Trauma and stressor-related disorders	MGM	MGM studied by the VA has shown promise for decreasing PTSD symptoms in Iraqi war veterans, many of whom are still emerging adults.[75]
Anxiety disorders	FBCBT Facilitate exposure; parent coaching; efforts to reduce parental accommodation, oveprotective, and overinvolved behaviors[76]	Literature does not provide clear rationale for involving family or how to include parents in treatment or which family variables to target.[76] Anxiety-disordered youth with comorbid ADHD, however, benefited more from FBCBT than child-focused CBT.[77]

Abbreviations: ABFT, attachment-based family therapy; ADHD, attention-deficit/hyperactivity disorder; AIM, adults in the making; AN, anorexia nervosa; CBT, cognitive behavior therapy; EE, expressed emotion; FBCBT, family-based CBT; FBT, family-based treatment; FFT, family-focused therapy; MDD, major depressive disorder; MFT, multifamily therapy; MGM, multifamily group model; PTSD, posttraumatic stress disorder; RCT, randomized controlled trial; SFT, single-family therapy; TAU, treatment as usual; VA, Department of Veterans Affairs.

greatly reduced. As young adults gain autonomy, familial conflict may not affect their mood to the same extent, and therefore family interventions may be less effective.[78]

ETHICAL AND LEGAL ISSUES

Clinicians treating young adults face ethical and legal issues whenever family members are involved in treatment. These include core ethical principles, considerations of privacy and confidentiality, liability risks regarding potential for harm, and crisis management strategies.

Ethical dilemmas arise when the interests of patients conflict with the concerns of parents, especially when a patient's ability to function is compromised. Common areas of ethical ambiguity include self-injurious behavior, risk taking, substance use, and failure to meet academic expectations. Whenever significant risks to an individual's safety are present, clinicians are obliged to address their dual role as an individual's care provider and as a collaborator with the family. Ethical principles of beneficence and nonmaleficence are fundamental in this work.

Protection of confidentiality is a central concern when working with TAY who are dependent on their families or embedded in academic institutions. Although there may be pressure from family members or administrators to disclose clinical information, and although the clinician may agree that open communication is best, confidentiality must be maintained unless a patient has given consent or is at risk of harming self or others. Similarly, if young adults are not willing to engage in family meetings or family therapy, it is important to respect their decision and preserve the therapeutic alliance.

Legal bases for maintaining privacy and confidentiality include professional licensing requirements, ethical guidelines, and state and federal laws. In the wake of the Virginia Tech tragedy, several states passed laws requiring parental notification of dangerousness, expanding on the "duty to warn" precedent set by *Tarasoff v. Regents of the University of California* (1976). Federal laws, such as the Health Insurance Portability and Accountability Act and the Family Education Rights and Privacy Act, which pertains to the release of college academic records, also set standards for maintenance of confidentiality.

Clinicians caring for college students should be aware that mental health records used for purposes other than treatment may be considered a shared record and potentially disclosed to parents. Interactions between clinicians, parents, and administrators are an evolving area of jurisprudence, as the potential consequences of family involvement to both the individual and the community must be assessed by all involved parties. Ultimately, determining a patient's level of risk is a matter of professional judgment.[79]

Appreciating the complex legal and ethical issues of working with TAY with mental health disorders can help clinicians navigate challenges when negotiating aspects of safety, disclosure, and family involvement.

SUMMARY

Family dynamics have critical influences on TAY's developmental progression to adulthood. Recognizing and assessing the impact of family structure, relationships, history, and culture is necessary to incorporate the family system into the treatment of TAY with a mental health diagnosis. It is increasingly evident that engaging family is a significant contributor to outcomes for TAY, and clinicians need to consider familial functioning as it relates to both a youth's treatment and transition to adulthood. Although further research regarding the most effective approach, degree of involvement, and the diversity of this demographic is needed, family support and inclusion are most likely beneficial for the majority of TAY. Finally, psychiatry training programs should incorporate modules on working with families of TAY to prepare future practitioners to address complex systems and clinical care issues involved in treating this vulnerable patient population.[80]

REFERENCES

1. Schulenberg JE, O'Malley PM, Bachman JG, et al. Early adult transitions and their relation to well-being and substance use. Chicago: University of Chicago Press; 2005.

2. Szapocznik J, Kurtines WM. Family psychology and cultural diversity. Am Psychol 1993;48:400–7.

3. Arnett JJ. Conceptions of the transition to adulthood among emerging adults in American ethnic groups. New Dir Child Adolesc Dev 2003;(100):63–75.

4. Phinney JS, Ong A, Madden V. Cultural values and intergenerational value discrepancies in immigrant and non-immigrant families. Child Dev 2000;71(2): 528–39.

5. Sher-Censor E, Parke RD, Coltrane S. Parents' promotion of psychological autonomy, psychological control, and mexican–American adolescents' adjustment. J Youth Adolesc 2011;40(5):620–32.

6. Pumariega AJ, Rothe E, Mian A, et al. Practice parameter for cultural competence in child and adolescent psychiatric practice. J Am Acad Child Adolesc Psychiatry 2013;52(10):1101–15.

7. Pumariega AJ, Joshi SV. Culture and development in children and youth. Child Adolesc Psychiatr Clin N Am 2010;19(4):661–80.

8. DiLillo D, Damashek A. Parenting characteristics of women reporting a history of childhood sexual abuse. Child Maltreat 2003;8:319–33.

9. Mendelson T, Letourneau EJ. Parent-focused prevention of child sexual abuse. Prev Sci 2015;16(6):844–52.

10. Arnett JJ. Emerging adulthood. A theory of development from the late teens through the twenties. Am Psychol 2000;55(5):469–80.

11. White LK, Riedmann A. Ties among adult siblings. Social Forces 1992;71:85–102.

12. Youness J, Smollar J. Adolescent relations with mothers, fathers, and friends. Chicago: University of Chicago Press; 1985.

13. O'Connor TG, Allen JP, Bell KL, et al. Adolescent-parent relationships and leaving home in young adulthood. New Dir Child Dev 1996;(71):39–52.

14. Vespa J, Lewis JM, Kreider RM. America's families and living arrangements: 2012. Available at: https://www.census.gov/library/publications/2013/demo/p20-570.html. Accessed January 8, 2017.

15. Bedford VH, Volling BL, Avioli PS. Positive consequences of sibling conflict in childhood and adulthood. Int J Aging Hum Dev 2000;51:53–69.

16. Conger KJ, Little WM. Sibling relationships during the transition to adulthood. Child Dev Perspect 2010;4(2):87–94.

17. Milevsky A, Smoot K, Leh M, et al. Familial and contextal variables and the nature of sibling relationships in emergeing adulthood. Marriage Fam Rev 2005;37: 123–41.

18. Guan SSA, Fuligni AJ. Changes in parent, sibling, and peer support during the transition to young adulthood. J Res Adolesc 2015;26(2):286–99.

19. Dunn J, Munn P. Sibling quarrels and maternal intervention: individual differences in understanding and aggression. J Child Psychol Psychiatry 1986;27(5):583–95.

20. Waters E, Weinfield NS, Hamilton CE. The stability of attachment security from infancy to adolescence and early adulthood: general discussion. Child Dev 2000; 71(3):703–6.

21. Whitbeck L, Hoyt DR, Huck SM. Early family relationships, intergenerational solidarity, and support provided to parents by their adult children. J Gerontol 1994; 49(2):S85–94.

22. Conger RD, Conger KJ. Resilience in Midwestern families: selected findings from the first decade of a prospective, longitudinal study. J Marriage Fam 2002;64: 361–73.

23. Cline FW, Fay J. Parenting with love and logic: teaching children responsibility. Colorado Springs (CO): Pinon Press; 1990.

24. Luebbe AM, Mancini KJ, Kiel EJ, et al. Dimensionality of helicopter parenting and relations to emotional, decision-making, and academic functioning in emerging adults. Assessment 2016. [Epub ahead of print].

25. Padilla-Walker LM, Nelson LJ. Black Hawk down? Establishing helicopter parenting as a distinct construct from other forms of parental control during emerging adulthood. J Adolesc 2012;35(5):1177–90.

26. Schiffrin HH, Miriam L, Miles-McLean H, et al. Helping or Hovering? The effects of helicopter parenting on college students' well-being. J Child Fam Stud 2014; 23(3):548–57.

27. Swartz TT, Kim M, Uno M, et al. Safety nets and scaffolds: parental support in the transition to adulthood. J Marriage Fam 2011;73(2):414–29.

28. Aquilino W. Family relationships and support systems in emerging adulthood. In: Arnett J, Tanner JL, editors. Emerging adults in the America: coming of age in the 21st century. Washington, DC: American Psychological Association; 2006. p. 193–217.

29. Fingerman KL, Cheng Y-P, Wesselmann ED, et al. Helicopter parents and landing pad kids: intense parental support of grown children. J Marriage Fam 2012;74(4): 880–96.

30. Belkin L. Unhappy helicopter parents. N Y Times Mag 2010.

31. Mitchell BA. Changing courses: the pendulum of family transitions in comparative perspective. J Comp Fam Stud 2006;37(3):325–43.

32. Furstenberg FF. Will marriage disappear? Proc Am Philos Soc 2015;159(3): 241–6.

33. Fry R. For first time in modern era, living with parents edges out other living arrangements for 18- to 34-year-olds. Pew Res Cent Social Demographic Trends 2016. Accessed May 24.

34. Otters RV, Hollander JF. Leaving home and boomerang decisions: a family simulation protocol. Marriage Fam Rev 2015;51(1):39–58.

35. Burn K, Szoeke C. Boomerang families and failure-to-launch: commentary on adult children living at home. Maturitas 2016;83:9–12.

36. Nikolaev B. Living with mom and dad and loving it...or Are you? J Econ Psychol 2015;51:199–209.

37. Kins E, Beyers W, Soenens B, et al. Patterns of home leaving and subjective well-being in emerging adulthood: the role of motivational processes and parental autonomy support. Dev Psychol 2009;45(5):1416–29.

38. Dor A. Don't stay out late! Mom, I'm twenty-eight: emerging adults and their parents under one roof. Int J Soc Sci Stud 2013;1(1):37–46.

39. Lebowitz ER. "Failure to launch": shaping intervention for highly dependent adult children. J Am Acad Child Adolesc Psychiatry 2016;55(2):89–90.

40. Fass P. The end of American childhood: a history of parenting from life on the frontier to the managed child. Princeton (NJ): Princeton Univeristy Press; 2016.

41. Akre C, Suris J-C. From controlling to letting go: what are the psychosocial needs of parents of adolescents with a chronic illness? Health Educ Res 2014;29(5): 764–72.

42. Kloep M, Hendry LB. Letting go or holding on? Parents' perceptions of their relationships with their children during emerging adulthood. Br J Dev Psychol 2010; 28(Pt 4):817–34.

43. Shiner RL, Masten AS. Transactional links between personality and adaptation from childhood through adulthood. J Res Pers 2002;35:580–8.

44. Masten AS, Coatsworth JD. Competence, resilience, and psychopathology. In: Cicchetti D, Cohen DJ, editors. Developmental psychopathology: vol. 2. Risk, disorder, and adaptation, vol. 2. New York: Wiley; 1995. p. 715–52.

45. Cicchetti D. A developmental psychopathology perspective on drug abuse. In: Glantz MD, Hartel CR, editors. Drug abuse: origins and interventions. Washington, DC: American Psychological Association; 1999. p. 97–117.

46. Shulman S, Kalnitzki E, Shahar G. Meeting developmental challenges during emerging adulthood: the role of personality and social resources. J Adolesc Res 2009;24:242–67.

47. Holahan CJ, Valentiner DP, Moos RH. Parental support and psychological adjustment during the transition to young adulthood in a college sample. J Fam Psychol 1994;8:215–23.

48. Preyde M, Cameron G, Frensch K, et al. Parent–child relationships and family functioning of children and youth discharged from residential mental health treatment or a home-based Alternative. Residential Treatment for Children & Youth 2011;28(1):55–74.

49. McGoldrick M, Garcia Preto NA, Carter BA. The expanding family life cycle: individual, family, and social perspectives. 5th edition. New York: Pearson; 2015.

50. Gioia G, Isquith PK, Guy SC, et al. Test review: behavior rating inventory of executive function. Child Neuropsychology 2000;6(3):235–8.

51. Barkley RA. Deficits of executive functioning scale (BDEFS for adults). New York: Guilford Press; 2013.

52. Przeworski A, Zoellner LA, Franklin ME, et al. Maternal and child expressed emotion as predictors of treatment response in pediatric obsessive-compulsive disorder. Child Psychiatry Hum Dev 2012;43(3):337–53.

53. Wedig MM, Nock MK. Parental expressed emotion and adolescent self-injury. J Am Acad Child Adolesc Psychiatry 2007;46(9):1171–8.

54. Mohapatra D. Expressed emotion in psychiatric disorders: a review. 2009. Available at: https://www.academia.edu/4041130/Expressed. Accessed September 15, 2016.

55. Barkley RA. Executive functions: what they are, how they work and why they evolved. New York: Guilford Press; 2012.

56. Peris TS, Miklowitz DJ. Parental expressed emotion and youth psychopathology: new directions for an old construct. Child Psychiatry Hum Dev 2015;46(6): 863–73.

57. Glick ID, Rait DS, Heru AM, et al. Couples and family therapy in clinical practice. 5th edition. New York: Wiley-Blackwell; 2015.

58. Goldenberg H, Goldenberg I. Family therapy: an overview. 8th edition. Belmont (CA): Cengage Learning; 2012.

59. Miklowitz DJ, Chung B. Family-focused therapy for bipolar disorder: reflections on 30 Years of research. Fam Process 2016;55(3):483–99.

60. Ougrin D, Tranah T, Leigh E, et al. Practitioner review: self-harm in adolescents. J Child Psychol Psychiatry 2012;53(4):337–50.

61. O'Brien MP, Miklowitz DJ, Candan KA, et al. A randomized trial of family focused therapy with populations at clinical high risk for psychosis: effects on interactional behavior. J Consult Clin Psychol 2014;82(1):90–101.

62. Pitschel-Walz G, Leucht S, Bäuml J, et al. The effect of family interventions on relapse and rehospitalization in schizophrenia: a meta-analysis. Schizophr Bull 2001;27(1):73–92.

63. Bird V, Premkumar P, Kendall T, et al. Early intervention services, cognitive-behavioural therapy and family intervention in early psychosis: systematic review. Br J Psychiatry 2010;197(5):350–6.

64. Koutra K, Vgontzas AN, Lionis C, et al. Family functioning in first-episode psychosis: a systematic review of the literature. Soc Psychiatry Psychiatr Epidemiol 2014;49(7):1023–36.

65. Ost LG, Riise EN, Wergeland GJ, et al. Cognitive behavioral and pharmacological treatments of OCD in children: a systematic review and meta-analysis. J Anxiety Disord 2016;43:58–69.

66. Storch EA, Geffken GR, Merlo LJ, et al. Family-based cognitive-behavioral therapy for pediatric obsessive-compulsive disorder: comparison of intensive and weekly approaches. J Am Acad Child Adolesc Psychiatry 2007;46(4): 469–78.

67. Steketee G, Van Noppen B. Family approaches to treatment for obsessive compulsive disorder. Rev Bras Psiquiatr 2003;25(1):43–50.

68. Dimitropoulos G, Freeman VE, Allemang B, et al. Family-based treatment with transition age youth with anorexia nervosa: a qualitative summary of application in clinical practice. J Eat Disord 2015;3(1):1.

69. Dimitropoulos G, Farquhar JC, Freeman VE, et al. Pilot study comparing multi-family therapy to single family therapy for adults with anorexia nervosa in an intensive eating disorder program. Eur Eat Disord Rev 2015;23(4): 294–303.

70. Tanner-Smith EE, Wilson SJ, Lipsey MW. The comparative effectiveness of outpatient treatment for adolescent substance abuse: a meta-analysis. J Subst Abuse Treat 2013;44(2):145–58.

71. Baldwin SA, Christian S, Berkeljon A, et al. The effects of family therapies for adolescent delinquency and substance abuse: a meta-analysis. J Marital Fam Ther 2012;38(1):281–304.

72. Horigian VE, Anderson AR, Szapocznik J. Family-based treatments for adolescent substance use. Child Adolesc Psychiatr Clin N Am 2016;25(4): 603–28.

73. Brody GH, Yu T, Chen YF, et al. The Adults in the Making program: long-term protective stabilizing effects on alcohol use and substance use problems for rural African American emerging adults. J Consult Clin Psychol 2012;80(1): 17–28.

74. Diamond GS, Reis BF, Diamond GM, et al. Attachment-based family therapy for depressed adolescents: a treatment development study. J Am Acad Child Adolesc Psychiatry 2002;41(10):1190–6.

75. Sherman MD, Perlick DA, Straits-Troster K. Adapting the multifamily group model for treating veterans with posttraumatic stress disorder. Psychol Serv 2012;9(4): 349–60.

76. Taboas WR, McKay D, Whiteside SPH, et al. Parental involvement in youth anxiety treatment: conceptual bases, controversies, and recommendations for intervention. J Anxiety Disord 2015;30:16–8.

77. Maric M, van Steensel FJ, Bogels SM. Parental involvement in CBT for anxiety-disordered youth revisited: family CBT outperforms child CBT in the long term for children with comorbid ADHD symptoms. J Atten Disord 2015. [Epub ahead of print].

78. Galambos NL, Barker ET, Krahn HJ. Depression, self-esteem, and anger in emerging adulthood: seven-year trajectories. Dev Psychol 2006;42(2):350–65.

79. Foundation TJ. Student Mental Health and the Law: A Resource for Insitutions of Higher Education; 2008. Available at: https://www.jedfoundation.org/wp-content/uploads/2016/07/student-mental-health-and-the-law-jed-NEW.pdf. Accessed January 8, 2017.
80. Derenne J, Martel A. A model CSMH curriculum for child and adolescent psychiatry training programs. Acad Psychiatry 2015;39(5):512–6.

Social Media as It Interfaces with Psychosocial Development and Mental Illness in Transitional Age Youth

Brian A. Primack, MD, PhD[a],*, César G. Escobar-Viera, MD, PhD[b]

KEYWORDS

- Social media • Depression • Anxiety • Facebook • Emotional contagion
- Cognitive neuroscience • Sleep • Social networks

KEY POINTS

- Social media has grown substantially, with more than 2 billion new users worldwide in the past 20 years.
- Nearly all transitional age youth use social media, and most use it daily.
- Large, cross-sectional, nationally representative studies demonstrate consistent, linear associations between social media use and depression and anxiety among young adults.
- However, social media networks also may be leveraged to identify individuals with mental health concerns and engage transitional age youth in treatment.
- Future research will be important to determine best practices for optimal use of social media to retain its benefits but minimize its drawbacks.

INTRODUCTION

Definition and Scope of Social Media

Social media (SM) can be defined as "a group of Internet-based applications that allow the creation and exchange of user-generated content."[1] This includes formation of online communities and sharing of information, ideas, opinions, messages, images, and videos. Therefore, although all online video games would not necessarily count as SM, video games that allow for substantial sharing of information

Disclosure Statement: The authors have nothing to disclose.
[a] Center for Research on Media, Technology, and Health, University of Pittsburgh School of Medicine, 230 McKee Place #600, Pittsburgh, PA 15213, USA; [b] Center for Research on Media, Technology, and Health, Health Policy Institute, University of Pittsburgh School of Public Health, 230 McKee Place #600, Pittsburgh, PA 15213, USA
* Corresponding author.
E-mail address: bprimack@pitt.edu

and development of online communities would fit this definition. SM has become an integral component of how people worldwide connect with friends and family, share personal content, and obtain news and entertainment.[2,3] Use of SM is particularly prevalent among transitional age individuals, who are at critical junctures around developmental tasks such as identity development and establishment of social norms.[4]

Currently, the most commonly used SM platform is Facebook[5,6]; however, there are many other commonly used SM sites, such as Twitter, Google+, Instagram, Tumblr, SnapChat, Vine, and Reddit.[7,8] Furthermore, different SM platforms lend themselves to different types of communication and different applications.[9] For example, many transitional age individuals maintain Facebook accounts but use them primarily for posting photos and receiving information from formal groups, such as college-related activities. These individuals may use SnapChat instead for private conversations with close friends. Meanwhile, Twitter and Reddit are common sources of news, whereas LinkedIn can be important for occupational social networking. Finally, sites such as Pinterest tend to be more popular among individuals with artistic and or craft-related aspirations.

Growth of Social Media

It is difficult to overstate the rapid growth of SM use. Many people consider the birth of modern SM to be in the mid to late 1990s, with a platform called SixDegrees. The subsequent decade was marked by the success of MySpace and the emergence of multiple other platforms. However, it was not until the mid-2000s that today's most frequently used sites, such as Facebook and Twitter, became more mainstream. In 2015, it was estimated that 2.2 billion individuals used SM worldwide. This brief history suggests that the number of SM users increased from zero to more than 2 billion in less than 2 decades.

Use has been particularly high among transitional age individuals. For example, in the United States, approximately 90% of young adults use SM, and most users visit these sites at least once a day (in the cited document, young adults were defined as those ages 18–29 years).[8] However, use in other age groups is also substantially increasing. For example, use among adults ages 65 and older in the United States more than tripled, from 11% to 35%, between 2010 and 2015.[8] Overall, SM use accounts for approximately 20% of time online on personal computers and 30% of time online via mobile devices.[7]

Facebook currently maintains approximately 1.6 billion users, which makes its population approximately 4 times that of the United States. Facebook adds approximately 500,000 new users each day. However, other sites, such as Twitter, Instagram, and SnapChat, are growing even more quickly. For example, daily SnapChat views increased from 8 billion videos per day to 10 billion videos per day in just 2 months (from February to April of 2016).[10] At this point, it is estimated that it would take nearly 160 years to watch just 1 day's worth of SnapChat stories.[11]

Social Media, Mental Illness, and the Purpose of This Review

Any rapid social and behavioral change such as this is likely to influence mental health. Despite the relative recency of this phenomenon, there has been a fair amount of initial research exploring how SM interfaces with both psychosocial development and mental health conditions among young adults. We aim in this article to broadly summarize major understandings that have been gleaned to date and to summarize important future directions for research.

PUBLISHED LITERATURE AROUND SOCIAL MEDIA, DEVELOPMENT, AND MENTAL HEALTH
Neuroscience and Developmental Psychology Around Social Media

The rapid growth of SM, as well as several studies showing an increasing time spent on SM sites among adolescents and young adults, have generated interest in the potential impact of SM on the developing brain of adolescents and young adults.[7,8,10,11]

However, few rigorous studies have focused on this area to date. A recently published review found only 7 articles covering the topic, with most of the studies conducted among Facebook users.[12] Additionally, a recent study used functional MRI to analyze social cognition and social influences.[13] Researchers measured activity in neural regions of adolescents while they were looking at a simulated Instagramlike feed of images. The findings showed that adolescents were more inclined to "like" photos that already had been "liked" many times. Additionally, there was a positive association between the number of "likes" seen and activity of neural regions usually linked to attention, imitation, social cognition, and reward processing.[13] According to the investigators, these findings suggest that SM may trigger a unique type of peer pressure through quantifiable social endorsement, which in turn might reinforce the importance of self-presentation during adolescence, including on SM.

Although little work has focused specifically on SM in this context, there are a number of observations from related work that may be highly relevant.[14] For example, because of its mobility and tendency to provide interruptions, SM use may be associated with increased multitasking, which has been associated in the past with negative cognitive and mental health outcomes.[15,16] For example, multitasking has been related to decreased ability to sustain attention,[17,18] poor academic performance,[19–21] decreased subjective well-being,[22] and higher levels of depression and anxiety.[23,24] It will be valuable for future research to examine more closely associations between SM use and pathways to these outcomes via multitasking.

Another issue is that SM messages tend to be brief and to link to multiple other sources. This may affect the ability to pay attention, which has also been associated with negative outcomes related to mental health. Because individuals in the United States use SM for approximately 2 to 3 hours per day,[25] this may present a substantial challenge, especially for youth who already tend toward attention problems.

Additionally, other research has linked increased use of technology and Internet to aggression and desensitization to pain and suffering. For example, one study used functional MRI to evaluate the impact of Internet use and video games in older adolescents.[26] Because their findings showed suppressed activation of the amygdala during portrayal of violent imagery, the investigators surmise that exposure to these messages may be associated with an increase in aggressive behavior during adulthood.[26] It is not clear whether these speculations extend to SM as well.

On the other hand, video games have been associated with certain improvements in visual, cognitive, attention, and motor skills.[27] For example, avid video game players were found to exhibit better visual memory and were flexible in switching between tasks.[27] Therefore, it will be valuable for future work to determine if these related findings extend to SM in terms of its potential for affecting both positive and negative developmental and cognitive outcomes.

Benefits and Concerns Around Social Media to Provide Mental Health Treatment

SM may present opportunities to augment traditional mental health treatment. For example, researchers have used publicly available SM data to provide surveillance and determine if patients are exhibiting suicidal and/or psychotic behavior.[28–31]

However, this type of surveillance also has been criticized in terms of potential invasion of patients' privacy.

In addition, it may be valuable to use SM and other Internet tools to provide mental health care as an alternative to traditional care. This is particularly the case because factors such as stigma, logistics, and finances have been identified as important barriers to mental health care. Thus, especially for those of transitional age who are highly accustomed to using SM, accessing care in this way may help alleviate those barriers.

However, others are concerned about the provision of mental health care using SM. For example, therapeutic relationships formed over SM networks may be inferior to those developed using person-to-person interactions.[32] Second, therapists are trained to use many nonverbal cues and language in their assessments. Other important issues are related to professional liability ramifications tied to the provision of treatment over SM. Finally, it will ultimately be important and practical for mental health professionals to understand reimbursement models and billing requirements for these services.

Benefits and Concerns Around Social Media to Provide Social Support and Education Among Individuals with Mental Illness

SM may facilitate forming connections among people with potentially stigmatizing health disorders, including depression, anxiety, schizophrenia, and autism spectrum disorders (ASDs).[33–37] This may happen over traditional SM sites, such as Facebook, Reddit, and Tumblr. However, there are also specialized SM sites related to mental health, such as Big White Wall (www.bigwhitewall.com) and Half of Us (www.halfofus.com). These sites, which offer the ability for individuals with mental health concerns to support each other, emphasize factors such as respecting privacy and confidentiality.[38]

SM can also facilitate self-disclosures that can provide education, support, and comfort to individuals with mental health concerns. The average user will generally not self-disclose potentially stigmatizing information. such as struggling with a mental illness.[6,39] However, there are a growing number of individuals who post self-disclosures around mental illness.[39–41] The information these individuals post may provide high-quality resources around mental health and spark valuable conversations.[39–41]

These messages can come from ordinary users or from virtual celebrities: individuals who make their livelihood by posting online material. Because these videos can have millions of views, when the information provided in these videos is accurate, they can be valuable to the public for 3 reasons. First, they may provide information to individuals who do not have access to health care professionals, either for logistical reasons or due to embarrassment. Second, peer-to-peer education and support are known to be potentially motivating, affording opportunities for persons with a mental illness to both challenge stigmatization and access online programs for improving their mental and physical well-being.[42] Third, these messages can demystify these previously stigmatizing conditions.[43]

Despite the potential value of these self-disclosures for education and motivation, however, there remain concerns if the information provided is not accurate.[32] A high-profile example of this is the damage that was done by a prominent celebrity who prominently displayed unsubstantiated concerns regarding vaccines and autism.[44] Additionally, self-disclosures during acute crises of some mental disorders may lead to "oversharing," with potential consequences, such as increased stigmatization and cyberbullying.[45] Moreover, use of temporary SM accounts, which provide some degree of anonymity, can be associated with problematic outcomes, such as higher negativity, cognitive bias, self-attention–seeking posts, and decreased self-esteem.[46] These investigators concluded that semi-anonymity of Reddit accounts allowed greater disinhibition among users. This may fulfill a unique need, allowing users to express views and thoughts about a topic, such as depression, that is usually considered highly sensitive.

There is also the potential for individuals to use SM to form bonds with each other around emotional concerns. It is an important developmental task of youth and young adulthood to form peer relationships, and SM may facilitate this. However, there also are questions as to whether online social contact with family members or close friends is a more productive way to approach the development of social relationships than with strangers and acquaintances.[37]

Population-Level Monitoring of Mental Health Concerns

Researchers have capitalized on readily available SM data to learn about human behavior and social phenomena. For example, SM data show promise for prediction of political election results[47] and outcomes of professional football games.[48] SM data also have been useful in monitoring health-related issues, such as disaster response to earthquakes[49] and outbreaks such as influenza.[50–54] Therefore, there has been some interest in leveraging these tools to better understand mental health. For example, some researchers have used SM data to better understand factors surrounding suicide attempts.[55–57] A recent systematic review identified current evidence on utilization of SM as a tool for suicide prevention. After analyzing 30 studies, the investigators found most studies were descriptive or qualitative and that no studies had reported on actual interventions. Although underscoring the need for more empirical research, the investigators concluded that SM platforms can be accessed by a large number of otherwise difficult-to-engage participants, providing an anonymous, yet accessible and nonjudgmental environment. Ultimately, this may allow interventions to be conducted after an expression of suicidal ideation is made online.[58]

Data from focus groups conducted among SM users with and without depression suggest that there is a wide range of reactions to this type of research. Although many individuals appreciate the value of using public domain information as a resource to improve mental health monitoring, others are concerned about issues related to privacy and lack of oversight.[59]

Another study analyzed a random sample of 2000 tweets to assess depression-related content. Researchers found that although 40% of the chatter consisted of supportive or helpful tweets, 32% disclosed feelings of depression. More than 65% of all tweets contained one or more DSM-5 symptoms necessary for the diagnosis of major depressive disorder. These findings underline the potential avenue that SM offers for prevention and awareness messages campaigns.[57]

Emotional Contagion

Traditional research has demonstrated that in-person interaction can be a powerful purveyor for "emotional contagion," resulting in the potential exacerbation and/or amelioration of emotional states. It is an important task of adolescence and young adulthood to develop identity based on shared interests and experiences.

However, there has been interest in determining whether this contagion effect applies in the SM milieu. One large study suggested that emotional states can be transferred among participants of SM via observation of others' positive experiences.[60] The investigators conducted an experiment among real Facebook users without their knowledge. They altered the amount of emotional material that was presented in certain users' News Feed and observed whether there were changes in participants' person-to-person interactions. They found that, when positively valenced expressions were reduced, participants spontaneously produced fewer positive posts and more negative posts. They also found that when negative expressions were reduced, there were fewer negative posts and more positive posts. The investigators concluded that in-person interaction and nonverbal cues are not strictly necessary for emotional contagion.[60]

Research also suggests that the likelihood of feeling happy after reading a positive post on Facebook is significantly related to strength of the relationship between the 2 individuals.[61] Although this may seem intuitive, these findings are important because they suggest potential avenues for intervention. For example, if individuals can be encouraged to increase positive posts through intervention, this may decrease overall negative cognitions.

Social Media and Mental Health Outcomes Among Young Adults

There is controversy as to whether, among young adults, overall SM use is associated with mental health outcomes. Some studies suggest that SM users may experience an increase in social capital, perceived social support, and life satisfaction.[62,63] Similarly, use of SM may provide opportunities for keeping in touch with family and friends, as well as other social interactions that may increase social capital and alleviate mental health concerns, such as depression and anxiety.[62,64,65] However, large-scale cross-sectional epidemiologic studies conducted among this population tend to find associations between increased SM use and negative outcomes related to mental health, such as depression, anxiety, poor sleep, eating concerns, and poor emotional support.

Depression

A nationally representative study based in the United States looked at individuals ages 19 to 32. It found consistent, linear associations between quartile of SM use and degree of depression as measured with the Patient-Reported Outcomes Measurement Information System (PROMIS) brief depression scale.[66] Results were consistent whether SM use was approximated by self-reported time spent on SM or by a frequency of use measure based on the Pew Internet Research study. For example, compared with those in the lowest quartile, individuals in the highest quartile of SM site visits per week had significantly increased odds of depression (adjusted odds ratio [AOR] 2.74, 95% confidence interval [CI] 1.86–4.04).[66]

Similar findings have been reported internationally. For example, a study of 340 Lebanese medical students suggested that there was a significant association between depression and Facebook use, including the specific use of Facebook-related tools, such as the "like" and "add friend" buttons.[67] Additionally, a study of 467 Scottish adolescents, which examined SM use and its association with sleep, anxiety, and depression, found that those who used more SM had lower sleep quality, worse self-esteem, increased anxiety, and increased depression.[68]

Because these studies are cross-sectional, they do not help determine causality. For example, it may be that individuals who are depressed turn to SM so as to self-soothe. On the other hand, there are conceptual reasons why depressive cognitions may be triggered in frequent SM users. For example, frequent SM users may substitute SM for potentially more valuable face-to-face social interactions.[69,70] Alternatively, frequent exposure to highly curated, unrealistic portrayals on SM may give people the impression that others are living happier, more connected lives, which may make people feel more depressed in comparison.[25]

Studies also suggest value in studying SM around depression. In a systematic review that explored whether youth use SM to share ideas and thoughts about deliberate self-harm, depressive language was present in 19% of participants.[71] This review also found a number of beneficial suggestions that were shared among SM users, such as ideas for formal treatment and advice on how to stop self-harming behavior. However, some concerning ideas were also shared, such as normalization of self-harming behavior, concealment of suicidal plans or ideas, and live enactments of self-harm acts.[71]

Anxiety

The population-based study of Scottish adolescents also found associations between increased SM use and anxiety.[68] Also, an online survey conducted in Norway among 23,533 individuals 16 years and older found a positive and significant association between symptoms of anxiety and obsessive compulsive disorder and potentially addictive use of SM.[72] Another study based in the United States involved a sample of 243 college students. These researchers found that there were significant associations between problematic use of Facebook, social anxiety, and the need for social assurance.[73]

Poor sleep

Researchers examined a nationally representative sample of young adults and found that increased SM use was independently associated with poor sleep.[74] Sleep disturbance was assessed using the brief PROMIS sleep disturbance measure. In models that adjusted for all sociodemographic covariates, participants with higher SM use volume and frequency had significantly greater odds of having sleep disturbance. For example, compared with those in the lowest quartile of SM use per day, those in the highest quartile had an AOR of 1.95 (95% CI 1.37–2.79) for sleep disturbance. Similarly, compared with those in the lowest quartile of SM use frequency per week, those in the highest quartile had an AOR of 2.92 (95% CI 1.97–4.32) for sleep disturbance. All associations demonstrated a significant linear trend.[74]

Research has found consistent results among 467 Scottish adolescents; again increased SM use was associated with poor sleep.[68] In this study, the researchers also found that nighttime-specific SM use was associated with poorer sleep, even when models controlled for related mental health factors, such as anxiety, depression, and self-esteem.[68]

Eating concerns

Multiple concerns have been raised in the literature regarding the availability on SM sites of problematic content that encourages disordered eating behaviors. For example, there are many so-called "pro-anorexia" communities on SM that encourage eating behaviors that physical health professionals would consider extremely problematic and dangerous, such as severe calorie restriction.[75] However, it also has been noted in the literature that there is also a growing community of individuals on SM who post "anti–pro-anorexia" messages.[76] Therefore, it is valuable for clinicians who work with individuals who have eating disorders to understand the complex dynamic environment of SM around this particular issue. It has also been noted that pro-anorexia SM content can be influential with regard to male body image issues.[77]

One large, nationally representative study examined this issue on a population level instead of focusing on those with specific eating disorder criteria.[78] In particular, the researchers examined overall SM use and the likelihood of having more eating and body image–related concerns in general. They found that, compared with those in the lowest quartile, participants in the highest quartiles for SM use volume and frequency had significantly greater odds of having eating concerns (AOR 2.18, 95% CI 1.50–3.17 and AOR 2.55, 95% CI 1.72–3.78, respectively). There were significant positive overall linear associations between the SM use variables and eating concerns (P < .001).[78] Although this was a cross-sectional study and directionality could not be established, these findings suggest that unhealthy messages around body image and eating behaviors may be a concern even in general SM environments and not only in the more extreme cases.

Autism spectrum disorders

The literature regarding ASD and SM is still emerging. Most studies are descriptive in nature.[37,79–81] Additionally, data have primarily been obtained from parents or caregivers, and most of these studies have focused solely on reporting prevalence of SM among people living with ASD.[37,79–81] In general, these studies have found that although young adults with ASD spend most of their free time using television or video games, only a small fraction uses SM in general.[37,79–81] One study among adolescents with ASD reported a significant and positive association between use of SM and greater security in their friendships.[37]

Emotional support

Some relatively small and localized studies indicate that frequent use of SM may be associated with declines in subjective well-being, life satisfaction, and real-life community.[5,82] These data are borne out in larger studies as well. For example, a nationally representative study of US young adults found that increased daily time devoted to SM use was independently associated with lower perceived emotional support. In particular, the researchers' multivariable model including all sociodemographic covariates and accounting for survey weights demonstrated that, compared with the lowest quartile of time on SM, being in the highest quartile was significantly associated with decreased odds of having higher perceived emotional support (AOR 0.62, 95% CI 0.40–0.94). Interestingly, however, this same study did not find a significant association with emotional support when SM was operationalized in terms of number of sites visited per week.[25]

FUTURE DIRECTIONS
Need for Longitudinal Research

Because most data linking SM use and mental health outcomes have been cross-sectional, the directionality of this association is not clear. When a study finds that there is a broad association between SM use and depression, for example, this may indicate that individuals with depression tend to use more SM; depressed individuals with a diminished sense of self-worth may turn to SM-based interactions for validation.[83,84] Subsequently, individuals may suffer from continuous rumination and guilt surrounding Internet use, while feeling compelled to continue the cycle due to low self-efficacy and negative self-appraisal.[83,85] Due to the high accessibility of SM and the possibility of socialization in a controlled setting, individuals with underlying depression and anhedonia may be more drawn to SM interactions rather than face-to-face interactions.[86,87]

However, it also may be that those who use increased amounts of SM subsequently develop or increase depressive symptoms. Multiple studies have linked SM use with declines in subjective mood, sense of well-being, and life satisfaction.[5,82,88] For example, passive consumption of SM content, as opposed to active communication, has been associated with decrease in bonding and bridging social capital and increase in loneliness.[89] One explanation may be that exposure to highly idealized representations of peers on SM elicits feelings of envy and the distorted belief that others lead happier and/or more successful lives.[90,91] Consequently, these envious feelings may lead to a sense of self-inferiority and depression over time.[92] It is also possible that the feeling of "time wasted" by engaging in activities of little meaning on SM negatively influences mood.[88] Moreover, in a nationally representative survey that assessed general health among college-age students, Internet use and computer games have consistently been identified among the top 5 factors impacting their academic performance.[93] Additionally, the substantial rise in the amount of time young individuals spend on the Internet, particularly on SM, has led some to call for the recognition of "Internet addiction" as a distinct psychiatric condition that is closely associated with depression.[94,95] Finally, it is possible that increased SM exposure may increase the risk of cyberbullying, which also may increase symptoms of depression.[96,97]

Need for Clinically Based Research

Because most research in this area has focused on community-based populations, it will be valuable for future work to involve clinical populations so as to facilitate discoveries with clinically relevant conclusions. For example, discovery of associations between SM use and mental disorders suggests that it may be valuable for clinicians to assess SM use among depressed individuals to probe for maladaptive patterns of use, which may be contributing to mood dysregulation. However, clinicians are extremely busy, and the actual value of this additional history has not been systematically studied. Still, because SM use is so common and integral to transitional age youth, bringing up a discussion of SM use would seem to have potential value simply in getting to know a patient better.

However, because SM has become an integrated component of human interaction, it is important for clinicians interacting with young adults to recognize the important balance to be struck in encouraging potential positive use, but redirecting from problematic use. Although much of the high-profile research has found overall associations between SM use and mental health problems, suggesting major limitation of use may be viewed by patients as insensitive or misguided.

Use of Social Media to Screen for Mental Health Problems

There may be useful ways of leveraging SM to decrease stigma of depression and identify individuals at risk, such as detecting self-disclosures of depression on SM.[39] The teams behind some SM sites have already begun to reach out to users who show signs of mental disorders. When one searches blog site Tumblr for tags indicative of a mental health crisis, such as "depressed," "suicidal," or "hopeless," the search function redirects to a message that begins with "Everything okay?" and provides links to pertinent resources.[98] Similarly, in early 2015, Facebook tested a feature by which users' friends could easily and anonymously report worrisome posts.[99] Authors of problematic content received pop-up messages on their next visit to the site voicing concern and encouraging them to speak with a friend or helpline worker. Although this button has since been removed, Facebook still accepts reports of suicidal content via an online form. Continued research into the factors that relate SM and depression will allow sites to refine their procedures and reach out to those with greatest need.

Understanding Nuances of Different Types of Social Media Use

It will be an important task of future qualitative and quantitative research to more comprehensively assess content and contextual elements related to SM use. Much of the previous research has grouped multiple different ways of using SM together. By parsing out different contextual factors associated with SM use, it will ultimately be easier to determine best practices around SM use.

Active versus passive social media use

Time on SM may be primarily spent viewing profiles, or it may be spent as an active participant, and these distinct patterns of use may have differential associations with mood conditions. Those who primarily observe are sometimes called "lurkers." It may be that those who are more active users feel more engaged and derive more sense of social capital from SM interactions.[62,100] However, it also may be that active users are more prone to having negative exposures, which can affect self-cognitions. Therefore, active versus passive character of SM interaction and its effect on mood may be valuable to assess in the future.

Emotional valence of social media use

Additionally, it will be important to assess the overall emotional valence of SM interactions. Some individuals may primarily spend time "liking" others' posts, wishing friends happy birthday, and making positive comments. Others, however, may be prone to posting negative status updates or engaging in contentious interactions, which may be detrimental to relationship-building and lead to depression.[101]

Personality characteristics and social media use

People with different personality characteristics might have substantially different experiences with SM as it relates to mental disorders. For example, personality characteristics, such as extraversion, neuroticism, and openness, have been associated with increased online communication and SM use.[102,103] Therefore, it is possible that people with these characteristics might obtain more benefit from SM use. As a trait, extraversion is associated with high levels of engagement with the outside world, energy, and sociability, and this tendency may carry into the world of SM.[104] Neuroticism is associated with anxiety, negative affect, and self-consciousness, all of which also may impact how individuals interact in a context related to SM.[104] Conscientiousness is associated with organization, diligence, and impulse control.[104] These qualities similarly may be relevant to how an individual approaches social interaction online. Finally, agreeableness is associated with altruism, consideration, and caring for others, all of which may be relevant to how individuals interact in SM-related situations.[104] It would be valuable to more systematically assess how SM and personality characteristics interact so as to develop targeted interventions and recommendations.

Online and offline use

It would be valuable for future work to more comprehensively address associations between online and offline use. Some previous research has suggested that there may be a substitution effect; those who commit more time and attention to online activities may subsequently develop fewer close and meaningful offline relationships.[69,70] However, other studies suggest that those with increased online activities did not have any decrease in the quality of offline relationships.[105] Therefore, these will be important areas for further research. Ultimately, for example, it would be useful to know under what circumstances online interactions may be leveraged to improve offline support. This is especially true because individuals living with mental disorders may find it relatively easy to begin to engage in the online milieu, even when they have anhedonia, lack of energy, anxiety, and/or other symptoms preventing them from immediately engaging with the "real" world. This research is also important to help us in better understanding how to generate support for transitional age youth with regard to relationship development. For example, among young adults 18 to 24 and 25 to 34 years of age, 27% and 22% reported to use online dating sites to find potential sentimental partners, which represents a threefold increase from 2013.[106]

Use of multiple platforms

Associations between SM use and self-reported depression and anxiety also may be related to the use of multiple SM platforms. The number of different SM platforms used is rising substantially. For example, use of 2 or more platforms increased by 10% in just 1 year, from 2013 to 2014.[107] On one hand, increased use of multiple platforms may be associated with an increase in one's social capital and social support, which subsequently may be related to improvement of depression and anxiety symptoms.[62,108] However, use of multiple platforms also may involve multitasking, which as noted previously has been associated in the past with negative cognitive and mental health outcomes.[15,16] Use of multiple SM platforms also may be related to negative mental health outcomes even if the different platforms are not all used at once. For example, the use of multiple platforms can lead to identity diffusion, which has been related to poor emotional health in the past.[109] This may be related to additional opportunities for online misunderstandings, negative interactions, and/or feelings of being left out, each of which may be associated with negative mood states.[110]

Balance of Risks and Opportunities for Use of Social Media in Treatment of Mental Health Conditions

There are both potential benefits and risks around using SM in the treatment of mental health conditions. Identified benefits include the ability to form therapeutic relationships even when there are barriers to seeking care, such as stigma, finances, or logistics. However, patient-provider relationships formed over SM may be inferior to those developed in person. Therefore, an important task of future research will be to determine under what circumstances and for whom SM-mediated mental health care is most valuable. For example, it may be useful to leverage SM in cases in which the barriers to in-person care are particularly profound. Similarly, there may be a role for the use of SM in the prevention of relapse. For example, SM could be leveraged to include medication reminders.

SUMMARY

In summary, SM has rapidly become an integral component of how transitional age individuals connect with others. Although literature around the influence of SM on development is still emerging, SM may facilitate a unique type of peer pressure through quantifiable social endorsement. There are potential benefits of using SM to alleviate mental health concerns, such as facilitation of connecting individuals with conditions such as depression, anxiety, and schizophrenia. Also, SM may be leveraged to provide mental health care and surveillance of mental health concerns. However, large cross-sectional epidemiologic studies suggest that increased SM use is linearly associated with prevalence of mental health concerns, such as depression, anxiety, and sleep disturbance. Future research should help to examine directionality of these associations and the role of contextual factors, such as style of SM use, personality, and the use of multiple platforms.

REFERENCES

1. Kaplan AM, Haenlein M. Users of the world, unite! the challenges and opportunities of Social Media. Bus Horiz 2010;53(1):59–68.
2. Subrahmanyam K, Reich SM, Waechter N, et al. Online and offline social networks: use of social networking sites by emerging adults. J Appl Dev Psychol 2008;29(6):420–33.

3. Fox S, Rainie L. The Web at 25 in the US. 2014. Available at: http://www.web citation.org/6eVfaSdN6. Accessed September 25, 2015.

4. Roisman GI, Masten AS, Coatsworth JD, et al. Salient and emerging developmental tasks in the transition to adulthood. Child Dev 2004;75:123–33.

5. Chou HTG, Edge N. "They are happier and having better lives than I am": the impact of using Facebook on perceptions of others' lives. Cyberpsychol Behav Soc Netw 2012;15(2):117–21.

6. Jelenchick LA, Eickhoff JC, Moreno MA. "Facebook depression?" Social networking site use and depression in older adolescents. J Adolesc Health 2013;52(1):128–30.

7. Nielsen. State of the media: The social media report 2012. 2012. Available at: http://www.webcitation.org/6bXTvRwTJ. Accessed June 8, 2016.

8. Pew Research Center. Social media update 2015. 2015. Available at: http://www.webcitation.org/6ajEhvS11. Accessed June 8, 2016.

9. Pantic I. Online social networking and mental health. Cyberpsychol Behav Soc Netw 2014;17(10):652–7.

10. Frler S. Snapchat User Stories Fuel 10 Billion Daily Video Views. Bloom Technol. 2016. Available at: http://www.bloomberg.com/news/articles/2016-04-28/snap chat-user-content-fuels-jump-to-10-billion-daily-video-views. Accessed August 30, 2016.

11. The Top 10 Snapchat Statistics You Need to Know in 2016. Mediakix. 2016. Available at: http://mediakix.com/2016/01/snapchat-statistics-2016-marketers-need-to-know/#gs.SzyZl0w. Accessed August 30, 2016.

12. Meshi D, Tamir DI, Heekeren HR. The emerging neuroscience of social media. Trends Cogn Sci 2015;19(12):771–82.

13. Sherman LE, Payton AA, Hernandez LM, et al. The power of the like in adolescence: effects of peer influence on neural and behavioral responses to social media. Psychol Sci 2016;27(7):1027–35.

14. Choudhury S, McKinney KA. Digital media, the developing brain and the interpretive plasticity of neuroplasticity. Transcult Psychiatry 2013;50(2):192–215.

15. Ophir E, Nass C, Wagner AD. Cognitive control in media multitaskers. Proc Natl Acad Sci U S A 2009;106(37):15583–7.

16. Chen Q, Yan Z. Does multitasking with mobile phones affect learning? A review. Comput Human Behav 2016;54:34–42.

17. Kiisel T. Is social media shortening our attention span? Forbes/Technology; 2012. Available at: http://www.forbes.com/sites/tykiisel/2012/01/25/is-social-media-shortening-our-attention-span/#4bfb2b486945. Accessed January 3, 2017.

18. Litsa T. How social media affects your attention span. Mountain View (CA): Linkedin; 2014. Available at: https://www.linkedin.com/pulse/20140519183028-114333012-how-social-media-affects-your-attention-span/. Accessed January 3, 2017.

19. Junco R, Cotten SR. The relationship between multitasking and academic performance. Comput Educ 2012;58(1):505–14.

20. Cain MS, Leonard JA, Gabrieli JDE, et al. Media multitasking in adolescence. Psychon Bull Rev 2016;23(6):1932–41.

21. Rosen L, Carrier LM, Cheever NA. Facebook and texting made me do it: media-induced task-switching while studying. Comput Human Behav 2013;29:948–58.

22. van der Schuur WA, Baumgartner SE, Sumter SR, et al. The consequences of media multitasking for youth: a review. Comput Human Behav 2015;53:204–15.

23. Becker MW, Alzahabi R, Hopwood CJ. Media multitasking is associated with symptoms of depression and social anxiety. Cyberpsychol Behav Soc Netw

2013;16(2):132–5. Available at: http://online.liebertpub.com/doi/pdf/10.1089/cyber.2012.0291. Accessed January 3, 2017.

24. Richards D, Caldwell PHY, Go H. Impact of social media on the health of children and young people. J Paediatr Child Health 2015;51(12):1152–7.

25. Shensa A, Sidani JE, Lin LY, et al. Social media use and perceived emotional support among US young adults. J Community Health 2016;41(3):541–9.

26. Mathiak K, Weber R. Toward brain correlates of natural behavior: fMRI during violent video games. Hum Brain Mapp 2006;27(12):948–56.

27. Bavelier D, Green CS, Dye MWG. Children, wired: for better and for worse. Neuron 2010;67(5):692–701.

28. Jashinsky J, Burton SH, Hanson CL, et al. Tracking suicide risk factors through Twitter in the US. Crisis 2013;35(1):51–9.

29. Larsen ME, Boonstra TW, Batterham PJ, et al. We feel: mapping emotion on Twitter. IEEE J Biomed Heal Inform 2015;19(4):1246–52.

30. Sueki H. The association of suicide-related Twitter use with suicidal behaviour: a cross-sectional study of young Internet users in Japan. J Affect Disord 2015; 170:155–60.

31. McManus K, Mallory EK, Goldfeder RL, et al. Mining Twitter data to improve detection of schizophrenia. AMIA Jt Summits Transl Sci Proc 2015;2015:122–6.

32. Cox-George C. The changing face(book) of psychiatry: can we justify "following" patients' social media activity? BJPsych Bull 2015;39(6):283–4.

33. Välimäki M, Athanasopoulou C, Lahti M, et al. Effectiveness of social media interventions for people with schizophrenia: a systematic review and meta-analysis. J Med Internet Res 2016;18(4):e92.

34. Merolli M, Gray K, Martin-Sanchez F. Health outcomes and related effects of using social media in chronic disease management: a literature review and analysis of affordances. J Biomed Inform 2013;46(6):957–69.

35. Merolli M, Gray K, Martin-Sanchez F. Therapeutic affordances of social media: emergent themes from a global online survey of people with chronic pain. J Med Internet Res 2014;16(12):e284.

36. Evans WD. Social marketing campaigns and children's media use. Future Child 2008;18(1):181–203.

37. Kuo MH, Orsmond GI, Coster WJ, et al. Media use among adolescents with autism spectrum disorder. Autism 2014;18:914–23.

38. Dosani S, Harding C, Wilson S. Online groups and patient forums. Curr Psychiatry Rep 2014;16(11):507.

39. Moreno MA, Jelenchick LA, Egan KG, et al. Feeling bad on Facebook: depression disclosures by college students on a social networking site. Depress Anxiety 2011;28(6):447–55.

40. Whitehill J, Brockman L, Moreno M. "Just talk to me": communicating with college students about depression disclosures on Facebook. J Adolesc Health 2013;52(1):122–7.

41. De Choudhury M, De S. Mental health discourse on Reddit: self-disclosure, social support, and anonymity. Proc Eight Int AAAI Conf Weblogs Soc Media held at Ann Arbor, MI, May 27–29, 2015.

42. Naslund JA, Aschbrenner KA, Marsch LA, et al. The future of mental health care: peer-to-peer support and social media. Epidemiol Psychiatr Sci 2016;25(2): 113–22.

43. Betton V, Borschmann R, Docherty M, et al. The role of social media in reducing stigma and discrimination. Br J Psychiatry 2015;206(6):443–4.

44. Kata A. Anti-vaccine activists, Web 2.0, and the postmodern paradigm – an overview of tactics and tropes used online by the anti-vaccination movement. Vaccine 2012;30(25):3778–89.

45. Torous J, Keshavan M. The role of social media in schizophrenia. Curr Opin Psychiatry 2016;29(3):190–5.

46. Pavalanathan U, De Choudhury M. Identity management and mental health discourse in social media. Proc 24th Int Conf World Wide Web Companion. 2015. p. 315–21.

47. Digrazia J, McKelvey K, Bollen J, et al. More tweets, more votes: social media as a quantitative indicator of political behavior. PLoS One 2013;8(11):e79449.

48. Sinha S, Dyer C, Gimpel K, et al. Predicting the NFL using Twitter. In: ECML/PKDD 2013 workshop on matching learning and data mining for sports analytics held at Prague (Czech Republic), September 27, 2013. Available at: https://dtai.cs.kuleuven.be/events/MLSA13/papers/mlsa13_submission_10.pdf. Accessed January 3, 2017.

49. Doan S, Vo B, Collier N. An analysis of Twitter messages in the 2011 Tohoku earthquake. In: Kostkova P, Szomszor M, Fowler D, editors. Electronic healthcare: fourth international conference, eHealth 2011. Lecture notes of the institute for computer sciences, social informatics and telecommunications engineering, vol. 91. Berlin: Springer; 2012. p. 58–66.

50. Achrekar H, Gandhe A. Predicting flu trends using Twitter data. In: IEEE Conference on computer communications workshops (INFOCOM WKSHPS) held at Shanghai (China), April 10–15, 2011.

51. Aramaki E, Maskawa S, Morita M. Twitter catches the flu: detecting influenza epidemics using Twitter. Proceedings of the Conference on Empirical Methods in Natural Languge Processing (EMNLP '11), Edinburgh (UK), July 27–31, 2011.

52. Broniatowski DA, Paul MJ, Dredze M. National and local influenza surveillance through twitter: an analysis of the 2012-2013 influenza epidemic. PLoS One 2013;8(12):e83672.

53. Collier N, Son NT, Nguyen NM. OMG u got flu? Analysis of shared health messages for bio-surveillance. J Biomed Semantics 2011;2(Suppl 5):S9.

54. St Louis C, Zorlu G. Can Twitter predict disease outbreaks? Br Med J 2012;344: e2353.

55. Haas A, Koestner B, Rosenberg J, et al. An interactive web-based method of outreach to college students at risk for suicide. J Am Coll Health 2008;57(1): 15–22.

56. Won H, Myung W, Song G, et al. Predicting national suicide numbers with social media data. PLoS One 2013;8(4):e61809.

57. Cavazos-Rehg PA, Krauss MJ, Sowles S, et al. A content analysis of depression-related Tweets. Comput Human Behav 2016;54:351–7.

58. Robinson J, Cox G, Bailey E, et al. Social media and suicide prevention: a systematic review. Early Interv Psychiatry 2016;10(2):103–21.

59. Mikal J, Hurst S, Conway M. Ethical issues in using Twitter for population-level depression monitoring: a qualitative study. BMC Med Ethics 2016;17:22.

60. Kramer ADI, Guillory JE, Hancock JT. Experimental evidence of massive-scale emotional contagion through social networks. Proc Natl Acad Sci U S A 2014; 111(24):8788–90.

61. Lin R, Utz S. The emotional responses of browsing Facebook: happiness, envy, and the role of tie strength. Comput Human Behav 2015;52:29–38.

62. Ellison NB, Steinfield C, Lampe C. The benefits of Facebook "friends": social capital and college students' use of online social network sites. J Comput Commun 2007;12(4):1143–68.
63. Valenzuela S, Park N, Kee KF. Is there social capital in a social network site? Facebook use and college students' life satisfaction, trust, and participation. J Comput Commun 2009;14(4):875–901.
64. de la Pena A, Quintanilla C. Share, like and achieve: the power of Facebook to reach health-related goals. Int J Consum Stud 2015;39(5):495–505. Available at: http://ovidsp.ovid.com/ovidweb.cgi?T=JS&PAGE=reference&D=psyc11&NEWS=N&AN=2015-39457-011. Accessed January 3, 2017.
65. Bessière K, Pressman S, Kiesler S, et al. Effects of Internet use on health and depression: a longitudinal study. J Med Internet Res 2010;12(1):e6.
66. Lin LY, Sidani JE, Shensa A, et al. Association between social media use and depression among U.S. young adults. Depress Anxiety 2016;33(4):323–31.
67. Naja WJ, Kansoun AH, Haddad RS. Prevalence of depression in medical students at the Lebanese university and exploring its correlation with Facebook relevance: a questionnaire study. JMIR Res Protoc 2016;5(2):e96.
68. Woods HC, Scott H. #Sleepyteens: social media use in adolescence is associated with poor sleep quality, anxiety, depression and low self-esteem. J Adolesc 2016;51:41–9.
69. Marar Z. Intimacy: understanding the subtle power of human connection. Durham (United Kingdom): Acumen Publishing; 2012. Available at: http://ovidsp.ovid.com/ovidweb.cgi?T=JS&PAGE=reference&D=psyc9&NEWS=N&AN=2012-18831-000. Accessed January 3, 2017.
70. Baek YM, Bae Y, Jang H. Social and parasocial relationships on social network sites and their differential relationships with users' psychological well-being. Cyberpsychol Behav Soc Netw 2013;16(7):512–7.
71. Dyson MP, Hartling L, Shulhan J, et al. A systematic review of social media use to discuss and view deliberate self-harm acts. PLoS One 2016;11(5):e0155813.
72. Schou Andreassen C, Billieux J, Griffiths MD, et al. The relationship between addictive use of social media and video games and symptoms of psychiatric disorders: a large-scale cross-sectional study. Psychol Addict Behav 2016;30(2):252–62.
73. Lee-Won RJ, Herzog L, Park SG. Hooked on Facebook: the role of social anxiety and need for social assurance in problematic use of Facebook. Cyberpsychol Behav Soc Netw 2015;18(10):567–74.
74. Levenson JC, Shensa A, Sidani JE, et al. The association between social media use and sleep disturbance among young adults. Prev Med 2016;85:36–41.
75. Oksanen A, Garcia D, Rasanen P. Proanorexia communities on social media. Pediatrics 2016;137(1).
76. Oksanen A, Garcia D, Sirola A, et al. Pro-anorexia and anti-pro-anorexia videos on YouTube: sentiment analysis of user responses. J Med Internet Res 2015;17(11):e256.
77. Juarez L, Soto E, Pritchard ME. Drive for muscularity and drive for thinness: the impact of pro-anorexia websites. Eat Disord 2012;20(2):99–112.
78. Sidani JE, Shensa A, Hoffman B, et al. The association between social media use and eating concerns among US young adults. J Acad Nutr Diet 2016;116(9):1465–72.
79. Mazurek MO, Shattuck PT, Wagner M, et al. Prevalence and correlates of screen-based media use among youths with autism spectrum disorders. J Autism Dev Disord 2012;42(8):1757–67.

80. Mazurek MO, Wenstrup C. Television, video game and social media use among children with ASD and typically developing siblings. J Autism Dev Disord 2013; 43(6):1258–71.

81. Shane HC, Albert PD. Electronic screen media for persons with autism spectrum disorders: results of a survey. J Autism Dev Disord 2008;38(8):1499–508.

82. Kross E, Verduyn P, Demiralp E, et al. Facebook use predicts declines in subjective well-being in young adults. PLoS One 2013;8(8):e69841.

83. Caplan SE. Problematic Internet use and psychosocial well-being: development of a theory-based cognitive-behavioral measurement instrument. Comput Human Behav 2002;18(5):553–75.

84. Sanders CE, Field TM, Diego M, et al. The relationship of Internet use to depression and social isolation among adolescents. Adolescence 2000;35(138): 237–42.

85. Davis RA. Cognitive-behavioral model of pathological Internet use. Comput Human Behav 2001;17(2):187–95.

86. Morahan-Martin J, Schumacher P. Loneliness and social uses of the Internet. Comput Human Behav 2003;19(6):659–71.

87. Korkeila J. The relationships depression and Internet addiction. Duodecim 2012;128(7):741–8.

88. Sagioglou C, Greitemeyer T. Facebook's emotional consequences: why Facebook causes a decrease in mood and why people still use it. Comput Human Behav 2014;35:359–63.

89. Burke M, Marlow C, Lento T. Social network activity and social well-being. In: Proceedings of the 28th international conference on human factors in computing systems - CHI '10. New York: ACM Press; 2010. p. 1909–12.

90. Krasnova H, Wenninger H, Widjaja T, et al. Envy on Facebook: a hidden threat to users' life satisfaction? Presented at the 11th International Conference on Wirtschaftsinformatik Proc at Leipzig (Germany), February 27-March 1, 2013. Available at: http://wi2013.de/dateien/WI2013_Proceedings_Volume_2.pdf. Accessed January 3, 2017.

91. Tandoc EC, Ferrucci P, Duffy M. Facebook use, envy, and depression among college students: is Facebooking depressing? Comput Human Behav 2015; 43:139–46.

92. Smith RH, Kim SH. Comprehending envy. Psychol Bull 2007;133:46–64.

93. American College Health Association. American College Health Association-National College Health assessment II: reference group executive summary 2015. Hanover (MD): American College Health Association; 2016.

94. Block JJ. Issues for DSM-V: internet addiction. Am J Psychiatry 2008;165(3): 306–7.

95. Morrison CM, Gore H. The relationship between excessive Internet use and depression: a questionnaire-based study of 1,319 young people and adults. Psychopathology 2010;43(2):121–6.

96. O'Keeffe GS, Clarke-Pearson K. The impact of social media on children, adolescents, and families. Pediatrics 2011;127(4):800–4.

97. Pew Research Center. Cyberbullying. Washington, DC: 2007. Available at: http://www.webcitation.org/6eVgbqVbe. Accessed May 1, 2015.

98. Tumblr. "Everything Okay?" Message. 2014. Available at: http://www.webcitation.org/6nFPOjNAO. Accessed January 3, 2017.

99. Facebook Safety. Updates in Facebook Safety. 2015.

100. Burke M, Kraut R, Marlow C. Social capital on Facebook. In: Proceedings of the 2011 annual conference on human factors in computing systems - *CHI '11*. 2011:571.

101. Forest AL, Wood JV. When social networking is not working: individuals with low self-esteem recognize but do not reap the benefits of self-disclosure on Facebook. Psychol Sci 2012;23(3):295–302.

102. Mark G, Ganzach Y. Personality and Internet usage: a large-scale representative study of young adults. Comput Human Behav 2014;36:274–81.

103. Correa T, Hinsley AW, de Zúñiga HG. Who interacts on the Web? The intersection of users' personality and social media use. Comput Human Behav 2010; 26(2):247–53.

104. McCrae RR, John OP. An introduction to the five-factor model and its applications. J Pers 1992;60(2):175–215. Available at: http://search.ebscohost.com/login. aspx?direct=true&AuthType=ip,uid&db=aph&AN=9208170743&scope=site. Accessed January 3, 2017.

105. Park J, Lee DS, Shablack H, et al. When perceptions defy reality: the relationships between depression and actual and perceived Facebook social support. J Affect Disord 2016;200:37–44.

106. Lenhart A, Duggan M. Couples, the Internet and social media. Washington, DC: Pew Res Cent; 2014. Available at: http://www.pewinternet.org/files/2014/02/PIP_Couples_and_Technology-FIN_021114.pdf. Accessed January 3, 2017.

107. Duggan M, Ellison NB, Lampe C, et al. Social media update 2014. Washington, DC: Pew Res Cent; 2014. p. 1. Available at: http://www.pewinternet.org/2015/01/09/social-media-update-2014/. Accessed January 3, 2017.

108. Keitzmann JH, Hermkens K, McCarthy IP, et al. Social media? Get serious! Understanding the functional building blocks of social media. Bus Horiz 2011;54: 241–51.

109. Marcia JE. Identity in adolescence. In: Adelson J, editor. Handbook of adolescent psychology. New York: Wiley; 1980. p. 159–87.

110. Arnett JJ. Adolescents' uses of media for self-socialization. J Youth Adolesc 1995;24(5):519–33.

Proximal Influences on the Trajectory of Suicidal Behaviors and Suicide during the Transition from Adolescence to Young Adulthood

Aradhana Bela Sood, MD, MSHA*, Julie Linker, PhD

KEYWORDS

- Adolescence • Suicide • Youth brain development • Public health approach

KEY POINTS

- Transitional age youth (TAY) are at a unique risk for self-harm.
- Factors that increase risk for suicide in TAY are developmental tasks of transitioning from adolescence to adulthood, brain development, reactivity to stressors, and prior mental disorder.
- Institutions of higher learning, high schools, and employers should use a public health approach to reduce the incidence and prevalence of suicidal behavior in this age group.

INTRODUCTION

Adolescence is a bridge between childhood and adulthood beginning with the onset of sexual maturation and ending with the acquisition of adult responsibilities and roles.[1] It is characterized by a period of intense developmental changes in the body (hormones, secondary sexual characteristics), the negotiation of certain psychological and emotional tasks (delinking from parents, forming stronger peer relationships), intense brain architecture changes, increased independent decision making, and the launching of the independent self into the adult world. Because of the wide range in the chronologic age of physical changes, cultural differences in gaining psychological independence, and the effect of nutrition on the onset of puberty, adolescence is considered a long stage of transition that is intense, and is often a stressful period for individuals preparing for adulthood.[2] For this

Conflict: The authors have nothing to disclose.
Virginia Commonwealth University, 515 North 10th Street, Richmond, VA 23298, USA
* Corresponding author.
E-mail address: Bela.sood@vcuhealth.org

Child Adolesc Psychiatric Clin N Am 26 (2017) 235–251
http://dx.doi.org/10.1016/j.chc.2016.12.004
childpsych.theclinics.com
1056-4993/17/© 2016 Elsevier Inc. All rights reserved.

reason, the term transitional age youth (TAY) acknowledges this bridge age between childhood and adulthood[3] that is typically considered to be between 16 and 26 years.

Second only to early childhood, adolescence is a time of major central nervous system reconstruction characterized by reduction in gray matter and increases in white matter[4] and myelination of the axons in the brain. The active reconstruction of neuronal connections, pruning of excitatory synapses, and removal of unused synapses and connections fits with an evolutionary model for the goal of more efficient communication[5] and eventually a less reactionary and impulsive quality to thought and action processing for the individual. Although the visual cortex develops earlier in life, the frontal, parietal, and temporal areas go through active sculpting during adolescence and, along with the prefrontal cortex, are responsible for executive functioning of the brain; that is, the capacity to respond thoughtfully to stimuli with a well-integrated understanding of sensory input consistent with past experiences.[6] This capacity matures by the end of adolescence and is reflected in pragmatic rather than impulsive decision making.[7,8] All the structural changes in the brain coupled with hormonal changes are thus mirrored as emotional reactivity and behavioral changes. Various areas of the brain mature and reach their adult state in stages and so maturation does not occur in synchrony. As an example, the amygdala, the seat of emotional processing, matures much later than the prefrontal cortex, which is the place of organization and planning.[9] This discrepancy leads to poorly thought through decisions in any perceived crisis that may appear impulsive. In addition, the changes in the type and quantity of hormones released during puberty occur in waves and therefore these factors combine to make this period of development potentially a phase of behavioral turmoil.[10] Early adolescence is characterized by a lack of emotional control and the later period of adolescence by increasing emotional stability. As TAY move into the adult world, temperamental differences, social supports, biologic changes, and life events may affect the way they handle mental health challenges. Presence of previous vulnerabilities may put them at risk for difficulty negotiating the challenges that the adult world and adult responsibilities pose for them, whether it is within institutions of higher education (IHE) or in the employment arena. Suicidal ideations are common in TAY; however, ideations do not always translate into actions.[11]

SUICIDE AND TRANSITIONAL AGE YOUTH
Definitions

Any discussion to reduce the incidence of suicide should be informed by knowledge of the correct definitions of suicide, and associated risk and protective factors, so that interventions can reduce risk and bolster protective factors.[12] The definition of suicide and suicidal behaviors has been complicated by the number of terms used in relation to the phenomenon, such as deliberate self-harm, self-injurious behavior (SIB), self-mutilation, and parasuicidal behavior. The National Center for Injury Prevention and Control of the Centers for Disease Control and Prevention[12] provides the following definitions, which are widely accepted:

1. Suicidal ideations: thinking about or considering or planning suicide.
2. Suicide attempt: a nonfatal, self-directed, potentially injurious behavior with an intent to die as a result of the behavior; might not result in injury.
3. Suicide: death caused by self-directed SIB with an intent to die as a result of that behavior.

Epidemiology of Suicide in Transitional Age Youth

Suicide is the second leading cause of death among persons aged 15 to 34 years; the highest among all age groups.[13] In 2013, a national survey showed that serious thoughts about suicide were highest among young adults aged 18 to 25 years (7.4%). Having made a suicide plan in the past year was also highest among adults aged 18 to 25 years (2.5%) compared with other age groups. These statistics highlight that, in TAY, the array of suicidal behaviors (which include ideation, plans, and attempts) is at a peak, thus making it a target of intervention and prevention efforts.

Public health researchers are alarmed about the recent growing rates of suicide in the college population. Deaths by suicide on college campuses may receive more attention because of there being an institutional body that has some presumed responsibility for the well-being of TAY, and there is a significant amount of literature about providing both prevention and intervention services to youth in college.[14] However, broader attention to this age group shows that efforts must extend beyond college campuses to meet the needs of individuals who are entering adulthood through other paths, because this is a time of high risk for both college students and nonstudents alike.[14] For young people aged 18 to 22 years, there are similar percentages of full-time college students and those who are the same age but not full-time students who had suicidal thoughts (8.0% and 8.7%, respectively) or had suicide plans (2.4% and 3.1%).[15] For those not attending college full time, suicidal behavior seems to be more severe. Full-time college students aged 18 to 22 years were less likely to attempt suicide (0.9% vs 1.9%) or receive medical attention as a result of a suicide attempt (suggesting more dangerous attempts) in the previous 12 months (0.3% vs 0.7%), compared with their same-aged peers.[13] The rate of completed suicides in the nonstudent population is double that of full-time students. The difference in these rates has been attributed to reduced access to firearms on college campuses, resulting in less lethal attempts.[16]

Risk Factors for Suicide in Transitional Age Youth

The literature on college students highlights many issues that put TAY at risk for suicide and can be applied to full-time students, part-time students, and nonstudents[17] in this age range. Rarely do suicidal ideations, behaviors, or gestures occur without context.[18] Mental health disorders such as depression or substance abuse and a high degree of prior aggression or impulsivity[15] are frequently predisposing factors to suicidal behavior in TAY and are discussed later. Life events that precipitate suicidality may be poor academic performance, disciplinary crises, relationship disappointments, perceived humiliation, and legal problems.[19] Other factors that could predispose a vulnerable population to suicidal behavior include living in a culture that does not approve of seeking mental health treatment and/or does not view suicide as a taboo behavior to manage stress[20]; ready access to lethal means of committing suicide (ie, firearms)[21]; and exposure to suicide in the media as a dramatic event, producing the potential of a contagion effect in the population.[22] All of the factors mentioned earlier can become particularly relevant to TAY whose world views and positive and negative experiences are expanding exponentially as they are exposed to the employment environment or IHE. Although college students experience academic demands and stressors, almost by definition, TAY are also experiencing many exciting but stressful life events. These events include moving into employment, leaving parents or redefining relationships with parents and family members to accommodate growing independence and expectations, changing social networks to go away to school or move into new living or work environments, demands of independent living, and the developmental salience and instability of romantic rela-tionships.[23] Considered normative and important to development, with cultural varia-tions, these life changes introduce serious stressors for young adults who may not yet have developed the coping skills to handle them, may no longer have access to their familiar social supports,[23] and may not have access to needed services because of a lack of availability, funding, knowledge, or acceptability to seek help.[17] Within this environment of independence, whether in IHEs or employment and independent living, TAY are faced with (1) reduced or absent parental supervision or support such as they had in high school; and (2) the freedom to set daily routines, which may involve making independent decisions regarding sleep, food, and social relation-ships.[23] Sleep deprivation is strongly connected to exacerbation of the mood disor-ders[24] that are strong predisposing factors for suicidal ideations/gestures. Developmentally, the psychological task of forming intimate relationships outside the nuclear family is important for TAY. Immaturity in making decisions relating to romantic relationships and the resulting consequences of loss can be serious for TAY[25] and is frequently associated with at least temporary feelings of depression that could progress to suicidal ideations and behavior, typically when in the context of significant risk factors. The need for autonomy and independence, although impor-tant developmentally,[23] can be a barrier for TAY to seek assistance from previous sup-port systems such as parents, extended family, or even close friends who they have left behind as part of their childhood. Many of these issues, although relevant at various stages in the lifespan, become even more intense for TAY because of body and brain changes, phase-of-life changes, and developmental needs that are rapidly altering. Combined with fewer supports than they had in high school, these issues may feel overwhelming to TAY.[23] Although specific prevalence rates of suicide secondary to gender dysphoria (GD) in TAY are not available, there is evidence that adults with GD are much more likely to complete suicide compared with adults without GD.[26,27] The literature cites suicidal thoughts in as many as 41%, with attempts at about 15% for youth with GD. LGBTQ (Lesbian, Gay, Bisexual, Transgender, Queer or Ques-tioning) youth have higher rates of suicidal ideations and suicide attempts.[28] The 2009 Youth Risk Behavior Surveillance[29] found that the rates of hopelessness and sadness in students self-identifying as heterosexual was 19.3% to 29% (suicidal thoughts, 9.9% to 13.2%; suicide attempts, 3.8%–9.6%). In youth identifying as lesbian and gay these percentages increased to 28.8% to 52.8% (suicidal thoughts, 18.8% to 43.4%; suicide attempts, 15.1%–34.3%) and in those identifying as bisexual rate were as high as 47.2% to 62.9%. One study reported suicide attempt rates in lesbian, gay, and bisexual (LGB) adolescents to be especially high among male African Amer-icans.[30] Among adults, suicide attempt rates have been reported to be highest among gay/bisexual men of lower socioeconomic status[31] and among LGB Latino men.[32] In a national probability study of Latino and Asian-American adults,[33] gay and bisexual men were more likely than heterosexual men to report a recent suicide attempt. Although still an area that is just beginning to be researched, these phenomena of increased suicidal ideations and attempts in LGBTQ youth seem to be related to discrimination and family rejection rather than to choice of sexual preference. The most accepted hypothesis is that the stressors of social ostracism secondary to bullying/being teased, poor peer relationships, feelings of isolation and burgeoning dysphoria[34–36] seem to put these individuals at higher risk for depression and anxiety, which then predispose them to feel suicidal and to attempt suicide. Factors that reduce risk in this situation are strong social supports and effective coping strategies.

The research data support the differing rates of suicide in individuals from different ethnicities: Native American and Alaskan men are at the highest risk for completed suicide in the United States, whereas women from the same background are at the highest risk for suicide attempts. Suicidal thoughts increase in Latino youth[37] as part of acculturative stress when they immigrate; the issue of shame and loss of face when they disappoint societal or parental expectations is common in suicidal east Asian youth.[38] Perception in African Americans that they are not at risk for suicide behavior may lead to underreporting or not seeking help for suicidal behavior in this population.[39] If a behavior is recognized as problematic but shaming, cultural factors may negatively affect a decision to seek help.[40] American Indian adolescents are less likely to seek assistance because of the stigma and embarrassment associated with seeking help when suicidal.[41] In addition, culture may influence the decision about the type of services or help to seek.[40] Recently immigrated Latino and Asian families may decide to solve problems within the family because of a lack familiarity with the health care system. Awareness of the interface of culture for the TAY and their capacity to seek help when needed is essential as systems build assessment and intervention services to cater to the needs of an increasingly diverse population of youth.

The presence of mental disorder, whether it persists beyond adolescence or first presents in young adulthood, is a powerful influence on suicidality. Mental disorder in TAY seems to be growing in both rate and severity, whereas individuals in this age range using mental health treatment services remains low.[42,43] Nearly one-half of TAY meet criteria for a Diagnostic and Statistical Manual of Mental Disorders, Fourth Edition[15] disorder. In the college population, the most common disorders were alcohol use disorders and personality disorder. For non–college students, the most common disorders were personality disorders and nicotine dependence. The prevalence of mood and anxiety disorders were similar (around 11% and 12%, respectively), but higher than in most other age ranges. In this age group, regardless of student status, risk factors for having a psychiatric disorder include:

- Being male
- Higher number of stressful life events in the last 12 months
- Loss of steady relationships
- Being widowed/divorced/separated
- Being US born
- Living in a rural setting
- Living away from parents

Being black, Asian, or Hispanic, being married or cohabitating, and being in overall good health were protective for psychiatric disorders.[15]

Note that TAY are experiencing easier access to substances, and can legally drink alcohol, or more easily obtain it. Binge drinking, which has been identified as a particular problem among college students, is strongly associated with suicidal thoughts and attempts, even in the absence of depression.[44]

Developmental Issues and Suicide in Transitional Age Youth

In addition to the developmental challenges that may precipitate suicidal behavior, for many transition aged youth, suicidal ideation that develops at an earlier age is a risk factor for poor outcomes. The prior experience of suicidal gestures may have habituated them to suicidal behaviors, putting them at increased risk of attempted or completed suicide as they move into adulthood.[45] After the age of 17 to 18 years, most suicide attempts are repeat attempts.[46] This literature suggests that the intent to die becomes more serious with number of attempts and increasing age, and that the lethality of attempts increases with age. As the number of attempts increases, the time between attempts decreases. Attempts in this high-risk profile of repeat attempters were not related to the amount of precipitating life stress, but to historical factors such as sexual abuse history and mental disorder.

Whether in relation to suicidal ideation, plans, or attempts, genetic factors have a strong influence on suicidal behaviors.[47] This influence seems to change through the lifespan. During childhood and adolescence, environmental factors, which include aspects of family, school, and neighborhood, have a stronger impact on suicidal behaviors.[48] These environmental risk factors include peer relationships and influences, poor parent-child interactions, parental mental disorder, abuse, and neglect.[49] However, as with other psychiatric problems, as youth move into young adulthood, these factors exert less influence, and long-term genetic influence becomes much more predominant.[50] Suicidal ideation in both adolescents and young adults has strong genetic and environmental links to depression and conduct disorder symptoms, suggesting the need for prevention and intervention strategies that address the role of both internalizing and externalizing symptoms in TAY at risk for suicide attempts.[48]

Challenges and Strengths of Suicidal Transitional Age Youth

Treatment rates for mental disorders and suicidal behaviors are disturbingly low in TAY. Even with the focus on reduction of suicide on college campuses, almost 80% of students who die by suicide did not receive counseling services.[51] For TAY with suicidal ideation, only 30% received mental health treatment in the past year, regardless of student status. Even in those who had ideation, a plan, and a previous attempt, less than 50% received mental health services in the past year.[17]

Rates for seeking treatment are lowest for substance abuse and highest for mood disorders; however, more than half of TAY with depression, and more than 80% with anxiety, did not seek treatment,[15] highlighting serious unmet mental health needs during a critical developmental period. These findings of high rates of mental disorder and low rates of service use are consistent in both college-attending individuals and their nonstudent peers. Although the type of psychiatric disorder may vary according to college status, overall risk for having a disorder does not.[15] What did vary was insurance coverage; although college students are often seen as privileged, they are less likely than their peers to have public insurance, and more likely to be uninsured. Reasons for not receiving mental health treatment, as self-reported by young adults 18 to 25 years old, were: inability to afford treatment, feeling like they could handle mental health problems on their own, not knowing where to go for treatment, and fear of being committed to treatment.[17]

Not all TAY with histories of serious suicidality as children go on to make suicide attempts. Although they may remain at risk for ideation, many resolve the issues that triggered the suicidality. Following hospitalization in adolescence, and tracked into adulthood, trajectories for ongoing suicidality varied, with some individuals experiencing increased risk (only 11%), some with a gradually decreasing risk from adolescence into adulthood (12%), some with more markedly decreasing risk (33%), and the rest remaining at fairly low risk following hospitalization (44%). Those in the 3 higher-risk categories had higher levels of trait anxiety. The highest risk class had more major depression and anxiety disorders, more likelihood of sexual abuse, and more hopelessness. Increased impulsivity and aggression in adulthood were also risk factors. Suicide risk was related to overall social adjustment difficulties and functional impairment of adult role performance, and impaired behavior toward others.[52] Although spanning a larger age range (10–55 years), the results of a recent Danish study indicate that individuals who present to an emergency room (ER) with a suicide attempt are at a high risk for repeat suicide attempt and suicide death, particularly within the first week of the index attempt,[53] suggesting major implications for treatment planning for suicidal patients discharged from an ER.

Suicide attempts in young people are prognostic of ongoing difficulties across domains through adulthood. Even after controlling for mental health conditions at the time of attempts, youth with attempts before the age of 24 years had ongoing difficulties with depression, substance dependence, and subsequent suicide attempts, higher rates of metabolic syndrome and other physical health problems, more violent behaviors, including violent crimes and intimate partner abuse, and were more likely to receive unemployment and welfare benefits.[54]

BEST PRACTICES IN THE ASSESSMENT OF SUICIDE RISK AND INTERVENTIONS IN THIS AGE GROUP

Consistent with most health care emergencies and their management in United States health systems, suicide and related behaviors are identified and treated once the crisis is set in motion within ERs and hospital clinics, the purpose being to reduce the secondary morbidity arising from the underlying causes identified earlier in this article and prevent death by suicide and/or future attempts.[55] This tertiary mode of assessment and intervention after the event occurs carries an economic and emotional cost.[56] Individuals who present to an ER with a suicide attempt are at an increased risk of a more serious repeat suicide attempt and even completed suicide.[53] Direct questions regarding suicide through tools such as the Patient Health Questionnaire can strongly and consistently predict suicide attempts/death by suicide up to 18 months.[57] This new knowledge can help build tertiary prevention models for suicide and can have a significant public health impact.

Because there is no single cause of suicide, it is difficult to build a prevention program that is effective or even lends itself to scientific study easily. As discussed earlier, suicidal behavior is complex and precipitated by a set of highly complex interactions involving genetics, environment, prevailing culture, temperament, life events, and co-morbid mental disorder. Prevention efforts therefore also need to be multilayered and complex. A major stressor for TAY is moving from one environment of living (ie, home) to IHEs, employment, or independent living. Public health prevention models are built[58] (1) to prevent people from entering a phase of risk (primary prevention); (2) if they are in the phase of risk, to enhance protective factors and reduce risk factors to prevent the illness (secondary prevention); and (3) once the event/illness has occurred to reduce the morbidity that arises from the disorder (tertiary prevention). Universal prevention strategies are predominantly under the classic primary prevention, selective prevention strategies under secondary prevention, and various indicated prevention strategies may be considered secondary or tertiary prevention.[59] Outcome studies that assess the impact of the interventions become vital because a public health prevention approach is costly and difficult to implement in the short term. However, it is vital for long-term health outcomes. Current tracking methods have reporting lags[60] and also missing information from large epidemiologic surveys.[61]

Primary Prevention Programs in Youth Suicide

Efforts to build protective factors within a youth start long before TAY move into this stage of life.[62] Keeping with the definitions of primary prevention, the development of protective factors relates to broad resilience-building programs that show promise or are backed by evidence and begin at elementary school age and go through high school. Targeting children before they enter the period of risk is the central premise of primary prevention. Although not targeting suicide per se, based on the discussion earlier the risk factors that predispose to self-harming behaviors include poor self-esteem, poor problem-solving skills, falling victim to bullying, being depressed, and aggression. Protective factors are social support, positive cognitive style, and positive school environment that builds resilience and reduces self-harm behaviors.[58] Prevention programs designed to prevent depression and anxiety, a more tangible construct on a universal level (ie, all students in school settings), seem to have an effect on the improvement of social and coping skills, reduction or modification of harmful thoughts and the use of positive problem-solving skills, enhancing positive cognitions, and overall improving school environment. These programs have been implemented as early as grade 3 and go up to grade 12. Examples of evidence-based programs with the support of randomized controlled studies include (1) beyondblue,[63] which teaches problem solving, adaptive cognitive styles, and social and coping skills and is implemented in school toward the end of eighth grade and covers 10 sessions; (2) Problem Solving for Life, which works on cognitive restructuring and problem-solving skills training over 8 sessions, and showed continued differences in problem-solving abilities in high-risk intervention versus control groups at risk for suicide[64]; and (3) The Good Behavior Game, developed in 1960 by Barrish and colleagues,[65] which has been used as early as the first grade and has been shown in randomized trials to inoculate against suicidal ideations.[66]

The development of primary prevention efforts at the college level and in the work environment is affected by the freedom of TAY as well as the stigma in discussing adjustment and mental health topics.[67,68] A systems of care approach has been outlined for TAY with preexisting mental illness who are transitioning from school to adulthood. The essential elements of the plan are that it should be intentional and involve key players in the young person's life who can provide the best input for a transition plan that considers developmental and treatment needs as early as the sophomore year of high school and minimizes risks and enhances the individual's natural abilities.

As critical incidents involving high-risk behaviors, accidents, and so forth occur on college campuses and also in communities involving TAY, there is growing awareness of the need for mental wellness programs in these settings. College and business leaders have a growing awareness of the importance of examining their values in viewing the work and education environments as part of a community and the realization that there is an interconnectedness between mental wellness, performance, and the quality of contributions of individuals to that community.[60,69,70] From the lens of collective wellness, a culture of inclusion, awareness of differences, and openness to differences in health status, both physical and mental, must guide the policies that support mental wellness, of which suicide prevention is a component.

The Suicide Prevention Resource Council (SPRC) offers safe messaging guidelines,[71] emphasizing that suicide can be prevented. SPRC stresses that most of those who die by suicide have a treatable psychiatric illness and/or substance abuse disorder, lists key warning signs and protective factors for suicide, and provides information on how to access treatment and where to find immediate assistance. Using nonclinical TAY to educate others about suicide leads to stigma reduction.[14] Trained student peers play an important role in promoting suicide prevention on college campuses. Groups such as Active Minds, peer educators, and student mental health advisory boards deliver paraprofessional services such as stress management workshops and biofeedback, outreach programs such as depression awareness days and wellness fairs, and marketing of educational materials. Peers are often more successful in intervening with those in distress than mental health professionals[14,72,73] and can recognize distress more adeptly and intervene.[74] However, prevention efforts are only as good as an informed persons' willingness to intervene when a peer is suicidal.[75] Research indicates that an understanding of students' attitudes[76] and their perceived behavioral control regarding their own capacities to perform the action determine whether they will intervene with a distressed peer.[75] Thus education of non-affected peers (ie, other students, employees, or employers) about suicide and warning signs becomes a form of gatekeeper training (discussed later).

Limiting means to committing suicide is considered one of the most effective primary prevention tools against suicide[77,78] and includes preventing access to firearms, detoxifying domestic fuels, using less lethal/toxic antidepressants, and building barriers in places that can be used to jump from.

With these factors in mind, the culture of any organization to which a TAY graduates determines mental wellness. This culture can be pivotal as a primary prevention tool. A culture/environment that supports the mental well-being of its community members, albeit not connected directly to suicide prevention, is essential to positive campus and workplace environments. These efforts should be guided by culturally competent, evidence-based, developmentally informed programming.[68] Examples of these mental wellness–promoting programs are listed in **Box 1**.

Secondary Prevention for Transitional Age Youth at Risk for Suicide

Secondary prevention strategies focus on identifying TAY at risk for suicide and referring them for assessment and treatment in order to prevent the behavior. The foundation of secondary prevention of suicide is to develop the knowledge, attitudes, and skills of those who come in contact with TAY around suicide and suicidal behaviors, to help them to know what to do once risk is identified, and to make appropriate referrals. Data from the National Surveys on Drug Use and Health 2013 underscore high rates for SIB in both college students and non–college-going peers.[17] The use of mental health treatment and self-perceived unmet treatment needs was examined in this population and there was a disturbing trend in that only 34.1% of young adults, in college or not in college, and high school students with SIB received mental health treatment, despite the availability of funding of suicide prevention programs for the 10-year-old to 24-year-old age group through the Garret Lee Smith Memorial Act[79] that is available to communities, colleges, and special populations and that has shown clear reduction in suicide rates.[79] The data are concerning in that more than 70% of TAY at

---

Box 1
Possible mental wellness programs on campus and in the workplace

- Formal curricula/programs in the workplace that foster open discussion of mental wellness, mental illness, and the teaching of positive psychology in interactive venues such as through blog posts and formal lectures[91]

- Venues to foster social connectedness (protective factor) on campus or in places of employment (JED Foundation)

- Acknowledgment of the importance of relationships as contributing to the well-being of TAY[23]

- Discussion and awareness of substance abuse as a risk factor for depression and suicide[92]

- Resources to teach skills to cope with academic pressures

- Introduction of self-efficacy interventions like yoga and guided meditation[93] in the work environment and college residence halls to prevent stress

- Strengthening protective factors by promoting positive adjustment of TAY to the workplace and college

risk for suicide, based on previous SIB, did not perceive a need for treatment and, of those who did accept need for treatment, 30% reported that they could handle the problem without treatment. The investigators tentatively suggested that TAY have a poor understanding of the effectiveness of mental health treatment and lack understanding of the predictive nature of suicidal behavior for future problems; this contributes to poor use of services. The importance of this study is that any secondary prevention programs, including those mentioned later, should take into account not only low treatment access but the lack of knowledge in TAY about the effectiveness of mental health treatment. The importance of (1) promoting public awareness about SIB in college students, non–college students, and high school students; (2) incorporating awareness of risk and protective factors; and (3) exposure to the effectiveness of mental health treatments could all be underscored in existing prevention programs for TAY. Continuity of care for youth who present to emergency departments should also be prioritized. Although not exhaustive, a few best-practice secondary prevention programs are listed in **Table 1**.

Tertiary Intervention and Prevention for Transitional Age Youth

If there is a crisis such as suicidal threats, plans, and behavior, the immediate focus is on crisis stabilization and a safety plan. As discussed earlier, a suicide attempt is a strong predictor of a repeat and more serious suicide attempt and even completed suicide. ER physicians must become adept at safety planning and fast tracking the individual to follow up care and ensure compliance with follow-up. Within the communities in which TAY live or work there should be formal or informal mechanisms to pick up warning signs, recognize a crisis, and provide a structured response to the suicidal/distressed TAY, including access to ER and mental health providers.

However, 80% of college students who die by suicide are not known to campus mental health professionals.[84] Limiting the access of suicidal TAY to lethal means such as firearms and high-toxicity prescription medications can be helpful to reduce further morbidity from suicidal ideations. In addition to institutional structures for oversight and follow-up, parents and family members play a crucial role in suicide prevention and support for the suicidal TAY. Using both qualitative and quantitative approaches, mtvU conducted a college mental health study [85]. Almost two-thirds (63%) of students turn to family in times of emotional distress, which is second only

Table 1 Best practice secondary prevention programs		
Program	**Description**	**Resource**
Interactive Screening Program, American Foundation for Suicide Prevention[80]	Interactive Web-based outreach to increase help-seeking	https://afsp.org/our-work/interactive-screening-program/
Gatekeeper Training Programs[79,81,82]	Psychoeducation to increase knowledge, encouragement of help seeking, and effective intervention skills	http://www.sprc.org/resources-programs/qpr-gatekeeper-training-suicide-prevention
Sources of Strength[83]	Use of student opinion leaders to increase help seeking	http://www.sprc.org/resources-programs/sources-strength

to friends (69%). Although not stratified by ethnicity, this study underscores the importance of parent and family outreach programs that provide information for parents of students with existing mental health conditions on entering college for adjustment to college life, how to notice distress in a relative, and campus mental health resources. The Health Insurance Portability and Accountability Act and Family Educational Rights and Privacy Act, which prevent the sharing of information with parents about their child after age 18 years, do not apply when there is an imminent safety risk, which suicide poses.[86] Presence of parents allows supervision, compliance with follow-up, and a support for the young person that mitigates imminent risk for self-harm in a period of grave vulnerability.

Treatment of the underlying cause of the suicide becomes paramount. Psychotherapy, specifically cognitive behavior therapy (CBT) and dialectical behavior therapy (DBT), has shown good results in depressed and suicidal individuals in many randomized controlled trials[87] even if only for short periods.[88] In practical terms, transitioning youth may be physically separated but not psychologically delinked from their distressed parents and this must be a clinical consideration for the intervention to be effective. College counseling centers should offer standard CBT, DBT, and DBT with skills training, which seems to reduce morbidity from suicidal behavior.[89]

Pharmacologic interventions include selective serotonin reuptake inhibitors, which are the standard treatment to address moderate to severe underlying depression and anxiety in suicidal TAY. However, lithium is a useful agent for overall mood stabilization and has shown effectiveness in reducing and preventing suicidal thoughts.[90] Severe recalcitrant depression may require referral for electroconvulsive therapy and transcranial magnetic brain stimulation. Access to such treatments for TAY are based on not only the adequacy of the university counseling center or the primary care physician for rapid intervention but also rapid access to mental health specialists. Suicide being a high-crisis behavior, memoranda of understanding should exist for rapid consultation and treatment between the IHE or PCP/pediatrician (for non–college-attending TAY or high school students) and a mental health specialist.

SUMMARY

Suicidal ideations and risk of death by suicide in TAY are high. Developmental transitions, rapid sculpting of the brain, cultural challenges, psychological tasks of forming identity, and individual differences in response to life events are some of the reasons for the emotional turmoil that make this age group particularly vulnerable to risk-taking and self-harm behavior. Growing interest in this age group and research initiatives are generating more information about risk and protective factors relating to suicide. Suicide is an eminently preventable event in this age group. A public health approach is an effective framework to systematically surveil the phenomena, reduce risk, enhance protective factors, and develop the capability for adequate access to effective and evidence-based treatments in the venues where TAY live and work.

RESOURCES

JED Foundation (https://jedfoundation.org/)
American Foundation for Suicide Prevention (https://afsp.org/)
Active Minds (http://www.activeminds.org)
National Alliance for Mental Illness (NAMI) On Campus (http://www.nami.org/#)
http://www.halfofus.com (MTV and JED Foundation)
Ulifeline (http://ulifeline.com) (JED Foundation)
Suicide Prevention Resource Center (http://www.sprc.org)

REFERENCES

1. Dahl RE. Adolescent brain development: a period of vulnerabilities and opportunities. Keynote address. Ann N Y Acad Sci 2004;1021(1):1–22.
2. Evans DL, Seligman ME. Introduction. Treating and preventing adolescent mental health disorders: what we know and what we do not know. In: Evans D, Foa EB, Gur RE, et al, editors. Commission chairs of the Anenberg Foundation Trust. New York: Oxford University Press; 2005. p. XXiX.
3. Pickles A, Pickering K, Simonoff E, et al. Genetic clocks and soft events: a twin model for pubertal development and other recalled sequences of developmental milestones, transitions, or ages at onset. Behav Genet 1998;28(4):243–53.
4. Spear L. The adolescent brain and age-related behavioral manifestations. Neurosci Biobehav Rev 2000;24(4):417–63.
5. Rakic P, Bourgeois J-P, Goldman-Rakic PS. Synaptic development of the cerebral cortex: implications for learning, memory, and mental illness. Prog Brain Res 1994;102:227–43.
6. Luna B, Garver KE, Urban TA, et al. Maturation of cognitive processes from late childhood to adulthood. Child Dev 2004;75(5):1357–72.
7. Casey B, Giedd JN, Thomas KM. Structural and functional brain development and its relation to cognitive development. Biol Psychol 2000;54(1–3):241–57.
8. Giedd JN, Blumenthal J, Jeffries NO, et al. Brain development during childhood and adolescence: a longitudinal MRI study. Nat Neurosci 1999;2:861–3.
9. Giedd JN. Structural magnetic resonance imaging of the adolescent brain. Ann N Y Acad Sci 2004;1021(1):77–85.
10. Dorn LD, Hitt SF, Rotenstein D. Biopsychological and cognitive differences in children with premature vs on-time adrenarche. Arch Pediatr Adolesc Med 1999; 153(2):137–46.
11. Nock MK, Green JG, Hwang I, et al. Prevalence, correlates, and treatment of lifetime suicidal behavior among adolescents. JAMA Psychiatry 2013;70(3):300–10.
12. Crosby AE, Ortega L, Melanson C. Self- directed violence surveillance: uniform definitions and recommended data elements, version 1.0. Atlanta (GA): Centers for Disease Control and Prevention; National Center for Injury Prevention and Control; 2011.
13. Substance Abuse and Mental Health Services Administration. Results from the 2013 national survey on drug use and health: mental health findings, NSDUH series H-49, HHS publication no. (SMA) 14-4887. Rockville (MD): Substance Abuse and Mental Health Services; 2014. Available at: http://www.samhsa.gov/data/sites/default/files/NSDUHmhfr2013/NSDUHmhfr2013.pdf.
14. Drum D, Brownson C, Denmark A, et al. New data on the nature of suicidal crises in college students: shifting the paradigm. Prof Psychol Res Pr 2009;40:213–22.
15. Blanco C, Okuda M, Wright C, et al. Mental health of college students and their non-college-attending peers: results from the national epidemiologic study on alcohol and related conditions. Arch Gen Psychiatry 2008;65(12):1429–37.
16. Schwartz A. College student suicide in the United States: 1990-1991 through 2003-2004. J Am Coll Health 2006;54:341–52.
17. Han B, Compton W, Eisenberg D, et al. Prevalence and mental health treatment of suicidal ideation and behavior among college students aged 18-25 years and their non-college-attending peers in the United States. J Clin Psychiatry 2016; 77(6):815–24.
18. Shaffer D, Craft L. Methods of adolescent suicide prevention. J Clin Psychiatry 1999;60:70–4.

19. Serafini G, Muzio C, Piccinini G, et al. Life adversities and suicidal behavior in young individuals: a systematic review. Eur Child Adolesc Psychiatry 2015; 24(12):1423–46.
20. Goldston D, Molock S, Whitbeck L, et al. Cultural considerations in adolescent suicide prevention and psychosocial treatment. Am Psychol 2008;63(1):14–31.
21. Miller M, Barber C, White RA, et al. Firearms and suicide in the United States: is risk independent of underlying suicidal behavior? Am J Epidemiol 2013;178(6): 946–55.
22. Haw C, Hawton K, Niedzwiedz C, et al. Suicide clusters: a review of risk factors and mechanisms. Suicide Life Threat Behav 2013;43(1):97–108.
23. Cleary M, Walter G, Jackson D. "Not always smooth sailing": mental health issues associated with the transition from high school to college. Issues Ment Health Nurs 2011;32:250–4.
24. Winsler A, Deutsch A, Vorona RD, et al. Sleepless in Fairfax: the difference one more hour of sleep can make for teen hopelessness, suicidal ideation, and substance use. J Youth Adolesc 2015;44(2):362–78.
25. Price M, Hides L, Cockshaw W, et al. Young love: romantic concerns and associated mental health issues among adolescent help-seekers. Behav Sci (Basel) 2016;6(2) [pii:E9].
26. Aitken M, Vanderlaan DP, Wasserman L, et al. Self-harm and suicidality in children referred for gender dysphoria. J Am Acad Child Adolesc Psychiatry 2016; 55(6):513–20.
27. Asscheman H, Giltay EJ, Megens JA, et al. A long-term follow-up study of mortality in transsexuals receiving treatment with cross-sex hormones. Eur J Endocrinol 2011;164:635–42.
28. Haas AP, Eliason M, Mays VM, et al. Suicide and suicide risk in lesbian, gay, bisexual, and transgender populations: review and recommendations. J Homosex 2011;58(1):10–51.
29. Centers for Disease Control and Prevention. Youth risk behavior surveillance summaries. MMWR Surveill Summ 2010;59(5):1–142.
30. Remafedi G. Suicidality in a venue-based sample of young men who have sex with men. J Adolesc Health 2002;31(4):305–10.
31. Paul JP, Cantania J, Pollack L, et al. Suicide attempts among gay and bisexual men: lifetime prevalence and antecedents. Am J Public Health 2002;92(8): 1338–45.
32. Meyer IH, Dietrich J, Schwartz S. Lifetime prevalence of mental disorders and suicide attempts in diverse lesbian, gay, and bisexual populations. Res Pract 2007; 97(11):9–11.
33. Cochran SD, Mays VM, Alegria M, et al. Mental health and substance use disorders in Latino and Asian-American lesbian, gay and bisexual adults. J Consult Clin Psychol 2007;75(5):785–94.
34. Zucker KJ, Wood H, VanderLaan DP. Models of psychopathology in children and adolescents with gender dysphoria. In: Kreukels BPC, Steensma TD, de Vries ALC, editors. Gender dysphoria and disorders of sex development: progress in care and knowledge. New York: Springer; 2014. p. 171–92.
35. Zucker KJ. Gender identity disorder in girls. In: Bell DJ, Foster SL, Mash EJ, editors. Handbook of behavioral and emotional problems in girls. New York: Kluwer Academic/Plenum Publishers; 2005. p. 285–319.
36. Zucker KJ. Psychosocial and erotic development in cross-gender identified children. Can J Psychiatry 1990;35:487–95.

37. Hovey J, King C. Acculturative stress, depression, and suicidal ideation among immigrant and second-generation Latino adolescents. J Am Acad Child Adolesc Psychiatry 1996;35:1183–92.

38. Zane N, Mak W. Major approaches to the measurement of acculturation among ethnic minority populations: a content analysis and an alternative empirical strategy. In: Chun K, Organista P, Marin G, editors. Acculturation: advances in theory, measurement, and applied research. Washington, DC: American Psychological Association; 2003. p. 39–60.

39. Morrison L, Downey D. Racial differences in self-disclosure of suicidal ideation and reasons for living: implications for training. Cultur Divers Ethnic Minor Psychol 2000;6:374–86.

40. Cauce AM, Domenech-Rodriguez M, Paradise M, et al. Cultural contextual influences in minority mental health help seeking: a focus on ethnic minority youth. J Consult Clin Psychol 2002;70:44–55.

41. Freedenthal S, Stiffman A. "They might think I was crazy": young American Indians' reasons for not seeking help when suicidal. J Adolesc Res 2007;22:58–77.

42. Hunt J, Eisenberg D. Mental health problems and help-seeking behavior among college students. J Adolesc Health 2010;46:3–10.

43. Copeland WE, Shanahan L, Davis M, et al. Increase in untreated cases of psychiatric disorders during the transition to adulthood. Psychiat Serv 2015;66:4.

44. Glasheen C, Pemberton M, Lipari R, et al. Binge drinking and the risk of suicidal thoughts, plans, and attempts. Addict Behav 2015;43:42–9.

45. Joiner T, Conwell Y, Fitzpatrick K, et al. Four studies on how past and current suicidality related even when "everything but the kitchen sink" is covariated. J Abnorm Psychol 2005;114:291–303.

46. Goldston D, Daniel S, Erkanli A, et al. Suicide attempts in a longitudinal sample of adolescents followed through adulthood: evidence of escalation. J Consult Clin Psychol 2015;83(2):253–64.

47. Statham D, Heath A, Madden P, et al. Suicidal behavior: an epidemiological and genetic study. Psychol Med 1998;28:839–55.

48. Linker J, Gillespie N, Maes H, et al. Suicidal ideation, depression, and conduct disorder in a sample of adolescent and young adult twins. J Suicide Life threat 2012;42:426–36.

49. Hawton K, Fortune S. Suicidal behavior and deliberate self-harm. In: Rutter M, Bishop D, Pine D, et al, editors. Rutter's child and adolescent psychiatry. Oxford (United Kingdom): Blackwell Publishing Limited; 2008. p. 648–69.

50. Eaves J, Hatemi P, Heath A, et al. Modeling the biological and cultural inheritance of social and political behavior in twins and families. In: Hatemi PK, McDermott R, editors. Man is by nature a political animal. Chicago: University of Chicago Press; 2010. p. 114–75.

51. Kisch J, Leino E, Silverman M. Aspects of suicidal behavior, depression and treatment in college students: results from the spring 2000 National College Health Assessment Survey. Suicide Life-Threat 2005;35:3–13.

52. Goldston D, Erkanli A, Daniel S, et al. Developmental trajectories of suicidal thoughts and behaviors from adolescence through adulthood. J Am Acad Child Psychiatry 2016;55:400–7.

53. Fedyszyn IE, Erlangsen A, Hjorthøj C, et al. Individuals with a first emergency department contact for attempted suicide. J Clin Psychiatry 2016;77(6):832–40.

54. Goldman-Mellor S, Caspi A, Harrington H, et al. Suicide attempt in young people: a signal for long-term health care and social needs. J Amer Med Assoc 2014; 71(2):119–27.

55. Betz M, Wintersteen M, Boudreaux E, et al. Reducing suicide risk: challenges and opportunities in the emergency department. Ann Emerg Med 2016;68:758–65.

56. Shepherd DS, Gurewich D, Lwin AK, et al. Suicide and suicidal attempts in the United States: costs and policy implications. Suicide and life threatening behavior. Wiley Periodicals 2016;46(3):1–11.

57. Simon GE, Coleman KJ, Rossom RC, et al. Risk of suicide attempt and suicide death following completion of the patient health questionnaire depression module in community practice. J Clin Psychiatry 2016;77(2):221–7.

58. Mrazek PJ, Haggerty RJ. Reducing risks for mental disorders: frontiers for preventive intervention research. Washington, DC: National Academy Press; 1994.

59. U.S. Department of Health and Human Services. Mental health: a report of the Surgeon General. Rockville, MD: U.S. Department of Health and Human Services, Substance Abuse and Mental Health Services Administration, Center for Mental Health Services, National Institutes of Health, National Institute of Mental Health; 1999.

60. Andrews G, Issakidis C, Sanderson K, et al. Utilizing survey data to inform public policy: comparison of the cost-effectiveness of treatment of ten mental disorders. Br J Psychiatry 2004;184:526–33.

61. Data and Surveillance Task Force of the National Action Alliance for Suicide Prevention. Improving national data systems for surveillance of suicide-related events. Am J Prev Med 2014;47:S122–9.

62. Gould M, Greenberg T, Velting D, et al. Youth suicide risk and preventive interventions: a review of the past 10 years. J Am Acad Child Adolesc Psychiatry 2003; 42(4):386–405.

63. Sawyer MG, Harchak TF, Spence SH, et al. School-based prevention of depression: a 2 year follow-up of a randomized controlled trial of the beyondblue schools research initiative. J Adolesc Health 2010;47(3):297–304.

64. Spence SH, Sheffield JK, Donovan CL. Preventing adolescent depression: an evaluation of the Problem Solving for Life program. J Consult Clin Psychol 2003;71(1):3–13.

65. Barrish HH, Saunders M, Wolfe MD. Good behavior game: effects of individual contingencies for group consequences and disruptive behavior in a classroom. J Appl Behav Anal 1969;2:119–24.

66. Wilcox HC, Kellam SG, Brown CH, et al. The impact of two universal randomized first- and second-grade classroom interventions on young adult suicide ideation and attempts. Drug Alcohol Depend 2008;95:S60–73.

67. Bathje GJ, Pryor JB. The relationships of public self-stigma to seeking mental health services. J Ment Health Couns 2011;33(2):161–76.

68. Martel AL, Sood AB. National models for college student mental health. In: Sood AB, Cohen R, editors. The Virginia Tech Massacre. Strategies and challenges for improving mental health in the college campus and beyond. New York: Oxford University Press; 2015. p. 93–126.

69. Kakuma R, Minas H, van Ginneken N, et al. Human resources for mental health care: current situation and strategies for action. Lancet 2011;378(9803):1654–63.

70. Mojtabai R, Olfson M, Sampson NA, et al. Barriers to mental health treatment: results from the National Comorbidity Survey Replication (NCS-R). Psychol Med 2011;41(8):1751–61.

71. U.S. Department of Health and Human Services (HHS) Office of the Surgeon General and National Action Alliance for Suicide Prevention. 2012 National strategy for suicide prevention: goals and objectives for action. Washington, DC: HHS; 2012.

72. Fortune S, Sinclair J, Hawton K. Help-seeking before and after episodes of self-harm: a descriptive study in school pupils in England. BMC Public Health 2008;8: 369–82.

73. Freedenthal S, Stiffman A. Suicidal behavior in urban American Indian adolescents: a comparison with reservation youth in a southwestern state. Suicide Life Threat Behav 2004;34:160–71.

74. Owens C, Owen G, Lambert H, et al. Public involvement in suicide prevention: understanding and strengthening lay responses to distress. BMC Public Health 2009;9:308–18.

75. Aldrich RS. Using the theory of planned behavior to predict college students' intention to intervene with a suicidal individual. Crisis 2015;36(5):332–7.

76. Barksdale CL, Molock SD. Perceived norms and mental help seeking among African American college students. J Behav Health Serv Res 2008;36(3):285–99.

77. Florentine JB, Crane C. Suicide prevention by limiting access to methods: a review of theory and practice. Soc Sci Med 2010;70:1626–32.

78. Mann JJ, Apter A, Bertolote J, et al. Suicide prevention strategies: a systematic review. JAMA 2005;294:2064–74.

79. Walrath C, Garraza LG, Reid H, et al. Impact of the Garrett Lee Smith youth suicide prevention program on suicide mortality. Am J Public Health 2015;105(5):986–93.

80. Haas A, Koestner B, Rosenberg J, et al. An interactive web-based method of outreach to college students at risk for suicide. J Am Coll Health 2008;57(1):15–22.

81. Wyman PA, Brown CH, Inman J, et al. Randomized trial of a gatekeeper program for suicide prevention: 1-year impact on secondary school staff. J Consult Clin Psychol 2008;76(1):104–15.

82. Sareen J, Isaak C, Bolton SL, et al. Gatekeeper training for suicide prevention in first nations community members: a randomized controlled trial. Depress Anxiety 2013;30:1021–9.

83. LoMurray M. Sources of strength facilitators guide: suicide prevention peer gatekeeper training. Bismarck (ND): The North Dakota Suicide Prevention Project; 2005.

84. Gallagher, RP. National survey of counseling center directors. 2009. Available at: http://www.iacsinc.org/2009%20 National%20Survey.pdf. Accessed March 17, 2010.

85. mtvU. Available at: http://cdn.halfofus.com/wp-content/uploads/2013/10/2006-mtvU-College-Mental-Health-Study-Executive-Summary-Final.pdf. Accessed January 5, 2013.

86. Sood AB, Martel A. Failures in the campus mental health system 2015. In: Sood AB, Cohen R, editors. The Virginia Tech Massacre. Strategies and challenges for improving mental health in the college campus and beyond. New York: Oxford University Press; 2015. p. 65–92.

87. Brown GK, Jager-Hyman S. Evidence-based psychotherapies for suicide prevention: future directions. Am J Prev Med 2014;47:S186–94.

88. Slee N, Garnefski N, van der Leeden R, et al. Cognitive-behavioural intervention for self-harm: randomised controlled trial. Br J Psychiatry 2008;192:202–11.

89. Linehan MM, Korslund KE, Harned MS, et al. Dialectical behavior therapy for high suicide risk in individuals with borderline personality disorder: a randomized clinical trial and component analysis. JAMA Psychiatry 2015;72:475–82.

90. Jacobs DG, Baldessarini RJ, Conwell Y, et al. Practice guideline for the assessment and treatment of patients with suicidal behaviors. Arlington (VA): American Psychiatric Association; 2010.

91. Shatkin J. Transition to college: separation and change for parents and students. New York: NYU Child Study Center; 2010.

92. Pedrelli P, Nyer M, Yeung A, et al. College students: mental health problems and treatment considerations. Acad Psychiatry 2015;39(5):503–11.
93. Barnhofer T, Duggan D, Crane C, et al. Effects of meditation on frontal a-asymmetry in previously suicidal individuals. Neuroreport 2007;18:709–12.

Challenges and Gaps in Understanding Substance Use Problems in Transitional Age Youth

Oscar G. Bukstein, MD, MPH

KEYWORDS

- Transitional age youth • Substance use disorder • Substance abuse • Screening
- Treatment

KEY POINTS

- Risk factors for the persistence of substance use problems and disorders into adulthood mirror those for the development of problems and disorders in adolescents.
- Early screening of both college students and noncollege high-risk youth in the community is critical to early and effective intervention.
- Brief interventions using motivational techniques are effective for many transitional age youth, particularly for those in early stages of problem use on college campuses.
- Professionals should be aware of evidence-based treatments and providers for substance use disorders in the community as well as the developmental nuances of this period.

INTRODUCTION

Transitional age youth (TAY), those approximately 16 to 26 years of age and covering the period between and encompassing late adolescence and early adulthood, are the target of increasing attention by health care providers and policymakers. TAY have a number of psychosocial and developmental challenges that portend the emerging challenges of adulthood. Despite obtaining the age of legal majority at age 18, successful achievement of adult tasks in this age group is complicated by incomplete cognitive maturation; continued dependency on parents and/or other adults for housing, education, and financial stability; the continued need for education and/or training to enter and succeed in the 21st-century job market; and the continued increased rates of psychopathology.[1,2] Another major challenge for TAY is substance use and substance use disorders (SUDs). For many TAY, substance use and SUDs emerged earlier in adolescence and, for others, the increased independence and decreased

The author has nothing to disclose.
Department of Psychiatry, Boston Children's Hospital, 300 Longwood Avenue, Boston, MA 02115, USA
E-mail address: oscar.bukstein@childrens.harvard.edu

Abbreviations	
ADHD	Attention deficit hyperactivity disorder
BASCIS	Brief Alcohol Screening and Intervention of College Students
BI	Brief intervention
EBT	Evidenced-based therapy
FRAMES	Feedback, responsibility, advice, menu, empathy, self-efficacy
MI	Motivational interviewing
SBIRT	Screening, brief intervention, and referral to treatment
SUD	Substance use disorder
TAY	Transitional age youth

supervision after high school allows for increased exposure to substance use and is fertile ground for the development of SUDs. TAY have the highest rates of substance use and SUDs of any age group.[3] By their late 20s, nearly two-thirds (63%) of today's young adults have tried an illicit drug, and about 4 in 10 (37%) have tried some illicit drug other than marijuana, usually in addition to marijuana.[4]

This article reviews what is known about the prevalence and course of substance use and SUDs in TAY and provides guidance on screening, and brief and comprehensive treatment approaches. Although most definitions of TAY include youth who are still adolescents (ie, <18 years old) and those who are young adults, the focus is on TAY 18 years and older. Although there are continuities in the younger and older TAY groups, the differences are more salient to most clinicians.

TAY are a heterogeneous group, particularly as manifested by their level of educational attainment—that is, whether they graduate from high school, attend vocational training programs, community colleges or 4-year colleges or universities. Those who do not graduate high school or go on to college are different in important ways from those who go to college and those who complete college. Similarly, those who attend postsecondary vocational schools or community colleges may differ from the other 2 groups. Predictors of low educational attainment include lower socioeconomic status, increased familial stressors, and psychopathology; these attributed also constitute many of the risk factors for the development of SUDs.[5] Certainly youth who attend college are not immune from the development of SUDs, but rather SUDs often occur in a different context (eg, fraternities, sororities, or dormitories), an important consideration for educators, clinicians, and social service agencies.

Many of the risk and protective factors associated with problem substance use in young adulthood are the same as those that predict adolescent substance use.[6] These shared risk factors are listed in **Box 1**. The consequences of TAY alcohol use include deaths, injuries, and, among college students, academic problems, fighting, and sexual behavior problems.[7] The most common causes of mortality among TAY are injury-related causes, including poisoning, motor vehicle/traffic-related deaths, and firearm-related deaths, which are often substance involved.[8] Environmental factors in young adulthood also affect future substance use. For example, in 1 study of young adults, the transition into marriage predicted decreases in alcohol consumption, and this effect was consistent across gender and age.[9] Conversely, divorce predicted increased alcohol consumption, particularly for men.

TRANSITIONAL AGE YOUTH BRAIN DEVELOPMENT AND BEHAVIOR

Successful adult functioning requires cognitive maturity and the development of self-control over behavior and emotions, which is an aspect of executive functions. Executive functions are generally defined as cognitive processes and include planning, working memory, attention, problem solving, verbal reasoning, inhibition, mental

| Box 1 |
| Risk factors for problem substance use in young adulthood |
| Peer substance use |
| Favorable attitudes and norms toward substance use |
| Male gender |
| Externalizing behavior disorders during adolescence |
| Low social conformity |
| Low commitment to school |
| Low school achievement |
| Early adolescent substance use |
| Parental substance use and favorable attitudes toward use |

flexibility, multitasking, and initiation and monitoring of actions.[10] Brain maturation involving neurobehavioral systems underlying executive functions in the prefrontal cortex is among the last region of the brain to achieve full functional maturation. The late adolescent–young adult brain is not fully mature when they are having to make adult goal-directed decisions. The imbalance between the earlier developing limbic system, which governs emotional reward, and the later maturing prefrontal cortex often results in risk-taking behaviors. The mismatch of impulse versus cognitive control is fertile ground for the early onset of substance use and a more rapid and early onset of problems related to use.

EPIDEMIOLOGY
Substance Use

According to the annual Monitoring the Future survey,[4] which now includes surveys of college students, for nearly all categories of illicit drugs, college students show lower levels of use than their same-age peers who are not in college. However, for a few categories of drugs—including any illicit drug, marijuana, and hallucinogens—college students show annual usage levels that are about average for all high school graduates their age. (College students are about average on the index of any illicit drug use owing to average levels of marijuana use, which constitutes most of the illicit drug use. Although college-bound 12th graders have generally had below-average levels of use on all of the illicit drugs while they were in high school, these students' eventual use of some illicit drugs attained equivalence with, or even exceeded, the levels of their age-mates who do not attend college.

- Marijuana use: College student and young adult levels of daily marijuana use showed an overall increased from 2007 to 2015, from 3.5% to 4.6% among college students and from 5.0% to 6.8% among young adults (including both those attending college and those not attending).[4]
- Prescription drug misuse: For stimulants, 7.7% and 1.8% of young adults endorsed dextroamphetamine plus amphetamine (eg, Adderall) and methylphenidate (Ritalin) use without medical supervision in the previous 12 months in 2015. Young adults are the biggest abusers of prescription opioid pain relievers, attention deficit hyperactivity disorder (ADHD) stimulants, and antianxiety drugs. In 2014, more than 1700 young adults died from prescription (mostly opioid) overdoses.[11] The use of acetaminophen plus hydrocodone (Vicodin) by young

adults has declined significantly and steadily from 9.1% in 2008 to 3.8% in 2015. For the group of narcotics other than heroin, 5.2% of all young adults reported use within the preceding 12 months.

- College students who report nonmedical prescription stimulant use (ie, misuse) are more likely than other students to be heavy drinkers and users of other illicit drugs. Academically successful students are less likely to misuse prescription stimulants. Although academic enhancement is 1 motivation for prescription stimulant misuse, many students use these drugs recreationally (eg, to enhance their experience of partying and getting high on other substances). Compared with nonusers, students who misuse prescription drugs are more likely to meet criteria in the *Diagnostic and Statistical Manual of Mental Disorders*, 4th edition, for dependence on alcohol and marijuana, skip class more frequently, and spend less time studying.[12–14]

- Alcohol use: From 1980 to 1993, according to the Monitoring The Future Study[4] college students reported less of a decrease in monthly prevalence of alcohol use (82% to 70%) than did 12th graders (72% to 51%), and also less of a decrease in occasions of heavy drinking (from 44% to 40%) than either 12th graders (41% to 28%) or their noncollege age-mates (41% to 34%). Since 1993, binge alcohol use has not changed much among college students with their level of binge drinking in 2015 being 32%. The level among noncollege age-mates was 24% in 2015 (and 30% in 2012), down from 34% in 1993.

- Cigarette use: In 2015, smoking one-half pack or more per day was 5 times as prevalent among the non–college-bound 12th graders as among the college-bound students (5.5% vs 1.1%). Among respondents of college age (1 to 4 years past high school), those not in college also show dramatically higher levels of one-half-pack-per-day smoking than those who are in college—9.1% versus 1.4%, respectively.[4]

- Compared with those attending college, non–college-attending young adults with at least or less than a high school degree had a higher prevalence of past-year nonmedical use of prescription opioids, yet lower prevalence of pre-scription stimulant use.[15] Among users, regardless of drug type, non–college-attending youth were more likely to have past-year disorder secondary to use. As for gender effects, females who completed high school but were not enrolled in college had a significantly greater risk of opioid disorder (compared with female college students) than the same comparison for men. Among Hispanics, there was no difference in the risk for nonmedical use of prescription opioids across educational attainment groups.

Substance Use Disorders

Approximately 4.3 million young adults (12.3%) aged 18 to 25 in 2014 had an alcohol use disorder in the past year.[3] The percentage of all young adults with an alcohol use disorder (*Diagnostic and Statistical Manual of Mental Disorders*, 4th edition) in 2014 was lower than the percentages in 2002 to 2012. Approximately 2.3 million young adults (6.6%) aged 18 to 25 in 2014 had an illicit drug use disorder in the past year, which represents a lower percentages than in 2002 to 2012. Approximately 1.7 million young adults (4.9%) aged 18 to 25 in 2014 had a marijuana use disorder in the past year.[3]

Racial/Ethnic Differences

Generally, research in college students supports the highest rates of drug use and drug use–related problems among Hispanic students, especially when compared with Asian and African American college students.[16] White students have higher rates of illicit drug use than African American and Asian college students, including marijuana and several classes of prescription drugs. Trajectories of substance use show that Hispanic youth had higher initial rates of substance use, whereas Caucasian adolescents showed higher rates of change and had the highest levels of substance use from mid-adolescence through the early 30s.[17] Racial/ethnic differences largely disappeared after age 30, except that African Americans showed higher final levels of smoking and marijuana use than the other racial/ethnic groups. African Americans generally had a later age of onset of alcohol problems.[18]

COURSE

Many TAYs begin their alcohol or other drug use before young adulthood or even before late adolescence. Many of the same risk factors that predict SUD in adolescents, such as earlier age of use and SUDs, and family history of SUDs, also predict persistence into young adulthood and beyond.[2] Persistence of alcohol dependence into later adulthood was predicted by family psychiatric history, TAY and adult externalizing and internalizing problems, TAY and adult substance use, adult quality of life, and coping strategies. The prospective predictors that distinguish those with persistence of alcohol dependence into later adulthood and those who no longer are dependent on alcohol involved family liability, TAY negative affectivity, daily alcohol use, and frequent marijuana use.[2] TAY who developed the persistent subtype of alcohol dependence were distinguished from the developmentally limited subtype by an inability to reduce drinking and by continued use despite problems, already by age 18. For drug use, risk factors for the persistence into adulthood include high school use, unemployment, and noncustodial parenthood. Lower use was associated with being female, a college graduate, a professional, married, or a custodial parent.[10]

SCREENING

Assessment is the foundation of clinical management. Assessment often begins with screening to identify TAY at risk for having drug or alcohol problems, and may include a comprehensive evaluation of the severity and range of problems associated with TAY substance use or SUDs. Assessment defines the problem(s). If multiple problems exist, what should be the focus? For TAY, assessment at its simplest level becomes: Does the TAY use alcohol or other illicit drugs, and how does this use impact the TAY's psychosocial functioning? For screening and assessment of TAY with substance use problems and disorders, the clinician must understand not only the content of any level of assessment, but should also be familiar with the process of both screening and comprehensive assessment, including such issues as engagement and confidentiality.

Many systems interface with TAY regarding screening and intervention for SUDs. These systems include medical settings (eg, primary care settings, emergency department), social service agencies, and schools (college and vocational training). SBIRT, which consists of screening, brief intervention (BI), and referral to treatment, was developed, implemented, and tested in a wide range of populations.[19,20] One of the principles underlying SBIRT is that screening may reveal varying levels of substance use involvement, ranging from abstinence to dependence, and should result in commensurate responses or interventions ranging from advice to specific SUD treatment. **Table 1** lists several well-studied screening measures.

At colleges, those responsible for screening may include staff from diverse disciplines, such as student health, counseling services, or even wellness departments.

Table 1
Useful drug and alcohol screening tools

Screening Tool	Substance		Self-Administered	Clinician-Administered
	Alcohol	Drugs		
Alcohol Use Disorders Identification Test-(AUDIT) –C and full[21]	X		x	X
NIDA Drug Use Screening Tool and Quick Screen[22]		X	x	X
Opioid Risk Tool[23]		X	x	
Drug Abuse Screening Tool (DAST)[24]		X	x	
NIDA-Modified ASSIST (APA) Pre- and general screen[25]	X	X	X	

Wellness coaches and others trained in screening may then hand off positive screens to specific medical or behavioral health staff. In emergency departments, nursing or social work staff are often trained to handle screening assignments. For those TAY not involved in higher education, social agency staff, probation officers, and other legal staff may be assigned to screen clients systematically for substance use problems. Particularly with TAY, and regardless of whether the task is screening or a more comprehensive assessment, the clinician should assume a nonjudgmental attitude and ask questions in a respectful, empathic, honest, and supportive manner, using open-ended questions to let the TAY define the problem. Regardless of age and family involvement, the clinician should maintain strict attention to confidentiality.

COMPREHENSIVE ASSESSMENT

A positive screen results in either referral for a more comprehensive assessment or, in case of lower severity problems, in a BI. A comprehensive assessment includes an inquiry into the history of substance use for all major categories of substances as well as age of first use, frequency, amount of use, psychiatric symptoms, history of treatment for both substance abuse and mental health problems, and medical, social, developmental history. Detailing the consequences of use is critical. Impairment in functioning owing to substance use is the hallmark of substance use pathology; thus, the clinician enquires about level of functioning in several psychosocial domains. In addition to the broad areas listed, the clinician should ask about legal problems, peer and social relationships, educational/vocational functioning, and family issues including family history of SUDs and/or psychiatric disorders.

TAY often present with a wider range of possible functioning domains. Some may be still residing at home and dealing regularly with their family of origin. Some may be married or reside with a partner, or even have children. For example, TAY may be completing high school, attending a community or 4-year college (or graduate school), attending a trade or vocational program, or be gainfully employed. Evaluation of the medical domain may require a full history and physical examination in addition to laboratory studies as needed. Eventually, the clinician should be able to make a diagnostic formulation using criteria set forth in the *Diagnostic and Statistical Manual of Mental Disorders*, 5th edition. A comprehensive assessment is usually completed by a substance abuse treatment or mental health professional and as part of a treatment program.

A final step of the assessment process involves treatment planning. For less severe presentations, advice or a BI may be sufficient. For TAY with more severe problems or a past history of treatment with subsequent relapse, referral for specific ambulatory treatment, including intensive outpatient treatment or residential treatment may be indicated.

BRIEF TREATMENT

Assessment, treatment planning, and intervention with TAY with substance use and SUDs intersect at BIs. BIs typically consist of 1 to 4 sessions. BIs can be standalone interventions or the beginning of ongoing care that could include any evidence-based interventions such as cognitive–behavioral therapy or family approaches. Almost always, BIs for SUDs include a motivational component, which may emphasize increasing motivation for the TAY's choice of abstinence from substance use, decreasing use, or motivation to participate in a more intensive level of treatment. A knowledge of motivational interviewing (MI) and its constituent principles and techniques is almost essential for administering BIs.[26–28] Bien and colleagues[29] describe several important characteristics of effective BIs using the acronym FRAMES (feedback, responsibility, advice, menu, empathy, self-efficacy). Although FRAMES is an excellent acronym, these components are not listed in chronologic order of likely use (**Box 2**).

CHANGE PLAN

Although not part of the FRAMES acronym, the elements of FRAMES, especially advice and menu, result ultimately in discussion of a change plan. A change plan is a summary of MI and BI efforts. After summarizing reasons for changing substance use or other behavior(s), the clinician and TAY set goals for change, consider options, outline specific steps (what the TAY will do and when), identify potential obstacles and how they might be overcome, and how the TAY and others will evaluate his or her progress.

The Brief Alcohol Screening and Intervention of College Students (BASICS), a harm reduction approach, is a preventive intervention for college students 18 to 24 years old.[30] BASICS targets students who drink alcohol heavily and have experienced or are at risk for alcohol-related problems such as poor class attendance, missed assignments, accidents, sexual assault, and violence. BASICS is designed to help students make better alcohol use decisions based on a clear understanding of the genuine risks associated with problem drinking, enhanced motivation to change, and the development of skills to moderate drinking. The program is conducted over the course of 2 brief sessions that seek to prompt and motivate students to change their drinking patterns. The program's style is empathetic, nonconfrontational or nonjudgmental, and aims to[1] reduce alcohol consumption and its adverse consequences,[2] promote healthier choices among young adults, and[3] provide important information and coping skills for risk reduction. The results of a metaanalysis examining the efficacy of BASICS indicate that this BI is more efficacious in reducing both heavy drinking and alcohol-related problems among at-risk college students in comparison with control groups after 12 months of follow-up.[31] A counselor-administered MI plus feedback may be preferred as a first-line intervention for college students who drink heavily. Other similar programs include Alcohol eCHECKUP TO GO,[32] an interactive web survey that allows college and university students to enter information about their drinking patterns and receive feedback about their use of alcohol, and Cannabis Screening and Intervention for College Students.[33] However, such BIs seem to be limited to students

Box 2
Frames approach to brief interventions

Feedback: Assessment of current status

Using an objective, noncoercive presentation, the clinician provides:
- Personalized information about the substance use and its effects, as pertains to the TAY
- Personalized normative feedback; factual details about the TAY's substance use and patterns in comparison with norms for use in similar-aged peer groups
- Objective data about consequences experienced by the TAY owing to substance use (eg, visit to emergency department for alcohol poisoning, school failure, possession of marijuana)
- Opportunity for TAY to give feedback about the feedback by asking questions "What do you make of this?" or "How does this fit or not fit with what you know about yourself?"

Responsibility: Personal decision to change

Cognizant of the value late adolescents and young adults place on autonomy, the clinician emphasizes the TAY's freedom of choice:
- "It's your choice when you are ready" "It's up to you; you're free to decide to change or not" "No one else can really decide for you or force you to change"

Advice: Recommend behavior change—cutting down or stopping substance use

Using a supportive, concerned tone, the clinician:
- Gives clear recommendations on need to change substance use behaviors
- Asks permission to offer advice: "Is it okay if I go over with you what options you have?"
- Gives advice on specific ways to change substance use

Menu: Alternative strategies or options to address substance use

Cognizant of the need to reinforce autonomy, and that TAY cannot be made to pursue a particular treatment or even treatment in general, if they truly do not want it, the clinician:
- Emphasizes TAY input and choice about treatment
- Attempts to elicit intervention options from the TAY
- If the TAY is unable to provide these options, asks permission to provide a variety of treatment options that the TAY may consider
- Provides a menu of treatment options for the TAY to choose from, essentially beginning treatment planning

Empathy: Being supportive and understanding about the TAY's situation

Using a supportive, nonjudgmental manner, the clinician:
- Uses techniques such as affirmations, reflections, and summaries to convey an understanding of patient's subjective experience
- Acknowledges the difficulty of addressing the problems of substance use as well as any perceived benefits from substance use that the TAY would be giving up. "Quitting is tough" "You've made a lot of hard decisions and changes in your life"

Self-efficacy: Reinforce hope and optimism

Using an optimistic tone and collaborative approach the clinician:
- Supports the patient's belief that he/she can successfully tackle changing substance use behaviors "I know that when you are ready that you will be able to do this"
- Working with the TAY, attempts to identify past successes and reframes prior failures as learning lessons "I know you have learned a lot about the kind of things that can trip you up" "You have been able to stay clean for quite a while in the past"

Abbreviation: TAY, transitional age youth.
    Adapted from Bien TJ, Miller WR, Tonigan JS. Brief interventions for alcohol problems: a review. Addiction 1993;88(3):315–35.

who have a lower severity of alcohol or marijuana use and/or are "at risk" for the development of SUDs. Students having moderate to severe SUDs will need referral for more comprehensive SUD treatment.

Outside of BIs administered in emergency departments, there is a paucity of studies examining BIs in non–college-attending TAY.

COMPREHENSIVE TREATMENT

For those TAY with longer, more severe histories of substance use or with substantial psychiatric comorbidities and impairment, clinicians may need to refer them for more comprehensive evaluation and treatment approaches than those afforded by SBIRT and BI interventions. Colleges, emergency departments, and primary care and behavioral health professionals should have identified SUD programs that offer higher levels of care for TAY for potential referral. Ideally, these programs use evidenced-based therapies (EBTs). EBTs for adolescents may also be useful into young adulthood (**Table 2**). Prominent EBTs for adults are listed in **Table 3**. EBTs for SUDs can be categorized into several target domains, making their selection by clinicians dependent on the TAY's specific situation, such as living with family or alone, the presence of high versus low motivation, and the presence or absence of specific skills for dealing with urges to use, and avoiding and dealing with cues prompting substance use.

Motivation-Based Therapies

MI and motivational enhancement therapy attempt to increase the individual's intrinsic motivation to change substance use behaviors. Contingency management

Table 2
Specific evidenced based interventions for adolescents with substance use disorders

Intervention	Type	Population
Adolescent Community Reinforcement Approach[34]	Family	Youth ages 13–17 Girls/boys Outpatient/home
Assertive adolescent outpatient and intensive outpatient treatment model[35]	Individual/group	Ages 12–18
Brief strategic family therapy[36]	Family	Youth ages 13–17 Girls/boys Outpatient/home
Family behavior therapy[37]	Family	Youth ages 13–17 Girls/boys Outpatient/home
Family support network[38]	Family	Youth ages 13–17 Girls/boys Outpatient/home
Functional family therapy[39]	Family	Youth ages 13–17 Girls/boys Outpatient/home
MET/CBT 5 or 12[38]	Individual/group	Youth ages 13–17 Girls/boys Outpatient/home
Motivational interviewing[40]	Individual/group	Youth ages 13–17
Multidimensional family therapy[41]	Family	Youth ages 13–17 Outpatient/home
Multisystemic therapy[42]	Brief Individual	Youth ages 13–17 home, school, or community
Teen Intervene[43]	Individual	Youth ages 12–19 outpatient, school, or juvenile detention setting

Abbreviations: CBT, cognitive–behavioral therapy; MET, motivational enhancement therapy.

Table 3
Prominent evidenced based treatments for adults with substance use disorders

Intervention	Population
12-Step facilitation therapy[44]	Adults
Behavioral self-control training[45,46]	Adults; young adults
Brief strategic family therapy[36]	Adults, adolescents
Cognitive–behavioral coping skills therapy[45]	Adults
Community reinforcement approach with vouchers[47]	Adults
Family behavior therapy[34]	Adults; adolescents
Matrix intensive outpatient program for the treatment of stimulant abuse[48]	Adults
Relapse prevention[49]	Adults
Motivational enhancement therapy (problem drinkers)[44]	Adults

interventions and/or motivational incentives involve giving patients tangible rewards to reinforce positive behaviors such as abstinence or attendance at treatment sessions.[50] Although studies of adults using contingency management for SUDs have included young adults and adolescents separately, the effectiveness for TAY with SUDs is specifically supported by studies with TAY.[51] The voucher-based reinforcement augments other community-based treatments by offering the patient a voucher for every drug-free urine sample and/or attendance at treatment sessions.[47] The voucher can be exchanged for food items, movie passes, or other goods or services that are consistent with a drug-free lifestyle. Community reinforcement approach plus vouchers is an intensive 24-week outpatient therapy for treating adults with SUDs by its use of a range of recreational, familial, social, and vocational reinforcers, along with material incentives, to make a non–drug-using lifestyle more rewarding than substance use.[44]

Skills-Based Therapies

The best known skills-based intervention for SUDs is cognitive–behavioral therapy. Patients are assisted in identifying and correcting problematic behaviors through the application of a range of different skills that can be used to stop substance abuse and to address a range of other problems that often co-occur with it, such as mood and anxiety disorders, and by developing effective coping strategies.[45] Specific techniques include exploring the positive and negative consequences of continued drug use, self-monitoring to recognize cues and cravings early, identifying situations that might put one at risk for use, and developing strategies for coping with cravings and avoiding those high-risk situations.

Family-Based Interventions

Family-based interventions are represented by several EBT for adolescents, including brief strategic family therapy, family support network, functional family therapy, multidimensional family therapy, and multisystemic therapy (see **Table 2**). The focus of family-based interventions is improving parent–adolescent communication and parent management skills, such as negotiating rules and consequences. Family behavior therapy has demonstrated positive results in both adults and adolescents and is aimed at addressing not only substance use problems but other co-occurring problems as well, such as conduct disorders, child mistreatment, depression, family conflict, and unemployment. FBT combines behavioral contracting with contingency management.

Twelve-Step Interventions

Although the use of peer support groups such as Alcoholics Anonymous and Narcotics Anonymous lack the evidence base seen with other EBT, 12-step facilitation therapy is an active engagement strategy designed to increase the likelihood of the affected patient becoming affiliated with and actively involved in 12-step self-help groups, thereby promoting abstinence.[52,53] TAY seem to benefit from such self-support groups by decreases in prodrinking social networks and self-efficacy in social situations as opposed to a wider range of mechanisms in older adults.[25]

Multimodal Interventions

The existence of EBT targeting different domains or aspects of TAY substance use and behaviors facilitating use suggests that multiple interventions can be used for the same TAY. For example, MI session(s) can use used to increase motivation for treatment to a cognitive-behavioral therapy–oriented group with attendance and abstinence supported by contingency management. Several EBTs often incorporate several modalities. Multisystemic therapy can include a variety of individual interventions within the context of an intensive family-based intervention. The matrix model, developed for the treatment of stimulant use disorder, includes elements of MI, relapse prevention, family and group therapies, drug education, and self-help participation.[48]

MEDICATION-ASSISTED TREATMENT

Medication-assisted treatment is the use of medications, almost always in combination with behavioral therapies, to provide a comprehensive approach to the treatment of SUDs.[54,55] Medication-assisted treatment is used primarily for the treatment of addiction to opioids such as heroin and prescription pain relievers that contain opiates. Some medications target alcohol use disorders. The prescribed medication operates to normalize brain chemistry, block the euphoric effects of alcohol and opioids, relieve physiologic cravings, and normalize body functions without the negative effects of the abused drug. Methadone, buprenorphine, and naltrexone are used to treat opioid dependence and addiction to short-acting opioids such as heroin, morphine, and codeine, as well as semisynthetic opioids like oxycodone and hydrocodone. People may safely take medications used in medication-assisted treatment for acute detoxification in the case of buprenorphine for opioids to longer term, maintenance treatment (buprenorphine for opioids and naltrexone for opioids or alcohol). Two studies support the use of buprenorphine in adolescents and TAY in short-term treatment,[56,57] although TAY show poorer rates of retention in buprenorphine programs.[58] The short-term use of naltrexone for alcohol use disorders in TAY is supported by a randomized, clinical trial showing improvements on percent days heavy drinking, percent days abstinent, and drinks per drinking day.[59] Although percent days heavy drinking showed improvements at both 8 weeks and 12 months compared with placebo, percent days abstinent and drinks per drinking day showed improvements over placebo only at 8 weeks; the use of other agents for TAY in alcohol use disorders such as acamprosate and topiramate is supported by adult studies.[60] Acamprosate may be used for TAY who have already stopped drinking alcohol and want to avoid drinking. The use of psychiatric drugs as serotonergic reuptake inhibitors should be reserved for TAY with depressive or anxiety disorder comorbidity with SUDs.

SPECIAL CONSIDERATIONS IN THE TREATMENT OF TRANSITIONAL AGE YOUTH WITH SUBSTANCE USE DISORDERS

Selection of the psychosocial treatment modality in TAY with SUDs depends largely on the individual TAY's living circumstances. For those in college or who are home-less, individual psychotherapeutic interventions are the most feasible. For TAY living at or near home, family-based interventions may be both practical and necessary. Owing to the frequent high level of resistance as well as the desire for autonomy, TAY preference often determine the intervention modality used. Multimodal interven-tions, combining individual modalities, or psychosocial modalities plus medication may be optimal, especially for those with psychiatric comorbidity.[61–63]

There are several very high-risk populations of TAY for the development of SUDs, including youth with comorbid psychiatric disorders, runaway and/or homeless youth, lesbian, gay, bisexual, transgender, and queer youth, and youth leaving the foster care and juvenile justice systems.[63–65] These TAY often have a variety of problems, including the lack of peer and parent supports and housing and the ex-istence of financial and educational/vocational problems, suggesting the need for SUD treatment programs that provide a variety of comprehensive services that target these problems.[66] Many TAY with SUDs have other psychiatric problems such as mood, anxiety, or psychotic disorders. Concurrent integration of psychiatric treatment with SUD treatment is an increasingly recognized and effective strategy for dealing with multiple problems.[66]

PREVENTION OF SUBSTANCE USE DISORDERS IN TRANSITIONAL AGE YOUTH

As with other populations at high risk for SUDs, TAY have a variety of salient risk fac-tors for the development and maintenance of SUDs, including family history (of SUDs), psychopathology, legal problems, school and occupational failure, and family and interpersonal discord. Clinicians, teachers, law enforcement professionals, and other social service agency professionals who come into contact with TAY should screen for these risk factor and refer, if indicated, for appropriate intervention. Secondary and tertiary prevention principles suggest that intervention in early adolescents may lessen the burden of suffering and prevalence of substance use problems in TAY.

To prevent problem alcohol use on college campuses, the National Institute on Alcoholism and Alcohol Abuse suggests a combination of individual-level and environ-mental strategies.[67] Strategies targeting individual students include focusing on those in higher risk groups, such as first-year students, student athletes, members of Greek organizations, and other mandated students. Such interventions are designed to change students' knowledge, attitudes, and behaviors related to alcohol so that they drink less, take fewer risks, and experience fewer harmful consequences. Types of individual-level interventions include (1) education and awareness programs, (2) cognitive–behavioral skills–based approaches, and (3) specific behavioral interven-tions by clinicians. Environmental-level strategies or those targeting the campus and surrounding community as a whole, are designed with a major goal of reducing the availability of alcohol, because reducing alcohol availability cuts consumption and harmful consequences on campuses. Generally, the approach to the prevention of marijuana use/abuse is similar to that of alcohol.

Prevention of the misuse of other prescription drugs college students consists of 2 major goals—to decrease the misuse by individual students and to reduce the diver-sion of such agents. For prescription opioids, individual interventions include those similar to alcohol prevention as well as careful screening of high-risk students. If college-based medical providers need to prescribe opioid analgesics, the providers should be familiar with guidelines for prescribing that minimize the opportunity for diversion or misuse (including overuse).[68]

For stimulants, intervention may occur for both those using stimulants under medical supervision (ie, have a documented diagnosis of ADHD) and those misusing. Clinicians should provide students needing stimulants for the treatment of ADHD with informed consent that cautions against sharing and/or selling of the prescribed stimulant. In addition, a detailed plan for use at college should include specific dosing (eg, which days on and off stimulants), where stimulants can be stored safely and securely while at college, provision for refills and new prescriptions, and strongly advising students not to tell other students lest they coerce the student into diverting the medication. The majority of stimulants being misused by college students originate from students being treated for ADHD who share and/or sell their stimulants to other students who desire them for nonmedical use.[12,14] Similarly, clinicians should caution parents to be aware of signs of diversion and/or misuse. The use of stimulants may be contraindicated in cases of concurrent SUDs or a history of stimulant abuse.

Clinicians working in college health services or counseling centers should be aware when students report a diagnosis of ADHD or symptoms without previous documentation. Having students be managed by clinicians outside the college campus and providing documentation of the diagnosis may decrease the possibility that college staff may be contributing inadvertently to the problem or misuse and/or diversion on campus.

RESEARCH GAPS AND FUTURE DIRECTIONS

Longitudinal research on the development and persistence of SUDs has focused on child and adolescent variables. Future research should include variables from the transitional period, including education and training status, peer and intimate relationships, and formation of families. Although sharing some similarities with adolescents and adults, TAY are different and may demand specific screening, comprehensive assessment, and intervention approaches that are tailored to the status and needs of TAY. Currently, there are few intervention approaches designed specifically for TAY and, as a result, few controlled clinical trials of such interventions. Adult research that includes TAY should break out age data for this group in their analyses and reports. To be relevant for TAY, such trials should include developmentally appropriate outcomes, such as attainment of adult developmental tasks and roles.

SUMMARY

Because substance use peaks during the TAY years, awareness of risk factors for the development and persistence of SUDs is critical. Both on college campuses and in the community, those in regular contact with TAY need to be aware of how to screen for SUDs, provide BIs, and, if necessary, refer for more comprehensive treatment. SUD treatment professionals need to be aware of the special needs of TAY and the unique developmental perspective of the transition into young adulthood.

REFERENCES

1. Wilens TE, Rosenbaum JF. Transitional aged youth: a new frontier in child and adolescent psychiatry. J Am Acad Child Adolesc Psychiatry 2013;52:887–90.
2. Brown SA, McGue M, Magge J, et al. A developmental perspective on alcohol and youths 16 to 20 years of age. Pediatrics 2008;121(Supplement 4):S290–310.

3. Substance Abuse and Mental Health Services Administration (SAMHSA). In: Behavioral Health Trends in the United States: Results from the 2014 National Survey on Drug Use and Health, 2015. Available at: http://www.samhsa.gov/data/sites/default/files/NSDUH-FRR1-2014/NSDUH-FRR1-2014.pdf. Accessed August 20, 2016.

4. Johnston LD, O'Malley PM, Bachman JG, et al. Monitoring the future. College Students & Adults Ages 19–55. In: Monitoring the Future, 2015. Available at: http://www.monitoringthefuture.org//pubs/monographs/mtf-vol2_2015.pdf. Accessed August 20, 2016.

5. Ou S-R, Reynolds AJ. Predictors of educational attainment in the Chicago Longitudinal Study. Sch Psychol Q 2008;23(2):199–229.

6. Stone AL, Becker LG, Huber AM, et al. Review of risk and protective factors of substance use and problem use in emerging adulthood. Addict Behav 2012; 37:747–75.

7. Wechsler H, Lee JE, Kuo M, et al. College binge drinking in the 1990s: a continuing problem: results of the Harvard School of Public Health 1999 College Alcohol Study. J Am Coll Health 2000;48:199–210.

8. Fingerhut LA, Anderson RN. The three leading causes of injury mortality in the United States, 1999–2005. National Center for Health Statistics: Health E Stats. Available at: www.cdc.gov/nchs/products/pubs/pubd/hestats/injury99-05/injury99-05.htm. Accessed September 4, 2016.

9. Kretsch N, Harden KP. Marriage, divorce, and alcohol use in young adulthood. Emerging Adulthood 2014;2:138–49.

10. Casey BJ, Jones RM. Neurobiology of the adolescent brain and behavior: implications for substance use disorders. J Am Acad Child Adolesc Psychiatry 2010; 49:1189–201.

11. National Institute on Drug Abuse. Abuse of Prescription (Rx) Drugs Affects Young Adults Most. Available at: https://www.drugabuse.gov/related-topics/trends-statistics/infographics/abuse-prescription-rx-drugs-affects-young-adults-most. Accessed September 10, 2016.

12. Arria AM, O'Grady KE, Caldeira KM, et al. Nonmedical use of prescription stimulants and analgesics: associations with social and academic behaviors among college students. J Drug Issues 2008;38:1045–60.

13. Arria AM, DuPont RL. Nonmedical prescription stimulant use among college students: why we need to do something and what we need to do. J Addict Dis 2010; 29(4):417–26.

14. Barrett SP, Darredeau C, Bordy LE, et al. Characteristics of methylphenidate misuse in a university student sample. Can J Psychiatry 2005;50:457–61.

15. Martins SS, Kim JH, Chen LY, et al. Nonmedical prescription drug use among US young adults by educational attainment. Soc Psychiatry Psychiatr Epidemiol 2015;50:713–24.

16. McCabe SE, Morales M, Cranford JA, et al. Race/ethnicity and gender differences in drug use and abuse among college students. J Ethn Subst Abuse 2007;6(2):75–95.

17. Chen P, Jacobson KC. Developmental trajectories of substance use from early adolescence to young adulthood: gender and racial/ethnic differences. J Adolesc Health 2012;50(2):154–63.

18. Chartier KG, Hesselbrock MN, Hesselbrock VM. Alcohol problems in young adults transitioning from adolescence to adulthood: the association with race and gender. Addict Behav 2011;36(3):167–74.

19. Mitchell SG, Gryczynski J, O'Grady KE, et al. SBIRT for adolescent drug and alcohol use: current status and future directions. J Subst Abuse Treat 2013; 44(5):463–72.

20. Substance Abuse and Mental Health Services Administration (SAMHSA). Screening, Brief Intervention, and Referral to Treatment (SBIRT). Available at: http://www.samhsa.gov/sbirt. Accessed August 20, 2016.

21. Bradley KA, Bush KR, Epler AJ, et al. Two brief alcohol-screening tests from the Alcohol Use Disorders Identification Test (AUDIT): validation in a female veterans' affairs patient population. Arch Intern Med 2003;163:821–9.

22. National Institute on Drug Abuse (NIDA). NIDA Drug Screening Tool. Available at: https://www.drugabuse.gov/nmassist. Accessed August 20, 2016.

23. Webster LR, Webster R. Predicting aberrant behaviors in opioid-treated patients: preliminary validation of the opioid risk too. Pain Med 2005;6(6):432.

24. Skinner HA. The drug abuse screening test. Addict Behav 1982;7(4):363–71.

25. National Institute on Drug Abuse. American Psychiatric Association Adapted NIDA Modified ASSIST Tools. Available at: https://www.drugabuse.gov/nidamed-medical-health-professionals/tool-resources-your-practice/screening-assessment-drug-testing-resources/american-psychiatric-association-adapted-nida. Accessed August 20, 2016.

26. Naar S, Suarez M. Motivational Interviewing with adolescents and young adults. New York: Guilford; 2011.

27. Miller WR, Rolinick S. Motivational interviewing – helping people change. 3rd edition. New York: Guilford; 2013.

28. Tanner-Smith EE, Lipsey MW. Brief alcohol interventions for adolescents and young adults: a systematic review and meta-analysis. J Subst Abuse Treat 2015;51:1–18.

29. Bien TJ, Miller WR, Tonigan JS. Brief interventions for alcohol problems: a review. Addiction 1993;88(3):315–35.

30. Dimeff LA, Baer JS, Kivlahan DR, et al. Brief alcohol screening and intervention for college students (BASICS): a harm reduction approach. New York: The Guilford Press; 1999.

31. Fachini A, Aliane PP, Martinez EZ, et al. Efficacy of brief alcohol screening intervention for college students (BASICS): a meta-analysis of randomized controlled trials. Subst Abuse Treat Prev Policy 2012;7:40.

32. Walters ST, Miller JE, Chiauzzi E. Wired for wellness: e-Interventions for addressing college drinking. J Subst Abuse Treat 2005;29:139–45.

33. Walters ST, Baer JS. Talking with college students about alcohol: motivational strategies for reducing abuse. New York: The Guildford Press; 2006.

34. Godley MD, Godley SH, Dennis ML, et al. The effect of Assertive Continuing Care (ACC) on continuing care linkage, adherence and abstinence following residential treatment for adolescents. Addiction 2007;102:81–93.

35. Godley SH, Garner BR, Passetti LL, et al. Adolescent outpatient treatment and continuing care: main findings from a randomized clinical trial. Drug Alcohol Depend 2010;110(1–2):44–54.

36. Santisteban DA, Suarez-Morales L, Robbins MS, et al. Brief strategic family therapy: lessons learned in efficacy research and challenges to blending research and practice. Fam Process 2006;45(2):259–71.

37. Donohue B, Azrin N, Allen DN, et al. Family behavior therapy for substance abuse: a review of its intervention components and applicability. Behav Modif 2009;33:495–519.

38. Dennis ML, Godley SH, Diamond G, et al. The cannabis youth treatment (CYT) study: main findings from two randomized trials. J Subst Abuse Treat 2004;27: 197–213.

39. Waldron HR, Slesnick N, Brody JL, et al. Treatment outcomes for adolescent substance abuse at 4- and 7-month assessments. J Consult Clin Psychol 2001;69: 802–13.

40. Barnett E, Sussman S, Smith C, et al. Motivational interviewing for adolescent substance use: a review of the literature. Addict Behav 2012;37(12):1325–34.

41. Liddle HA, Rowe CL, Dakof GA, et al. Multidimensional family therapy for young adolescent substance abuse: twelve month outcomes of a randomized controlled trial. J Consult Clin Psychol 2009;77:12–25.

42. Henggeler SW, Pickrel SG, Brondino MJ. Multisystemic treatment of substance-abusing and dependent delinquents: outcomes, treatment fidelity, and transportability. Ment Health Serv Res 1999;1(3):171–84.

43. Winters KC, Fahnhorst T, Botzet A, et al. Brief intervention for drug-abusing adolescents in a school setting: outcomes and mediating factors. J Subst Abuse Treat 2012;42:279–88.

44. Project MATCH Research Group. Matching alcoholism treatments to client heterogeneity: project MATCH posttreatment drinking outcomes. J Stud Alcohol 1997;58:7–29.

45. Carroll KM, Onken LS. Behavioral therapies for drug abuse. The American Journal of Psychiatry 2005;168:1452–60.

46. Schuster RM, Hanly A, Gilman J, et al. A contingency management method for 30-days abstinence in non-treatment seeking young adult cannabis users. Drug Alcohol Depend 2016;167:199–206.

47. Roozen HG, Boulogne JJ, van Tulder MW, et al. A systemic review of the effectiveness of the community reinforcement approach in alcohol, cocaine and opioid addiction. Drug Alcohol Depend 2004;74:1–13.

48. Rawson R, Shoptaw SJ, Obert JL, et al. An intensive outpatient approach for cocaine abuse: the Matrix model. J Subst Abuse Treat 1995;12:117–27.

49. Larimer ME, Palmer RS, Marlatt GA. Relapse prevention: Marlatt's cognitive-behavioral model. Alcohol Res Health 1999;23:151–60.

50. Stanger C, Budney AJ. Contingency management approaches for adolescent substance use disorders. Child Adolesc Psychiatr Clin N Am 2010;19:47–62.

51. Budney AJ, Moore BA, Rocha HL, et al. Clinical trial of abstinence-based vouchers and cognitive behavioral therapy for cannabis dependence. J Consult Clin Psychol 2006;74:307–16.

52. Donovan DM, Wells EA. "Tweaking 12-step": the potential role of 12-Step self-help group involvement in methamphetamine recovery. Addiction 2007; 102(Suppl 1):121–9.

53. Hoeppner BB, Hoeppner SS, Kelly JF. Do young people benefit from AA as much, and in the same ways, as adult aged 30+? A moderated multiple mediation analysis. Drug Alcohol Depend 2014;143:181–8.

54. Substance Abuse and Mental Health Services Administration (SAMHSA). Medication for the treatment of alcohol use disorder: a brief guide. Available at: http://store.samhsa.gov/product/SMA15-4907. Accessed August 25, 2016.

55. Center for Substance Abuse Treatment. Medication-assisted treatment for opioid addiction in opioid treatment programs. Rockville (MD): Substance Abuse and Mental Health Services Administration (US); 2005 (Treatment Improvement Protocol (TIP) Series, No. 43).

56. Marsch LA, Bickel WK, Badger GJ, et al. Comparison of pharmacological treatments for opioid-dependent adolescents: a randomized controlled trial. Arch Gen Psychiatry 2005;62:1157–64.
57. Woody G, Poole SA, Subramaniam GA, et al. Extended vs. short-term buprenorphine/naloxone for treatment of opioid-addicted youth: a randomized trial. JAMA 2008;300:2003–11.
58. Schuman-Olivier Z, Weiss RD, Hoeppner B, et al. Emerging adult age status predicts poor buprenorphine treatment retention. J Subst Abuse Treat 2014;47: 202–12.
59. Demartini KS, Gueorguieva R, Leeman RF, et al. Longitudinal findings from a randomized clinical trial of naltrexone for young adult heavy drinkers. J Consult Clin Psychol 2016;84:185–90.
60. Jonas DE, Amick HR, Feltner C, et al. Pharmacotherapy for adults with alcohol use disorders in outpatient settings: a systematic review and meta-analysis. JAMA 2014;311:1889–900.
61. Barrowclough C, Haddock G, Tarrier N, et al. Randomized controlled trial of motivational interviewing, cognitive behavior therapy, and family intervention for patients with comorbid schizophrenia and substance use disorders. Am J Psychiatry 2001;158:1706–13.
62. Miklowitz DJ. Family treatment for bipolar disorder and substance abuse in late adolescence. J Clin Psychol 2012;68:502–13.
63. Narendorf SC, McMillen JC. Substance use and substance use disorders as foster youth transition to adulthood. Child Youth Serv Rev 2010;32:113–9.
64. Foster EM, Gifford EJ. The transition to adulthood for youth leaving public systems: challenges to policies and research. In: Setterson RA, Furstenburg FF, Rumbant RG, editors. On the frontier of adulthood: theory, research, & public policy. Chicago: University of Chicago Press; 2005. p. 501–33.
65. Marshal MP, Friedman MS, Stall R, et al. Sexual orientation and adolescent substance use: a meta-analysis and methodological review. Addiction 2008;103: 546–56.
66. Cavanaugh DS, Goldman B, Friesen C, et al. Designing a recovery-oriented care model for adolescents and transition age youth with substance use of co-occurring mental health disorders, report from CSAT/CMHS/SAMSHA Consultative Session. Washington, DC: Georgetown University; 2009. November 13–14, 2008.
67. NIAAA, 2016. CollegeAIM: Alcohol Intervention Matrix. 2015. Available at: http://www.collegedrinkingprevention.gov/CollegeAIM/. Accessed September 1, 2016.
68. Centers for Disease Control (CDC). CDC Guideline for Prescribing Opioids for Chronic Pain — United States, 2016. Available at: https://www.cdc.gov/media/modules/dpk/2016/dpk-pod/rr6501e1er-ebook.pdf. Accessed September 15, 2016.

Multicultural Developmental Experiences
Implications for Resilience in Transitional Age Youth

Deborah Rivas-Drake, PhD[a],*, Gabriela Livas Stein, PhD[b]

KEYWORDS

- Ethnic minority • Racial minority • Ethnic identity • Racial identity • Discrimination
- Cultural stressors • Cultural assets

KEY POINTS

- Transitional age youth are more ethnically and racially diverse than ever before.
- Cultural stressors such as acculturative stress and discrimination are linked to adverse health and mental health outcomes among ethnic and/or racial minority youth.
- Cultural resilience factors, including adaptive ethnic-racial identity and endorsement of communalistic cultural values, protect young adults from the sequelae of cultural stressors.

Adolescents and young adults in the United States are becoming a more ethnically and racially diverse group than ever before. Ethnic and/or racial minorities currently comprise more than 40% of the population under the age of 18% and 40% of the population of young people ages 18 to 24 years. These numbers are only poised to increase because more than 50% of births in 2011 were to ethnic and/or racial minorities.[1,2] Over the next several decades, it is expected the white population will decline while all other ethnic minority groups increase significantly. Specifically, by 2060, minorities will increase to 56% of the population.[3] The United States will become a majority-minority nation for the first time in less than 30 years. Adolescents and young adults of today will ultimately live in a plurality of white, Latino, black, Asian, American Indian, and multiracial peers.

Today's youth were born into a world that is becomingly increasingly diverse as they are transitioning to adulthood. Due to immigration and internal migration patterns, most of the country has become more diverse; relatively few areas have not experienced

Disclosure Statement: The authors have nothing to disclose.
[a] Department of Psychology, School of Education, University of Michigan, 530 Church Street, Ann Arbor, MI 48109-1043, USA; [b] Department of Psychology, University of North Carolina at Greensboro, 296 Eberhart Building, Greensboro, NC 27412-5001, USA
* Corresponding author.
E-mail address: drivas@umich.edu

a change in their foreign-born populations. In other words, the country has become more diverse in more places outside the well-established areas of ethnic minority presence, including major urban centers such as Los Angeles, New York City, and Miami.[4] This increasing diversity presents challenges and opportunities to researchers and practitioners. There are disparities in the educational outcomes of Latino and African Americans relative to whites and Asian Americans that foreshadow a bifurcation in the life trajectories of these broad groups. For instance, by 2050, 31% of the working-age population (18–64 years) will be Latino[5] but because they are currently less likely to become highly educated they will collectively likely continue to be at an occupational and economic disadvantage in that future.

CHALLENGES FOR ETHNIC AND/OR RACIAL MINORITY YOUTH IN THE TRANSITION
Risk for Health, Mental Health, and Substance Use Problems

The transition to young adulthood brings increased risk across multiple domains of health, and many of these risks are exacerbated in ethnic and racial minority youth.[6–8] Alcohol, substance, and tobacco use risk is highest at this point in development but these outcomes show differential risk for ethnic and/or racial minority young adults.[9] Typically, for alcohol and substance use, Latino youth demonstrate similar risk to non-Latino whites but black youth demonstrate lower levels of risk for use and disorder.[9] Yet, American Indian or Native youth demonstrate high levels of risk across substance use outcomes. The risk for sexually transmitted diseases is also highest in young adulthood, with black youth demonstrating the greatest risk.[7] Obesity risk also increases from adolescence, and Latino and black young adults demonstrate greater risk compared with non-Latino white youth.[8] Mental health and substance use disorders demonstrate high cost in young adulthood, serving as the primary contributor to disability.[6] Most lifetime psychiatric disorders also show an onset before age 24 years, highlighting the importance of understanding mental health at this developmental stage.[10] Overall, ethnic and/or racial minority transitional adults do not demonstrate greater risk for diagnosed mental health conditions.[11] The risk of suicide triples in young adulthood, with non-Latino white and American Indian or Native youth demonstrating the greatest risk.[7] Increases in epidemiologic risks can be understood partly through reductions in healthy behaviors that coincide with the transition to adulthood, including decreases in exercise, healthy eating habits, and preventative health care that are accompanied by increases in health risk behaviors (ie, substance use, sexual risk-taking).[12] Although not universal across all health behaviors, overall, black and Latino young adults demonstrated greater risk in many of these behaviors compared with non-Latino white and Asian youth (ie, food consumption, exercise, sexually transmitted disease risk, health care coverage) but not necessarily in substance use except tobacco use, where black adolescents demonstrated a greater growth in risk compared with non-Latino whites.

This stage of development thus carries significant health risks for all young adults, with some unique risks for ethnic minority youth. These risks are coupled with other contextual experiences that likely shape the trajectories of health for ethnic minority transitional adults. First, this stage in development is unique in that, unlike adolescence in which most youth are enrolled in an educational setting, transitional adults have diverse educational, familial, and occupational experiences that vary across race and/or ethnicity. Black and Latino young adults are less likely to be enrolled in postsecondary education, especially men.[6] Black men are the most likely to be neither employed nor enrolled in school compared with other ethnic groups.[6] Additionally, for those transitional youth in the workforce, these occupations will likely not translate to upward mobility because these are low-skilled jobs. Second, Latino and black transitional adults are more likely than their white counterparts to engage in family-building behaviors (ie, cohabitating, marriage, parenting) before age 25 years.[6] In terms of transition to parenting, black and Latina women are more likely to transition to this role outside of marriage compared with non-Latino white and Asian women.[6] Yet, this racial and/or ethnic risk is mitigated in higher socioeconomic status minority women, suggesting that socioeconomic position plays a significant role in risk for childbearing outside of partnerships. Third, black and Latino male young adults show a significantly greater risk of incarceration and/or participation in the justice system compared with non-Latino white young adults, which has broad ramifications for family relationships and ethnic minority communities. Fourth, as in other stages of development, black and Latino young adults are over-represented in poverty and face significant structural barriers to socioeconomic success. The intersection of race and socioeconomic position in understanding risk faced by these communities cannot be overstated.

CULTURAL STRESSORS UNDERMINE HEALTH ADAPTATION

The challenges that ethnic and/or racial minority transitional age youth (TAY) encounter due their ethnic and/or racial minority status are often referred to as cultural stressors. Cultural stressors refer to experiences of marginalization due to one's ethnic and/or racial group membership. Two important cultural stressors are (1) acculturative stress among immigrant-origin youth due to cultural and linguistic barriers and (2) discrimination due to ethnic or racial group membership.

Acculturative Stress

Young adults who are children of immigrants often encounter situations in which they have had to contend with competing expectations and norms of immigrant and host society cultures. The extent to which individuals experience such cultural conflicts as a stressor is known as acculturative stress.[13,14] Studies find that acculturative stress is linked to substance use, mental and physical health problems, and psychiatric disorder.[15,16] For example, in a community sample of Mexican American young adults aged 18 to 30 years, those reporting greater acculturative stress were more likely than their counterparts with less acculturative stress to have experienced trauma and to have a post-traumatic stress disorder (PTSD) diagnosis[16] and to evince alcohol dependence, substance dependence, and anxiety disorders.[15]

Discrimination

Young adults experience ethnic or racial discrimination in educational, work, and community settings that underscore the salience of their social exclusion in the United States The best available evidence suggests that 50% of Latinos aged 18 to 24 years (from the National Latino and Asian American Study [NLAAS]) and 87% of African American adolescents aged 13 to 17 years (from the National Survey of American Life) report having experienced ethnic or racial discrimination. Data from the NLAAS, which included Asian American adults aged 18 years and older, indicate that roughly 63% of the sample had experienced ethnic and/or racial discrimination.[17] Smaller, community-based studies provide similar statistics, underscoring the prevalence of this sort of social exclusion among diverse groups, including African Americans, Latinos, Asian Americans, and Arab American youth.[18–20]

A large literature has documented the negative impact of discrimination on mental and physical health outcomes throughout life and across socioeconomic strata,[21–23] and its negative effects can be partly attributed to the heightened activation of the stress response system. Efforts have focused on understanding the physical tolls associated with discrimination as measured through allostatic load (ie, dysregulation of body's stress response regulatory systems).[24] In a sample of African American youth, those who perceived greater discrimination throughout adolescence had worse allostatic load profiles at 20 years old but the effect was buffered by high levels of perceived emotional support.[25] Hypothalamic-pituitary-adrenal (HPA) axis functioning is one indicator of allostatic load, and other research has linked experiences of discrimination to flatter cortisol slopes in ethnic minority young adults compared with non-Latino whites.[26] Discrimination is also known to interfere with sleep among young adults,[27] and youth who encounter more discrimination and report lower daily sleep quality experience more depressive symptoms over time.[28] Institutional discrimination (ie, policies supporting residential segregation) is also associated with poorer health outcomes in ethnic minority communities, underscoring the need to conceptualize the discrimination–health link broadly.[29,30] Although few studies have focused on the impact of discrimination on mental health diagnoses per se, a review indicated that these experiences indeed predict clinical levels of symptoms.[30]

CULTURAL ASSETS AS RESILIENCE FACTORS

Within a risk and resilience framework, it is important to consider processes that mitigate risk, thereby enhancing the potential for resilient outcomes among young people.[31–33] Decades of research demonstrate that cultural assets can serve as risk-reducing and resilience-enhancing mechanisms among ethnic and racial minority and immigrant youth.[32–36] Important cultural assets include the development of a healthy ethnic-racial identity[32,34,35,37,38] and maintenance of cultural values within families[32,34,36,39,40] (see later discussion).

Ethnic-Racial Identity

Identity development, generally, and ethnic-racial identity, in particular, evolves significantly during transitional age period as youth seek to solidify their place in the world.[41,42] Meta-analytic studies suggest that having a positive sense of ethnic-racial identity is linked to a host of positive psychosocial benefits, including better interpersonal functioning and mood; fewer depressive symptoms; fewer internalizing, externalizing, and antisocial behaviors; less substance use and exposure and intention to use; and less risky attitudes toward sex.[37,38] There is also some evidence that ethnic-racial identity may support adaptive endocrine and immune functioning. In a community sample of Latina and African American women, those who believed that society viewed their ethnic and/or racial group more positively experienced lower levels of basal interleukin-6 (IL-6), which is known to be sensitive to social stress.[43] In addition, Latina women in the study who felt positively about their identities experienced higher basal dehydroepiandrosterone (DHEA) levels, a steroidal hormone thought to promote cellular resilience to stress. Numerous studies with behavioral measures suggest ethnic-racial identity also helps mitigate the negative psychological and physical sequelae of discrimination for blood pressure, mental health, psychological distress, perceived stress, aggressive behavior, violent behavior, and criminal offending among African American[44–46] and Latino youth.[47]

Cultural Values

A second cultural resilience factor is the maintenance of cultural values within young adults' family contexts.[36,39,40] Adherence to communalistic values, in particular, confers important psychosocial and health benefits to ethnic and/or racial minority youth.

Among youth of immigrant heritage, familism, which is a sense of deference toward, mutual support, and respect for family members, is a cultural value that is associated with numerous adjustment outcomes, including better emotional well-being, greater emotional persistence, and higher grade point averages.[36,39,48–51] Further, familistic behaviors seem to activate neural reward systems for Latinos. Evidence from neuro-imaging studies suggests there are cultural differences in young adults' social rewards from familial versus personal monetary contributions.[52] Specifically, white young adults showed greater recruitment of the mesolimbic reward system, including the ventral striatum, dorsal striatum, and ventral tegmental area when making personal monetary gains compared with family contributions. By contrast, Latino young adults showed similar or greater recruitment of these areas when contributing to their families compared with making personal gains. Among African American young adults, racial discrimination was associated with higher diastolic blood pressure (DBP) among those with lower endorsement of Africentric values, whereas it was unrelated to DBP among those who strongly endorsed such values.[45]

CHALLENGES AND OPPORTUNITIES FOR TRANSITIONAL AGE YOUTH

The transitional age period is one in which youth are becoming more aware of how so-cial marginalization affects their life chances. Youths' cultural assets inform how they cope with social marginalization and the potential realization that racism and xeno-phobia may be a fact of daily life for individuals like them. Thus, it is a critical time in which to promote positive coping mechanisms, including further cultivating cultural resilience-enhancing processes. Supporting the development of an adaptive ethnic-racial identity and maintenance of salient cultural values and supports within the family are protective processes by which to support resilience in the face of social marginal-ization experiences.

BEST PRACTICES IN SUPPORTING ETHNIC AND/OR RACIAL MINORITY TRANSITIONAL AGE YOUTH

As the United States continues to become more diverse, mental health practitioners will need to prepare to provide services to a rapidly changing population. Across pro-fessions, mental health practitioners are calling for better training on the develop-mental needs of TAY.[53–55] For ethnic minority TAY, practitioners need to consider the role of culturally based stress and resilience processes in conceptualizing the mental health needs of this population. Best practices that have been identified for mental health services at this transition for ethnic minority youth include attending to issues of self-determination and autonomy, linking TAY to opportunities and re-sources, facilitating help-seeking and coping skills, on-campus support groups, providing resources and information to families with limited English skills, addressing discrimination, exploring ethnic identity, and building on cultural values and tradi-tions.[53,54,56] Cognitive-behavioral approaches have been shown to be useful in treat-ing mental health problems in TAY broadly,[57] and newer studies have found a benefit of incorporating technology.[58]

Assessment is also a critical starting point for culturally competent care[59] because it helps clinicians determine current functioning, conceptualize the case, and plan for treatment. Thus, clinicians need to incorporate questions that assess for cultural iden-tity, values, and beliefs of ethnic minority TAY to not only harness their protective ef-fects but also to inform how these shape the experiences of this transition. TAY may be negotiating their cultural identity and values as they enter adulthood[60] and this negotiation may pose a risk for mental health.[61] For example, balancing familial obligations with college expectations may bring stress to first-generation Latino TAY.[49,54] Or, similarly within Asian American populations, academic stress may incorporate conflicting desires rooted in interdependent vis-à-vis independent values.[62] Assessments should also attend to issues of discrimination and racism becuse these may pose unique challenges to ethnic minority TAY adapting to environments that may be predominantly white (ie, workplace, college). The intersection of discrimination and the transition to adult roles may also lead to perceived limitations to future potential that may serve as barriers to completion of education and fulfilling career trajectories fueling mental health symptoms and substance use.[63] The *Diagnostic and Statistical Manual of Mental Disorders*, fifth edition, provides an example of an interview that incorporates culturally grounded questions but it would be necessary to modify these to the unique developmental context of TAY.[59]

These assessments may be necessary as families of color anticipate the transition and clinicians may be able to address the intersection of mental health; cultural risk or resilience; and critical transitions in education, employment, and family domains.[6] Helping TAY and families understand these transitions through cultural and developmental lenses may be especially useful. A social-psychological intervention that framed difficulties associated with transition to college as transient and typical led to greater academic competencies for African American college students compared with non-Latino whites.[64] Another intervention focused on forming culturally sensitive career support groups on campus that provided a space to talk with other Latinos who were transitioning to college life. Together, the students discussed myriad pertinent issues such as financial, personal, cultural, and academic stressors and received referrals from the group facilitator to appropriate on-campus and off-campus services as needed.[54] These efforts suggest that how stigmatized groups' appraisals of their experiences at this transition point may be key to supporting adaptation. Providing opportunities for TAY to reflect on stressors and develop coping skills is consistent with cultural models of resilience that focus on appraisals and coping in the face of discrimination.[34] These same strategies can be leveraged during the transition, as well help TAY make life choices consistent with their values, beliefs, and cultural identity.

One family-centered prevention was specifically developed to promote positive adaptation in African American TAY.[25,65,66] The Adults In the Making was designed to buffer the negative effects of chronic life stress in rural, African American teens as they were transitioning to adulthood by targeting key interpersonal, developmental, and cultural processes. The intervention focused on increasing emotional support, providing vocational coaching, and incorporating racial socialization messages to support youth in the transition. Overall, the prevention program led to less engagement in risk behaviors and improved substance use outcomes by decreasing cognitions associated with risk-behavior engagement. However, this protective effect was strongest for youth with combined genetic and environmental risk.[67] More interventions tackling this risky transition point for ethnic minority TAY are needed to continue to understand how to facilitate an adaptive transition and mitigate risk at this important developmental window.[6]

GAPS IN RESEARCH AND POLICY

Risk at this transition is especially notable for vulnerable TAY, including those involved in systems geared for children and youth (ie, special education, juvenile justice, foster care) in which youth transition out of these systems into adult systems.[68] Ethnic minority youth are over-represented in these systems due to multiple risk factors, such as systemic racism and poverty that contribute to poorer outcomes in adulthood.[68]

Therefore, policies are needed to help youth with multiple vulnerabilities find appropriate supports and services, and these services need to be coordinated across systems.[6,68] In particular, the juvenile justice system may need to attend to mental health issues to foment adaptive life skills necessary to support a successful transition.[6] Integrated health systems can provide an important avenue for population-wide interventions aimed at attenuating the elevated health risk of ethnic minority TAY that are the result of heightened allostatic load due to experiences of discrimination.[69] In these health contexts, mental health clinicians can serve as the frontline in providing behavioral consultation to promote engagement in health behaviors in a culturally consonant fashion.[69] Policy recommendations center on the coordination of care across systems and health programs that target TAY.[6,52,68] More efforts are needed that target TAY who are not connected to larger systems and who are not college-enrolled and that can be delivered within work settings.[6] Finally, policies aimed at facilitating the transitions across the pediatric and adult health care settings will be critical in supporting the health of TAY youth.[6]

One of the primary differences between the child and adult mental health treatment is parental involvement; however, how best to integrate families into treatment is not well delineated at this phase in development. Given the collectivistic, familistic orientation of many communities of color, it is important for clinicians to continue to include families in treatment.[70] For the most part, the specific developmental needs of TAY youth of color has not been attention of clinical intervention research, and intervention studies specifically targeting the intersection of culture and this developmental stage are necessary to inform evidenced based practice.[6]

SUMMARY

Developmental science suggests multiple ways to support the positive life outcomes of racial minorities and immigrant heritage youth. Building on cultural assets in such youths' selves, families, and communities is an important step toward serving them well. Researchers and practitioners must strive to build their capacity to keep pace with the demographic shifts of the United States youth population.

REFERENCES

1. Table 10. Resident population by race, Hispanic origin, and age: 2000 and 2009. U.S. Census Bureau, Statistical Abstract of the United States: 2012. Available at: https://www.census.gov/prod/2011pubs/12statab/pop.pdf. Accessed December 31, 2016.
2. 2012 National Population Projections - People and Households - U.S. Census Bureau. Censusgov. 2016. Available at: http://www.census.gov/population/projections/data/national/2012.html. Accessed October 6, 2016.
3. 2014 National Population Projections - People and Households - U.S. Census Bureau. Censusgov. 2016. Available at: http://www.census.gov/population/projections/data/national/2014.html. Accessed October 6, 2016.
4. U.S. Census Bureau. Migration by race and Hispanic origin: 1995 to 2000. U.S. Washington, DC: Department of Commerce Economics and Statistics Administration; 2016.
5. 2008 National Population Projections - People and Households - U.S. Census Bureau. Censusgov. 2016. Available at: http://www.census.gov/population/projections/data/national/2008.html. Accessed October 7, 2016.
6. Bonnie R, Stroud C, Breiner H. Investing in the health and well-being of young adults. Washington, DC: National Academies Press; 2014.

7. Park M, Paul Mulye T, Adams S, et al. The health status of young adults in the United States. J Adolesc Health 2006;39(3):305–17.

8. Park M, Scott J, Adams S, et al. Adolescent and young adult health in the United States in the past decade: little improvement and young adults remain worse off than adolescents. J Adolesc Health 2014;55(1):3–16.

9. Johnston L, O'Malley P, Bachman J. Monitoring the future: national results on adolescent drug use: overview of key findings. FOCUS 2003;1(2):213–34.

10. Kessler R, Chiu W, Demler O, et al. Prevalence, severity, and comorbidity of 12-month DSM-IV disorders in the national comorbidity survey replication. Arch Gen Psychiatry 2005;62(6):617.

11. Breslau J, Aguilar-Gaxiola S, Kendler K, et al. Specifying race-ethnic differences in risk for psychiatric disorder in a USA national sample. Psychol Med 2005; 36(01):57.

12. Harris KM, Gordon-Larsen P, Chantala K, et al. Longitudinal trends in race/ethnic disparities in leading health indicators from adolescence to young adulthood. Arch Pediatr Adolesc Med 2006;160(1):74–81.

13. Gil A, Vega W, Dimas J. Acculturative stress and personal adjustment among Hispanic adolescent boys. J Community Psychol 1994;22(1):43–54.

14. Gil A, Wagner E, Vega W. Acculturation, familism, and alcohol use among Latino adolescent males: longitudinal relations. J Community Psychol 2000;28(4): 443–58.

15. Ehlers CL, Gilder DA, Criado JR, et al. Acculturation stress, anxiety disorders, and alcohol dependence in a select population of young adult Mexican Americans. J Addict Med 2009;3(4):227–33.

16. Ehlers C, Kim C, Gilder D, et al. Lifetime history of traumatic events in a young adult Mexican American sample: relation to substance dependence, affective disorder, acculturation stress, and PTSD. J Psychiatr Res 2016;83:79–85.

17. Chae D, Takeuchi D, Barbeau E, et al. Unfair treatment, racial/ethnic discrimination, ethnic identification, and smoking among Asian Americans in the national Latino and Asian American study. Am J Public Health 2008;98(3):485–92.

18. Thompson T, Kiang L, Witkow M. "You're Asian; You're supposed to be smart": adolescents' experiences with the Model Minority Stereotype and longitudinal links with identity. Asian Am J Psychol 2016;7(2):108–19.

19. Witherspoon D, Seaton E, Rivas-Drake D. Neighborhood characteristics and expectations of racially discriminatory experiences among African American adolescents. Child Dev 2016;87(5):1367–78.

20. Sirin S, Fine M. Hyphenated selves: Muslim American youth negotiating identities on the fault lines of global conflict. Appl Dev Sci 2007;11(3):151–63.

21. Syed M, Juan M. Discrimination and psychological distress: examining the moderating role of social context in a nationally representative sample of Asian American adults. Asian Am J Psychol 2012;3(2):104–20.

22. Williams D, Mohammed S. Discrimination and racial disparities in health: evidence and needed research. J Behav Med 2008;32(1):20–47.

23. Williams D, Neighbors H, Jackson J. Racial/ethnic discrimination, and health: findings from community studies. Am J Public Health 2003;93(2):200–8.

24. Schulkin J, editor. Allostasis, Homeostasis, and the costs of physiological adaptation. Cambridge (United Kingdom): Cambridge University Press; 2004.

25. Brody G, Lei M, Chae D, et al. Perceived discrimination among African American adolescents and allostatic load: a longitudinal analysis with buffering effects. Child Dev 2014;85(3):989–1002.

26. Zeiders K, Hoyt L, Adam E. Associations between self-reported discrimination and diurnal cortisol rhythms among young adults: the moderating role of racial-ethnic minority status. Psychoneuroendocrinology 2014;50:280–8.
27. Zeiders K, Updegraff K, Kuo S, et al. Perceived discrimination and Mexican-origin young adults' sleep duration and variability: the moderating role of cultural orientations. J Youth Adolesc 2016. http://dx.doi.org/10.1007/s10964-016-0544-9.
28. Yip T. The effects of ethnic/racial discrimination and sleep quality on depressive symptoms and self-esteem trajectories among diverse adolescents. J Youth Adolesc 2014;44(2):419–30.
29. Gee G. A multilevel analysis of the relationship between institutional and individual racial discrimination and health status. Am J Public Health 2002;92(4):615–23.
30. Mays V, Cochran S, Barnes N. Race, race-based discrimination, and health outcomes among African Americans. Annu Rev Psychol 2007;58(1):201–25.
31. Zimmerman M, Stoddard S, Eisman A, et al. Adolescent resilience: promotive factors that inform prevention. Child Dev Perspect 2013;7(4):215–20.
32. Coll C, Lamberty G, Jenkins R, et al. An integrative model for the study of developmental competencies in minority children. Child Dev 1996;67(5):1891.
33. Cameron C, Ungar M, Liebenberg L. Cultural understandings of resilience: roots for wings in the development of affective resources for resilience. Child Adolesc Psychiatr Clin N Am 2007;16:285–301.
34. Neblett E, Rivas-Drake D, Umaña-Taylor A. The promise of racial and ethnic protective factors in promoting ethnic minority youth development. Child Dev Perspect 2012;6(3):295–303.
35. Rivas-Drake D, Seaton E, Markstrom C, et al. Ethnic and racial identity in adolescence: implications for psychosocial, academic, and health outcomes. Child Dev 2014;85(1):40–57.
36. Stein G, Cupito A, Mendez J, et al. Familism through a developmental lens. J Latina/o Psychol 2014;2(4):224–50.
37. Rivas-Drake D, Syed M, Umaña-Taylor A, et al. Feeling good, happy, and proud: a meta-analysis of positive ethnic-racial affect and adjustment. Child Dev 2014; 85(1):77–102.
38. Smith T, Silva L. Ethnic identity and personal well-being of people of color: a meta-analysis. J Couns Psychol 2011;58(1):42–60.
39. Fuligni A, Pedersen S. Family obligation and the transition to young adulthood. Dev Psychol 2002;38(5):856–68.
40. Tseng V. Family interdependence and academic adjustment in college: youth from immigrant and U.S.-born families. Child Dev 2004;75(3):966–83.
41. Syed M, Azmitia M. Longitudinal trajectories of ethnic identity during the college years. J Res Adolesc 2009;19(4):601–24.
42. Rivas-Drake D, Witherspoon D. Racial identity from adolescence to young adulthood: does prior neighborhood experience matter? Child Dev 2013;84(6): 1918–32.
43. Ratner K, Halim M, Amodio D. Perceived stigmatization, ingroup pride, and immune and endocrine activity: evidence from a community sample of black and Latina women. Social Psychol Personal Sci 2012;4(1):82–91.
44. Sellers R, Caldwell C, Schmeelk-Cone K, et al. Racial identity, racial discrimination, perceived stress, and psychological distress among African American young adults. J Health Social Behav 2003;44(3):302.
45. Neblett E, Carter S. The protective role of racial identity and Africentric worldview in the association between racial discrimination and blood pressure. Psychosomatic Med 2012;74(5):509–16.

46. Caldwell C, Kohn-Wood L, Schmeelk-Cone K, et al. Racial discrimination and racial identity as risk or protective factors for violent behaviors in African American young adults. Am J Community Psychol 2004;33(1–2):91–105.

47. Umaña-Taylor A, Tynes B, Toomey R, et al. Latino adolescents' perceived discrimination in online and offline settings: an examination of cultural risk and protective factors. Dev Psychol 2015;51(1):87–100.

48. Rudolph B. Filial responsibility among Mexican American college students: a pilot investigation and comparison. J Hispanic Higher Educ 2005;4(1):64–78.

49. Sanchez B, Esparza P, Colon Y, et al. Tryin' to make it during the transition from high school: the role of family obligation attitudes and economic context for Latino-emerging adults. J Adolesc Res 2010;25(6):858–84.

50. Sy S. Family and work influences on the transition to college among Latina adolescents. Hispanic J Behav Sci 2006;28(3):368–86.

51. Stein G, Rivas-Drake D, Camacho T. Ethnic identity and familism among Latino college students: a test of prospective associations. Emerging Adulthood 2016. http://dx.doi.org/10.1177/2167696816657234.

52. Telzer E, Masten C, Berkman E, et al. Gaining while giving: an fMRI study of the rewards of family assistance among white and Latino youth. Social Neurosci 2010;5(5–6):508–18.

53. MacLeod K, Brownlie E. Mental health and transitions from adolescence to emerging adulthood: developmental and diversity considerations. Can J Commun Ment Health 2014;33(1):77–86.

54. Berríos-Allison A. Career support group for Latino/a college students. J Coll Couns 2011;14(1):80–95.

55. Derenne J, Martel A. A model CSMH curriculum for child and adolescent psychiatry training programs. Acad Psychiatry 2015;39(5):512–6.

56. Fuligni A, Hardway C. Preparing diverse adolescents for the transition to adulthood. Future Child 2004;14(2):98.

57. Christensen H, Pallister E, Smale S, et al. Community-based prevention programs for anxiety and depression in youth: a systematic review. J Prim Prev 2010;31(3):139–70.

58. Farrer L, Gulliver A, Chan JK, et al. Technology-based interventions for mental health in tertiary students: systematic review. J Med Internet Res 2013;15(5):e101.

59. Lewis-Fernández R, Aggarwal N, Bäärnhielm S, et al. Culture and psychiatric evaluation: operationalizing cultural formulation for DSM-5. Psychiatry Interpersonal Biol Process 2014;77(2):130–54.

60. Schwartz SJ, Unger JB, Zamboanga BL, et al. Rethinking the concept of acculturation: implications for theory and research. Am Psychol 2010;65(4):237.

61. Phinney JS. Ethnic identity exploration in emerging adulthood. In: Arnett JJ, Tanner JL, editors. Emerging adults in America: coming of age in the 21st century. Washington, DC: American Psychological Association; 2006. p. 117–34.

62. Kwan KLK. Counseling Chinese peoples: perspectives of filial piety. Asian J Couns 2000;7(1):23–41.

63. Hammack P. Toward a unified theory of depression among urban African American youth: integrating socioecologic, cognitive, family stress, and biopsychosocial perspectives. J Black Psychol 2003;29(2):187–209.

64. Walton G, Cohen G. A brief social-belonging intervention improves academic and health outcomes of minority students. Science 2011;331(6023):1447–51.

65. Brody G, Chen Y, Kogan S, et al. Buffering effects of a family-based intervention for African American emerging adults. J Marriage Fam 2010;72(5):1426–35.

66. Brody G, Yu T, Chen Y, et al. The adults in the making program: long-term protective stabilizing effects on alcohol use and substance use problems for rural African American emerging adults. J Consulting Clin Psychol 2012;80(1):17–28.

67. Brody G, Yu T, Beach S. A differential susceptibility analysis reveals the "who and how" about adolescents' responses to preventive interventions: tests of first- and second-generation Gene × Intervention hypotheses. DevPsychopathol 2015; 27(01):37–49.

68. Osgood D, Foster EM, Courtney ME. Vulnerable populations and the transition to adulthood. Future Child 2010;20(1):209–29.

69. Holden K, McGregor B, Thandi P, et al. Toward culturally centered integrative care for addressing mental health disparities among ethnic minorities. Psychol Serv 2014;11(4):357–68.

70. Sue DW, Sue D. Counseling the culturally diverse: theory and practice. Hoboken (NJ): John Wiley & Sons; 2012.

Special Populations

Transitioning to Adulthood from Foster Care

Terry Lee, MD[a],*, Wynne Morgan, MD[b]

KEYWORDS

- Foster care • Foster home care • Foster child • Child welfare • Youth
- Transition to adulthood • Transition age

KEY POINTS

- Foster youth do not usually receive the types of family support their nonfoster peers enjoy when transitioning to adulthood; foster youth often experience multiple adversities that increase their risk for negative outcomes.
- Foster care alumni are more likely to experience lower educational attainment, unemployment, poverty, homelessness, food insecurity, mental health and substance use challenges, health problems, early parenthood, and justice system involvement.
- Federal legislation recognizes a state responsibility to act in the parent role for state dependents transitioning to adulthood, and the need to provide transition services.
- Stakeholders are developing promising practices to improve foster youth transition to adulthood. More research is needed to assess the effectiveness and efficiency of existing programs, and to inform program development and improvement.
- Much more research of transition age foster youth is needed. Policies must support effective transition services that are developmentally appropriate, accessible, responsive, continuous, enduring, coordinated, and integrated.

INTRODUCTION

The transition from adolescence to young adulthood in the United States is increasingly lengthy and complicated. Transitional age youth (TAY) face more challenges than previous generations.[1] Many TAY benefit from emotional, pragmatic, and financial support from their parents and kin, but foster youth do not typically enjoy these types of family support.[2] Furthermore, many foster youth experience adverse events that increase risk for problematic emancipation, including neglect, abuse, trauma,

The authors have nothing to disclose.
[a] Division of Public Behavioral Health and Justice Policy, Department of Psychiatry and Behavioral Sciences, University of Washington School of Medicine, 2815 Eastlake Avenue East, Suite #200, Seattle, WA 98102, USA; [b] Department of Psychiatry, University of Massachusetts Medical School, 55 Lake Avenue North, Worcester, MA 01655, USA
* Corresponding author.
E-mail address: drterry@uw.edu

Child Adolesc Psychiatric Clin N Am 26 (2017) 283–296
http://dx.doi.org/10.1016/j.chc.2016.12.008
1056-4993/17/© 2016 Elsevier Inc. All rights reserved.

childpsych.theclinics.com

disrupted attachments, unstable housing, multiple placements, fragmented schooling, disrupted social networks, poverty, and gestational exposures. These realities increase the risk that foster care alumni will experience negative functional outcomes, including lower education attainment, unemployment, poverty, homelessness, food insecurity, mental health and substance use challenges, health problems, early pregnancy and parenthood, and involvement with the justice system.

CHILD WELFARE AND DEMOGRAPHICS

The federal 1997 Adoption and Safe Families Act established three national goals for child welfare: (1) safety, (2) well-being, and (3) permanency. The concept of well-being encompasses social-emotional health and medical and educational needs.[3] Permanency is a concept based on the value that youth grow up best in a family environment that is committed, long-lasting, nurturing, and stable. Despite child welfare agencies' mandates and efforts to establish permanent homes for youth in foster care, some youth emancipate from foster care when they turn 18 or 21 years old or achieve a high school diploma, sometimes referred to as "aging out." By definition, youth who age out of foster care did not achieve permanency. Approximately 700,000 youth are substantiated maltreatment victims each year.[4] On any given day, the number of youth in foster care hovers around 400,000 youth nationally, down from just more than 500,000 in 2002. The average length of stay is 22 months, and foster youth older than 12 are less likely to achieve permanency.[5] About 26,000 foster youth age out of services annually, most at age 18. Recent changes to federal law allow states to provide foster care to youth up to age 21, also known as extended foster care (EFC), and claim federal reimbursement. Among all foster youth, 30% are between the ages of 12 and 17 and 4% are between 18 and 21 years old. Most older youth in foster care entered care as adolescents. Reunification is the most common exit for foster youth of all ages, and around 40% of adolescent foster youth reunify with family.[6] African American and Native American youth have the highest rates of representation in the child welfare system at 17.4 and 14.1 per 1000 youth, respectively, compared with 5.8 for Hispanic, 4.6 for white youth, and 1.3 for Asian youth.[7,8]

TRANSITIONAL AGE FOSTER YOUTH BEHAVIORAL HEALTH CONCERNS

Upward of 80% of foster youth have developmental, behavioral, or mental health concerns.[9,10] Foster care alumni have higher rates of mental health disorders than the general population. For instance, posttraumatic stress disorder rates among foster care alumni are nearly five times that of the general population and exceed rates of war veterans; and posttraumatic stress disorder recovery rates for foster care alumni are 28%, compared with 47% for the general population.[11] Compared with nonfoster peers, foster youth and alumni also have higher rates of substance use disorders. More changes in foster placement and schools are associated with higher rates of alcohol use disorder.[12,13] Compared with other Medicaid-eligible youth, foster youth have higher rates of behavioral health expenditures.[14]

Foster youth are prescribed psychotropic medications at two to eight times the rate of other Medicaid-eligible youth.[15] Higher rates of foster youth mental health disorders may explain some degree of higher psychotropic prescription rates. However, foster youth are also at risk for inappropriate overprescription and underprescription of psychotropic medications. Foster youth are at risk for inappropriate prescribing because of limited access to youth behavioral health information and history; fragmented and/ or inadequately coordinated care; insufficient time for assessment, treatment, and collaboration; undiagnosed or misdiagnosed trauma-related conditions; limited access to effective psychosocial and psychiatric treatments; and ineffective advocacy for foster youth.[16]

UNIQUE CHALLENGES IN THE TRANSITION TO ADULTHOOD

Youth in the child welfare system have been exposed to traumatic events that are often chronic and cumulative. They often lack the protection and support of a parent or caregiver to help buffer the effects of trauma. Exposure to chronic trauma has a direct effect on youth mental and physical health. This phenomenon has been conceptualized as "toxic stress." Toxic stress chronically activates the body's neuroendocrine stress response system.[17] This activation has a direct negative effect on gene translation, immune system response, and neurodevelopment.[18] Chronic glucocorticoid exposure from the toxic stress response has a direct effect on key areas of the developing brain including the amygdala, hippocampus, and prefrontal cortex. These changes interfere with the development of emotion regulation, impulse control, concentration, and decision-making. An emerging body of research has shown toxic stress may impact the way genes are transcribed through epigenetic changes to DNA expression. These epigenetic changes may influence how the body responds to stress, and impact physical and mental health.[19] Toxic stress also has a direct effect on physical health. A large body of research shows that youth in foster care, compared with nonfoster peers, have increased rates of acute and chronic infections, asthma, and obesity. This is caused by the physical sequelae of trauma, but also directly related to toxic stress–induced chronic immune response and inflammation. Poor health outcomes persist into adulthood for foster care alumni, with higher risk of chronic health conditions.[20]

In addition to complex mental and physical health needs, transitional age foster youth also have complex social needs. Social supports are critical determinants of physical and mental health. Foster youth transitioning out of care often lack the support network so greatly used by their nonfoster peers as they take on more independence. Multiple moves and school settings make it difficult to form and maintain relationships. Disrupted social networks are linked to higher rates of emotional distress. These frequent moves and traumas can also instill a lack of trust in people.[21] A lack of social supports and connectedness increases the risk of negative outcomes.

If not already connected, youth transitioning out of care often reconnect with their family of origin. About 64% of transitional age foster youth reported feeling very or somewhat close to their birth mothers. If they were living with relatives, nearly 95% of youth reported feeling very or somewhat close to those relatives.[22] Although birth families can provide critical support during transition, reconnecting with families can also be stressful for youth. Before aging out, systems should be put in place to help foster youth make informed decisions around reconnecting, form realistic expectations, establish appropriate boundaries, navigate family of origin interactions, and develop skills to address possible negative interactions.

FOSTER CARE ALUMNI YOUNG ADULT OUTCOMES

Researchers have begun studying young adult outcomes of foster youth. The Northwest Foster Care Alumni Study combined case reviews and interviews of almost 500 foster care alumni ages 20 to 33 in Oregon and Washington, shedding light on the challenges for this vulnerable population.[11] More than half of the foster care alumni experienced at least one mental health problem in the previous year and more than 20% experienced homelessness within a year of exiting foster care. About 80% were employed (compared with 95% of the same-age general population), one-third had household incomes at or below the poverty level (three times the poverty rate of the general population), and one-third did not have health insurance (double the same-age national rate). The Midwest Study was undertaken to develop a more comprehensive view of foster youth transition to adulthood. In this study youth were followed from age 17 or 18 through 26 with five waves of data collection.[2] This study highlighted disparities in multiple domains. At age 26, former foster youth were three times more likely than same-age peers to not have a high school diploma or GED (20% vs 6%), whereas same-age peers were six times more likely to have a postsecondary degree (46% vs 8%) and nine times more likely to have a 4-year college degree (36% vs 4%). About 50% of female foster care alumni had been pregnant by age 19, a rate 2.5 times that of nonfoster peers.[23] At age 26, female foster care alumni were 7 to 10 times more likely to have been arrested (41% vs 5%), convicted (22% vs 3%), and incarcerated (33% vs 3%) since age 18, whereas male foster care alumni reported three-fold to seven-fold increases (68% vs 22%, 47% vs 11%, and 64% vs 9%, respectively).[2]

BEST PRACTICES SUPPORTING FOSTER YOUTH TRANSITION TO ADULTHOOD
Resiliency and Strengths Orientations

Child welfare systems value strengths-based approaches and resilience orientations.[16] Masten[24] defined resilience as a class of phenomenon characterized by good outcomes despite serious threats to adaptation or development, and emphasized that resilience is a common rather than extraordinary characteristic of individuals. Ungar[25] conceptualized resilience among maltreated youth as an interactive process between youth and their social ecology, which is influenced by youth individual characteristics (temperament and personality), the social determinants of health affecting youth and their caregivers, the quality of services provided by stakeholder agencies, and government policies addressing high-risk populations. Resilience is promoted by ensuring the availability and accessibility of social supports and formal services, and program flexibility to address individual youth-specific needs. A resilience orientation portends a strengths-based approach that identifies and enhances protective factors in a youth's ecology. Foster youth strengths often include persistence, resourcefulness, determination, grit, and self-reliance. Latent class analysis identified four subgroups of young adults in the Midwest Study. The subgroup termed "accelerated adults" who viewed themselves as "having to grow up fast" and "take on adult responsibilities" tended to have better outcomes, such as higher rates of employment and decreased involvement in the criminal justice system. This group comprised about one-third of the study participants and was mostly female.[26] The Midwest Study also found that foster youth with high school diplomas or GEDs were almost twice as likely to be employed as adults,[27] and placement stability correlated with high school graduation in the Casey Family Alumni Study.[28]

Encouraging mentoring relationships can promote success. Foster youth with a positive and significant relationship with at least one adult, compared with nonmentored foster youth, fare better on general health, feelings of stress, education attainment, physical aggression, suicidality, arrests, and sexually transmitted diseases.[21] Some supportive adults enter youths' lives through interactions with the child welfare system. Important qualities of the mentoring relationship include trust, consistency, empathy, and authenticity. Transitional age foster youth value mentors who are understanding and nonjudgmental, provide direct communication and advice, and have similar life experiences that they share.[29]

Federally Legislated Transitional Age Foster Youth Supports

Federal legislation, including the 1999 Foster Care Independence Act and the 2008 Fostering Connections to Success and Increasing Adoptions Act, establishes several services and practices to facilitate foster youth transition to adulthood. A transition plan must be developed 90 days before discharge from foster care. The transition plan must be youth-directed and address housing, health insurance, education, opportunities for mentors and continuing support services, and workforce supports and employment services. Federal legislation requires states to develop oversight practices and coordination of health care, including behavioral health, and encourages mechanisms for ensuring continuity of care and transition to adult health care systems. Federal legislation offers funding to states to help with education, employment, financial literacy, housing, life skills training, transition services, emotional support, and encouraging relationships with caring adults. The Affordable Care Act extends Medicaid eligibility to foster care alumni up to age 26.

The Education and Training Vouchers Program is a federal program providing financial assistance (currently up to $5000/year) to foster youth and alumni enrolled in college, university, vocational, or technical training programs. Youth must enroll before their 21st birthday and remain eligible until age 23. Some states provide additional financial assistance for foster or former foster youth postsecondary education.

Federal legislation also provides individual states the option to provide developmentally modified foster care services (EFC), to foster youth up to age 21. To qualify for EFC, youth must be in an education or training program; working; in a program to address barriers to schooling, training, or work; or suffering a disability that prevents schooling or work. The Midwest Study examined EFC effects. At the time of the study, Illinois offered foster care up to age 21, whereas Iowa and Wisconsin terminated foster care at age 18. At age 19, youth in Wisconsin and Iowa were 2.7 times more likely to be homeless than foster youth in Illinois,[30] and youth remaining in foster care were at least twice as likely to complete at least 1 year of college by age 21. Courtney, and colleagues[31,32] estimated that each dollar spent on EFC returned $2.40 in increased income, based on anticipated higher college graduation rates. To avoid disincentives to permanency, EFC, independent living programs (ILPs), and education and training supports can also be made available to youth exiting foster care through guardianship at age 16 or older.

Transition Readiness Assessment

The Casey Life Skills Web site contains resources for youth and coaches (providers or caregivers) to help foster youth achieve their long-term goals. The Casey Life Skills Assessment is a tool that helps youth to self-evaluate the behaviors and competencies necessary for successful transition to adulthood (casey.org-lifeskills). The competency domains are listed in **Table 1**.

After the Casey Life Skills Assessment, youth and coaches can use the Resources to Inspire Guide to develop a plan for acquiring needed skills. The guide contains suggestions for free or low-cost life skills training resources, and encourages searching for additional resources.

Promising Practices

The California Evidence-Based Clearinghouse for Child Welfare (cebc4cw.org) is an online resource whose mission is to "advance the effective implementation of evidence-based practices for children and families involved with the child welfare system." The site includes a program registry and ratings of the strength of evidence for

Table 1
Casey life skills domains

Life Skills	Competencies Assessed
Daily living	Nutrition, menu planning, grocery shopping, meal preparation, table manners, kitchen cleanup, food storage, home cleanliness, home safety, home repairs, computer and Internet basics, and leisure time
Self-care	Healthy physical and emotional development, health care, personnel benefits, personal hygiene, and sexuality
Relationships and communication	Developing and sustaining healthy relationships, personal development, communication skills, cultural competency, domestic violence, and permanent relations with caring adults
Housing and money management	Housing, budgeting and spending plan, banking and credit, and transportation
Work and study	Basics of employment, study skills, time management, personal development, income tax, and legal issues
Career and education planning	Planning for career and postsecondary education, work goals, employment, and work place communications
Looking forward	Youth's level of confidence and internal feelings important to their success
Permanency	Embedded within all of the skill areas are items that assess youth's connection to trusted adults, support network, and overall interdependent connections

From Casey Family Programs. Casey living skills assessment practitioners guide. Available at: http://www.casey.org/media/CLS_project_PracticeGuide.pdf. Used with permission.

specific programs and practices. Youth Transitioning into Adulthood is one topic area.[33] At this time, all Youth Transitioning into Adulthood programs are rated "Not Able to Rate" because of a lack of available research evidence. This highlights the need for more research and program evaluation. Some of these programs target individual functional domains, such as social supports, housing, education, employment, living skills, financial literacy, health, and mental health. Other programs are more comprehensive and target multiple domains. Some are child welfare–specific, whereas others target general high-risk TAY. These target domains were identified through interviews with foster care alumni and stakeholders, and research on long-term outcomes.

Mentoring

Relationships with caring nonfamilial adults can enhance youth resiliency.[21] The Caring Adults R Everywhere program is a manualized 12-week mentoring intervention designed to bolster social supports by developing and strengthening existing relationships between youth and supportive adults from the youth's natural ecology.[34,35] A master's-trained social worker (not the youth's child welfare worker), called an interventionist, meets with a youth aging out of foster care to identify an appropriate mentor. After screening and approval, mentors undergo training in adolescent development, the child welfare system, trauma-informed mentoring, practices of effective mentors, what to do with one's mentee, and establishing and maintaining boundaries. Youth and mentors participate in group activities and one-on-one sessions with the interventionist to strengthen and clarify expectations for the mentoring relationship.

Homelessness

Foster youth experience homelessness at much higher rates than their same age peers. The My First Place (MFP) program, located in the San Francisco Bay Area, targets transitional age foster youth at risk for homelessness.[36,37] The program typically lasts 18 to 24 months and is comprised of six core elements as follows:

1. Ongoing case management by a Youth Advocate, the primary case manager, and an Education and Employment Specialist. Foster youth work with both to achieve specific goals in the area of housing, education, employment, and healthy living.
2. MFP uses scattered site housing throughout the five-county region. The program seeks housing in safe neighborhoods near public transportation. MFP typically signs a master lease with landlords, and then subleases units to program participants. Youth receive training on tenancy.
3. MFP has a property management department that maintains relationships with landlords and affordable housing partners, rents apartments, manages subleasing, oversees move-ins, and manages rent payment. The department also deals with tenant issues, such as property damage, maintenance, and compliance with regulations.
4. A larger organization infrastructure provides administrative and clinical support.
5. The organizational culture focuses on the quality of on-the-ground implementation.
6. MFP collaborates with community partners, including referral sources for program youth, education and employment partners, and health and mental health provider agencies.

Financial Literacy

Limited financial knowledge and capabilities can undermine efforts to achieve financial stability. MyPath Saving is a financial knowledge and skills program for economically disadvantaged youth earning their first paychecks.[38,39] The program provides financial education, familiarizes youth to conventional financial products, and uses experiential teaching with peer learning and support. Topics and skills include direct deposit, checking and restricted savings accounts, and savings incentives. Youth are aided to open accounts, set up direct deposit, set a savings goal, and save a designated portion of each paycheck; and provided incentives to meet savings goals.

Postsecondary Education Support

Most foster youth aspire to attend college. However, foster youth enroll in and graduate from college at much lower rates than their nonfoster peers.[40] Foster youth often report that few people in their lives expect and/or encourage them to attend and succeed in college. In addition, foster youth experience several risk factors that negatively impact education, including disrupted schooling, few college preparatory classes, learning disabilities, behavioral health concerns, and poverty.[41] Several states are developing programs to support foster youth and alumni in postsecondary education, including college, community college, and vocational training. More than 30 states provide scholarships, grants, or tuition waivers to foster youth attending higher education.[42]

Casey Family Programs developed Supporting Success, a resource for improving higher education outcomes for students from foster care.[42] It identifies and discusses 12 core program elements for improving outcomes, listed in **Box 1**.

The Seita Scholars Program is a campus-based support program for foster youth and alumni attending Western Michigan University.[43,44] The program is named after Dr John Seita, a graduate of the Michigan child welfare system and Western Michigan

---

Box 1
Casey family programs improving higher education outcomes for students from foster care

Six Elements Necessary for Program Development
1. Designated leadership: Youth from foster care need a caring, trusted staff person or designated lead who has primary responsibility for identifying them and consistently providing guidance in navigating higher education.
2. Internal and external champions: Support champions within and outside of the college community provide direct and indirect program support through their influence and advocacy.
3. Collaborations with community agencies: College support programs should have strong connections with local social services agencies, foundations, and the independent living (IL) programs operated by state child welfare systems.
4. Data-driven decision making: Decisions on individual support and program development should be based on data collection and analysis.
5. Staff peer support and professional development: New and established support program staff benefit from belonging to a network of peers in other colleges who support youth from foster care.
6. Sustainability planning: Explicit planning should be undertaken to sustain successful support initiatives.

Three Elements to Provide Direct Student Support: Phase 1
7. Year-round housing and other basic needs: Youth from foster care need to have priority for available campus housing and access to year-round housing. For campuses without dormitories, they need assistance in finding stable, safe, affordable housing, transportation, and food services.
8. Financial aid: Youth from foster care need a financial aid package that maximizes funds to cover the cost of attendance and minimizes or eliminates the need for loans.
9. Academic advising, career counseling, and supplemental support: Youth from foster care benefit from frequent contact with knowledgeable academic and career counselors with whom they develop a trust relationship.

Three Additional Elements to Provide Direct Student Support: Phase 2
10. Personal guidance, counseling, and supplemental support: Personal guidance, mental health counseling, supplemental support, and health insurance are essential for youth coming from care because of their early independence, history of abuse, neglect, or abandonment.
11. Opportunities for student community engagement and leadership: Youth from foster care benefit from inclusion and engagement with campus activities. Some seek out opportunities to be with other youth from foster care, whereas others choose to avoid such association. Colleges should provide opportunities for students to engage in college life including developing a sense of community and developing leadership and advocacy skills.
12. Planned transitions, to college between colleges, from college to employment: Youth from foster care need assistance in planning for college, making application, and beginning their college careers. Once on track to complete an associate of arts degree, many require help transferring to a 4-year college. As they near completion of college, most students need help making a successful transition to a career. Each of these three transitions involves letting go of one academic home and adjusting to a new one. This adjustment has a different meaning for youth without family support.

From Casey Family Programs. Supporting success: a framework for program enhancement version 2.0. 2010. p. 13–4. Available at: http://www.casey.org/media/SupportingSuccess.pdf. Accessed September 12, 2016. Used with permission.

University. Coaches provide support to students in the program (Seita Scholars) with focus on lifespan development domains suggested by Casey Family Programs: academics, finances and employment, housing, physical and mental health care, social relationships and community connections, cultural and personal identity, and life skills. The program includes a scholarship at Western Michigan University. Students reside on campus and have access to 24-hour on-call support and emergency financial resources. The program uses trained Master's-level Campus Coaches, and provides training and certification for professionals working with college students who have been involved in the foster care system or other high-risk youth.

Independent Living Programs

Federal legislation provides funds to states to offer ILPs to assist foster youth and alumni transitioning to adulthood. Program components typically involve social-emotional supports, mentoring, housing, education and training, employment, daily living skills, health and behavioral health, and financial literacy.

The Orangewood ILP was developed by the Orangewood Foundation, and provides workshops, special events, mentoring, and case management to foster youth 16 to 21 years old to help prepare them for the transition to independence.[45] Each month the ILP focuses on one of four key areas (education, career, relationships, and daily living), providing workshops and take-home activities. Youth can earn ILP Dollars by participating in workshops and special events, and completing take-home assignments. Examples of take-home activities include writing an interview thank you letter (career), completing a change of address form or getting a credit report (daily living), completing a FAFSA application (education), and identifying one's core values or completing a roommate agreement (relationships). The ILP Dollars are tracked in an Orangewood bank account and ILP youth can purchase a maximum of one $50 gift certificate per month for use at stores for groceries, clothing, and general goods. ILP Dollars can also be used for bills and rent. Youth must plan the use of ILP Dollars, because processing requests may take up to 2 weeks and staff may discuss the youth's requests.

Foster care alumni who have successfully transitioned to independent living serve as peer mentors in the ILP. Peer mentors help establish program rapport and credibility with ILP youth, teach independent living skills, facilitate small group discussion during workshops, and serve as positive role models. Participants provide feedback at each workshop to assess interest and effectiveness.

Supportive individuals are invited to participate in the youth's transition plan and attend workshops. ILP also coordinates with other programs designed to serve transitional age foster youth, such as housing, scholarships, independent living specialists, and youth leadership opportunities.

Legal and Ethical Issues

Ethical, legal, and policy issues overlap because state responsibilities to foster youth should translate into policies and legislation. Given that most nonfoster youth require and receive social, pragmatic, and financial support from their parents well into their 20s and beyond, one can make the case that the state and society are ethically bound to provide comparable support for a similar duration to foster youth. Vast geographic disparities in public health and behavioral health care and child welfare systems require contemplation from child and adolescent behavioral health providers and stakeholders. It is imperative to advocate for changes within local, state, and federal governments to ensure access to the comprehensive services owed to this highly vulnerable population.

Behavioral health clinicians should provide and advocate for the appropriate use of psychiatric medications and psychosocial treatments. When working with youth who are in the care and protection of the state, providers should familiarize themselves with state laws around mental health treatment and psychotropic consent. Authority for psychotropic consent varies from state to state, and may rest with the biologic parents; a child welfare agency; or some other party, such as a court or state-appointed consent agent. Questions about a youth's legal status, consent, release of information, and legal authority should be directed to the child welfare worker.

Research and Policy Gaps

The Institute of Medicine and the Future of Children contemplated transition, including research and policy gaps relating to "marginalized" and "vulnerable" youth transitioning to adulthood.[46,47] Foster youth were included in these groups, along with youth involved with the juvenile justice, mental health, and special education systems, and youth with disabilities. More research on transitional age services for foster youth is needed. Existing research is typically more descriptive, report service delivery/utilization, and/or not well controlled. A more comprehensive understanding of transitional age foster youth and outcomes will inform policy and program development. Many existing programs seem promising, but more research is required to determine the effectiveness and cost-effectiveness of programs and inform quality improvement. States are given wide latitude to develop transition programs; differences in state transition services provide opportunities to compare implementation processes and functional outcomes. Databases must be expanded, strengthened, and linked to support more rigorous evaluation and outcome tracking. Administrative data may include relevant information, including secondary and postsecondary education performance, health and behavioral health care utilization and outcomes, employment, justice system involvement, and participation in public assistance programs.

Legislation and policies have begun to address the myriad challenges facing transitional age foster youth, but to sufficiently support foster youth emancipation and self-sufficiency, federal legislation and policies must be strengthened to expand the availability and breadth of transition services. Although recent federal legislation seeks to extend state responsibility to act as parents to foster youth beyond age 18, it does so mostly to age 21, too young given most foster youths' developmental needs. Most states provide transition services in a limited, interrupted, and piecemeal fashion, contrasted with the more comprehensive, continuous, and enduring supports many parents provide their children. Transitional age foster youth may be involved with multiple agencies because they have multiple needs, requiring integration and coordination of efforts. Moreover, federal legislation permits but does not require states to provide necessary transition services. For example, not all states offer EFC,[48] and those that do often offer more limited services than federal policies allow. In addition, although states must extend Medicaid eligibility to age 26 to foster youth from their own state, most states do not do so for foster alumni from other states.[49]

Existing programs are too bureaucratic, inaccessible, idiosyncratic, fragmented, poorly responsive, and stigmatizing.[46] Transitional age foster youth will benefit from policies promoting a youth-centered, family-focused, culturally sensitive, developmentally appropriate, accessible, responsive, comprehensive, and integrated and coordinated system of transition care. This care should be continuous and seamless from adolescence to early adulthood, trauma-informed, nonstigmatizing, and socially inclusive. Accountability for outcomes must be heightened to improve the well-being of foster care alumni.

SUMMARY

Transitional age foster youth do not typically receive the range of family supports that their nonfoster peers enjoy. Foster youth often experience multiple adversities that complicate successful transition, and negatively impact mental and physical health. Foster care alumni are at increased risk for negative outcomes in education, homelessness, employment, financial security, health, and behavioral health. Youth-serving public systems of care often end at age 18 or 21, or are discontinuous with adult approximations. The federal government, states, foundations, nongovernment organizations, families, and current and past foster youth have begun addressing transitional age foster youth needs. Many policies and programs seem to be promising. More research is needed to assess the effectiveness and efficiency of existing programs, and to inform program and policy development and quality improvement. Policies must be strengthened to increase accountability for developing youth self-sufficiency, and improve transition service availability, access, responsiveness, continuity, duration, and effectiveness.

REFERENCES

1. Settersten RA, Ray B. What's going on with young people today? The long and twisting path to adulthood. Future Child 2010;20:19–41.

2. Courtney ME, Dworsky A, Brown A, et al. Midwest evaluation of the adult functioning of former foster youth: outcomes at age 26. Chicago: Chapin Hall at the University of Chicago; 2011.

3. Wilson C. Integrating safety, permanency, and well-being: a view from the field. Children's Bureau, Health and Human Services. 2014. Available at: http://www.acf.hhs.gov/sites/default/files/cb/wp_overview.pdf. Accessed September 24, 2016.

4. US Department of Health and Human Services, Administration for Children and Families, Administration on Children, Youth, and Families, Children's Bureau. 2016. Child maltreatment. 2014. Available at: http://www.acf.hhs.gov/sites/default/files/cb/cm2014.pdf. Accessed September 24, 2016.

5. US Department of Health and Human Services, Administration for Children and Families, Administration on Children, Youth, and Families, Children's Bureau. Child welfare outcomes 2009-2012: report to congress. Available at: http://www.acf.hhs.gov/sites/default/files/cb/cwo09_12.pdf. Accessed September 24, 2016.

6. US Department of Health and Human Services, Administration for Children and Families, Administration on Children, Youth and Families, Children's Bureau, The AFCARS report for FY2014. 2015. Available at: http://www.acf.hhs.gov/sites/default/files/cb/afcarsreport22.pdf. Accessed September 24, 2016.

7. US Department of Health and Human Services, Administration for Children and Families, Administration on Children, Youth, and Families. Children's Bureau. Data brief 2013-1: recent demographic trends in foster care. 2013. Available at: http://www.acf.hhs.gov/sites/default/files/cb/data_brief_foster_care_trends1.pdf. Accessed September 24, 2016.

8. Bartholet E, Wulczyn F, Barth R, et al. Race and child welfare. Chicago: Chapin Hall at the University of Chicago; 2011.

9. Stahmer AC, Leslie LK, Hurlburt M, et al. Developmental and behavioral needs and service use for young children in child welfare. Pediatrics 2005;116:891–900.

10. McMillen JC, Zima BT, Scott LD, et al. Prevalence of psychiatric disorders among older youths in the foster care system. J Am Acad Child Adolesc Psychiatry 2005;44:88–95.

11. Pecora PJ, Kessler RC, Williams J, et al. Improving family foster care: findings from the northwest foster care alumni study. Seattle (WA): Casey Family Programs; 2005.

12. White CR, O'Brien K, White J, et al. Alcohol and drug use among alumni of foster care: decreasing dependency through improvement of foster care experiences. J Behav Health Serv Res 2008;35:419–34.

13. Braciszewski JM, Stout RL. Substance use among current and former foster youth: a systematic review. Child Youth Serv Rev 2012;34:2337–44.

14. dos Reis S, Zito JM, Safer DJ, et al. Mental health services for youths in foster care and disabled youths. Am J Public Health 2001;91:1094–9.

15. US Government Accountability Office. Foster children: HHS guidance could help states improve oversight of psychotropic prescriptions. GAO-12–270T. Washington, DC: Government Accountability Office; 2011. Available at: http://www.gao.gov/assets/590/586570.pdf. Accessed September 24, 2016.

16. Lee T, Fouras G, Brown R. Practice parameter for the assessment and management of youth involved with the child welfare system. J Am Acad Child Adolesc Psychiatry 2015;54:502–17.

17. Shonkoff JP, Garner AS, Committee on Psychosocial Aspects of Child and Family Health, et al. The lifelong effects of early childhood adversity and toxic stress. Pediatrics 2012;129:e232–46.

18. Anda RF, Felitti VJ, Bremner JD, et al. The enduring effects of abuse and related adverse experiences in childhood: a convergence of evidence from neurobiology and epidemiology. Eur Arch Psychiatry Clin Neurosci 2006;256:174–86.

19. Nugent NR, Goldberg A, Uddin M. Topical review: the emerging field of epigenetics: informing models of pediatric trauma and physical health. J Pediatr Psychol 2016;41:55–64.

20. Forkey H, Szilagyi M. Foster care and healing from complex childhood trauma. Pediatr Clin North Am 2014;61:1059–72.

21. Collins ME, Spencer R, Ward R. Supporting youth in the transition from foster care: formal and informal connections. Child Welfare 2010;89:125–43.

22. Courtney M, Terao S, Bost N. Midwest evaluation of former foster youth: conditions of youth preparing to leave state care. Chicago: Chapin Hall at the University of Chicago; 2004.

23. Dworsky A, Courtney M. The risk of teenage pregnancy among transitioning foster youth: implications for extending state care beyond age 18. Child Youth Serv Rev 2010;32:1351–6.

24. Masten AS. Ordinary magic: resilience processes in development. Am Psychol 2001;56:227–38.

25. Ungar M. Resilience after maltreatment: the importance of social services as facilitators of positive adaptation. Child Abuse Negl 2013;37:110–5.

26. Courtney ME, Hook JL, Lee JS. Distinct subgroups of former foster youth during the transition to adulthood: implications for policy and practice. Chicago: Chapin Hall at the University of Chicago; 2010.

27. Hook JL, Courtney ME. Employment of former foster youth as young adults: evidence from the Midwest study. Chicago: Chapin Hall at the University of Chicago; 2011.

28. Pecora P, Williams J, Kessler R, et al. Assessing the educational achievements of adults who formerly placed in family foster care. Child Fam Soc Work 2006;11:220–31.

29. Munson MR, Smalling SE, Spencer R, et al. A steady presence in the midst of change: nonkin natural mentor in the lives of older youth exiting foster care. Child Youth Serv Rev 2010;32:527–35.
30. Dworsky A, Courtney M. Assessing the impact of extending care beyond age 18 on homelessness: emerging findings from the Midwest study. Chicago: Chapin Hall at the University of Chicago; 2010.
31. Courtney ME, Dworsky A, Peters CM. California's fostering connections to success act and the costs and benefits of extending foster care to 21. Seattle (WA): Partners for Our Children; 2009.
32. Casey Family Programs. Casey life skills. 2013. Available at: http://www.casey.org/casey-life-skills-resources/. Accessed September 12, 2016.
33. California Evidence-Based Clearinghouse for Child Welfare. Youth transitioning into adulthood programs. Available at: http://www.cebc4cw.org/topic/youth-transitioning-into-adulthood/. Accessed September 12, 2016.
34. CEBC. Caring adults "r" everywhere. Available at: http://www.cebc4cw.org/program/caring-adults-r-everywhere/detailed. Accessed September 12, 2016.
35. Greeson JKP, Thompson AE, Kinnevy S. Natural mentoring of older foster care youths. Soc Work Today 2014;14:11–3.
36. California Evidence-Based Clearinghouse for Child Welfare. My first place. Available at: http://www.cebc4cw.org/program/my-first-place/detailed. Accessed September 12, 2016.
37. Public/Private Ventures. My first place, a program of first place for youth. Formative evaluation findings: June 2010 to March 2012. Available at: http://www.firstplaceforyouth.org/wp-content/uploads/2014/06/First-Place-Formative-Evaluation-Summary-Brief.pdf. Accessed September 12, 2016.
38. California Evidence-Based Clearinghouse for Child Welfare. MyPath Savings. Available at: http://www.cebc4cw.org/program/mypath-savings/. Accessed September 12, 2016.
39. Loke V, Choi L, Libby M. Increasing youth financial capability: an evaluation of the MyPath Savings initiative. J Consum Aff 2015;49:97–126.
40. Salazar AM, Roe SS, Ullrich JA, et al. Professional and youth perspectives on higher education-focused interventions for youth transitioning from foster care. Child Youth Serv Rev 2016;64:23–34.
41. Salazar AM. Supporting college success in foster care alumni: salient factors related to postsecondary retention. Child Welfare 2012;91:139–67.
42. Casey Family Programs. Improving higher education outcomes for students from foster care. Version 2.0. 2010. Available at: http://www.casey.org/supporting-success/. Accessed September 12, 2016.
43. California Evidence-Based Clearinghouse for Child Welfare. Seita scholars program. Available at: http://www.cebc4cw.org/program/seita-scholars-program/detailed. Accessed September 12, 2016.
44. Unrau YA. From foster care to college: the Seita scholars program at Western Michigan University. Reclaiming Child Youth 2011;20:17–20.
45. California Evidence-Based Clearinghouse for Child Welfare. Independent living program-Orangewood (ILP). Available at: http://www.cebc4cw.org/program/independent-living-program-orangewood/detailed. Accessed September 24, 2016.
46. IOM (Institute of Medicine) and NRC (National Research Council). Investing in the health and well-being of young adults. Washington, DC: The National Academies Press; 2015. Available at: http://nap.edu/18869. Accessed September 24, 2016.
47. Osgood DW, Foster EM, Courtney ME. Vulnerable populations and the transition to adulthood. Future Child 2010;20(1):209–29.

48. American Academy of Pediatrics. Covering extended foster care. Available at: https://www.aap.org/en-us/advocacy-and-policy/state-advocacy/Documents/Covering%20Extended%20Foster%20Care.pdf. Accessed November 9, 2016.

49. Child Information Gateway. Health-care coverage for youth in foster care—and after. 2015. Available at: https://www.childwelfare.gov/pubPDFs/health_care_foster.pdf. Accessed September 24, 2016.

Transitional Age Lesbian, Gay, Bisexual, Transgender, and Questioning Youth

Issues of Diversity, Integrated Identities, and Mental Health

Scott M. Rodgers, MD

KEYWORDS

- Sexual orientation • Gender identity • Lesbian • Gay • Bisexual • Transgender
- Questioning

KEY POINTS

- LGBTQ transitional age youth face heightened risk of victimization through bullying and discrimination in a variety of environments.
- Educational institutions, families, and churches, usually considered safe havens for people, are sometimes unsupportive of LGBTQ youth.
- Health and mental health of LGBTQ youth and young adults may be compromised by unsupportive environments and bullying/victimization.
- Changing the outcome for LGBTQ transitional age youth is possible through a variety of best practices.

INTRODUCTION

Many lesbian, gay, bisexual, transgender, and questioning (LGBTQ) youth do well as they make the transition from adolescence to adulthood, but research suggests that the population is at a higher risk for developing certain health, mental health, and social problems. These include, but are not limited to, sexually transmitted diseases, school difficulties, addiction, depression, and suicide.[1,2] These negative outcomes may be higher because of the discrimination, marginalization, and isolation that are associated with LBGTQ youth. LGBTQ youth experience bullying and victimization

Disclosure Statement: The author has nothing to disclose.
Department of Psychiatry and Human Behavior, University of Mississippi Medical Center, 2500 North State Street, Jackson, MS 39216, USA
E-mail address: srodgers@umc.edu

Child Adolesc Psychiatric Clin N Am 26 (2017) 297–309
http://dx.doi.org/10.1016/j.chc.2016.12.011   **childpsych.theclinics.com**
1056-4993/17/© 2016 Elsevier Inc. All rights reserved.

at higher rates than their heterosexual and cisgender peer group.[3–6] Additionally, LGBTQ youth sometimes lack the type of support that exists for most youth in such settings as the home environment, on campus, and in the workplace, and religion may become a source of distress if one's beliefs are in conflict with one's sexual identity.[2,7,8] Furthermore, LGBTQ youth with gender-nonconforming behaviors seem to be at higher risk for bullying and victimization than those with gender-conforming behaviors, and males seem to have heightened risk.[9,10] As these youth enter adulthood, bullying and victimization begin to decrease, and this results in overall improvement in health for some individuals. However, there remain persistent health disparities in LGBTQ young adults.[11] There are research-supported interventions that work to reduce the risk of poor health outcomes for LGBTQ youth as they make the transition to adulthood.[12–15]

HEALTH AND MENTAL HEALTH DATA

Compared with heterosexuals, members of sexual minority groups experience lower levels of self-esteem, higher levels of psychological stress, and a lower level of general well-being.[9,16–18] Additionally, those whose gender expression does not match typical masculine and feminine appearance and behaviors (also known as gender nonconformity) experience more stigmatization, rejection, and a lower level of well-being than those with a lower level of gender nonconformity.[8,18–20] Indeed, gender nonconformity seems to be a stronger predictor of a lower level of well-being and of greater stigmatization among sexual minorities than sexual orientation.[9] Stigmatization, in turn, may adversely affect the development of sexual minority youth, specifically by worsening their psychosocial adjustment and mental health, and by inducing more health risk behaviors.[8,21–23]

The lower level of psychological well-being among sexual minorities is understood by the minority stress model, as described by Meyer.[19,24] Several stressors exist for the LGBTQ community, including discrimination, expected homonegativity, concealing one's sexual orientation, and internalized homonegativity.[19,24] Discrimination involves experiencing prejudice events; for LGBTQ youth, bullying at school and being rejected by family and friends are prime examples.[11,23,25,26] A second type of stressor involves "expecting to experience prejudice events or rejection."[11] When LGBTQ youth experience discrimination, the result is an expectation that these experiences will recur, and this leads to heightened vigilance and greater stress.[11,19,27] Concealment is a third stressor; it involves attempting to conceal one's LGBTQ status. Concealment requires "constant self-monitoring" to ensure that one's behavior conforms to expected gender-based behaviors, and the stigma of concealment can have an adverse effect on mood and self-esteem.[11,28] Finally, members of the LGBTQ community sometimes internalize the negative societal views of LGBTQ people. When this happens, individuals begin to think less of themselves based on social stigma.[29] Greater levels of these stressors are associated with poor psychosocial health outcomes.[30,31]

"Coming out" is a process in which one chooses to disclose to others his/her sexual orientation and/or gender identity, and it is considered a key developmental milestone associated with better psychological well-being. In a study by Kosciw and colleagues,[32] outness was associated with higher levels of peer victimization, with rural youth experiencing more victimization than urban youth. However, outness was also associated with higher self-esteem and lower levels of depression. Being out may reflect resilience despite the higher risk of victimization and may promote well-being in other ways. Contextual factors, such as the level of support in school or in the community, play a role in influencing outcomes.[32]

SEXUAL BEHAVIOR AND RISK

In August 2016, the Centers for Disease Control and Prevention (CDC) released the first nationally representative study on the health risks of LGB high school students in the United States. Among their findings, they discovered that LBG students are significantly more likely to report being forced to have sex (18% LGB vs 5% heterosexual), experience sexual dating violence (23% LGB vs 9% heterosexual), and experience physical dating violence (18% LGB vs 8% heterosexual).[1] More research is needed to understand what places LGB youth at risk for this heightened level of victimization, but some prior studies have already begun to shed light on the problem.

Studies have shown that high school–aged LGBT youths tend to take more risk with regard to sexual behavior than do their heterosexual peers. Examples of heightened risk include having a higher number of sex partners and not using protection, such as condoms, during sex.[6,33,34] Homelessness is a problem that disproportionately affects LGBT youth, and some of these young people stay with strangers, putting them at risk for sexual exploitation.[35] Research has also established a potential link between victimization, for which LGBT youth face heightened risk, and sexual risk disparities between LGBT and heterosexual youths.[6,34]

According to Robinson and Espelage,[6] "victimization may lead to increased sexually risky behavior through several pathways." These include "heightened feelings of isolation leading to increased desires for sexual fulfillment, psychological distress leading to unprotected sex, and stigmatization leading to lack of knowledge about sexual-minority identity in turn leading to seeking out same-sex activities to navigate identity."[36–38] According to a recent retrospective study of LGBT young adults, "those who recalled greater peer victimization during their teenage years were more likely to have had a sexually transmitted disease and to have been at HIV risk in the past 6 months."[6,25] Recent CDC data have shown an increase in human immunodeficiency virus infection by 26% from 2008 to 2011 among young men who have sex with men aged 13 to 24 years, 56% of whom were black and 20% of whom were Hispanic/Latino.[39]

MENTAL HEALTH
Depression and Suicide

The previously mentioned CDC study showed that more than 40% of LGB students have seriously considered suicide, and 29% have attempted suicide in the past 12 months. A total of "60% of this same group has been so sad or hopeless that they stopped doing some of their usual activities."[1] Consistent with these CDC findings, another nationally representative study of adolescents in grades 7 to 12 found that LGB youth were more than twice as likely to have attempted suicide as their heterosexual peers.[40] Although more studies are needed to better understand the suicide risks among transgender youth, one study with 55 transgender youth found that approximately 25% reported suicide attempts.[3,41]

Teasing of LGB students seems to have a direct effect on rates of depression and suicide; those who did not experience homophobic teasing reported the lowest levels of depression and suicidal feelings of all student groups.[5,25,42,43] Interestingly, all students, regardless of sexual orientation, reported the lowest levels of depression, suicidal feelings, alcohol and marijuana use, and unexcused absences from school when they were in a positive school climate that expressly disallows homophobic teasing.[5,43–45] This suggests that the learning environment for all students improves when antibullying campaigns are inclusive of LGBT students.

One study by Birkett and colleagues[11] showed that "the psychological distress of LGBTQ adolescents does decrease across adolescence and into young adulthood." The "reduction in distress appears to be related to the co-occurring developmental decline in LGBTQ victimization." Some youth might experience greater victimization than others. Males, some racial/ethnic minorities, and transgender individuals reported greater victimization.[10]

Anxiety Disorders and Posttraumatic Stress Disorder

In an Australian study from 1999 of youth 14 to 21 years old, LGB youth were more likely to experience generalized anxiety disorder compared with heterosexual youth. A more recent US study of LGBT youth ages 16 to 20 revealed a rate of posttraumatic stress disorder at 11.3% in the previous 12 months, which is higher than a national rate of posttraumatic stress disorder at 3.9% for all youth.[46]

Alcohol and Illicit Drug Use

Sexual minority youth drink alcohol and engage in heavy episodic drinking more frequently than their heterosexual peers.[47–50] Among youth identifying as bisexual, 56% report past-month alcohol use, compared with 38% of their heterosexual peer group.[13,51] Lifetime prevalence rates of drug use, including heroin, inhalants, cocaine, and Ecstasy, among sexual-minority youth are also higher.[13,51] The previously cited 2016 CDC report showed that LGB students are up to five times more likely than other students to report using illegal drugs.[1]

As with heterosexual students, peer and social influences likely play a role in drug use with LGBT students. However, LGBT students face negative reactions to their sexual minority status, and they often lack support from family, peers, schools, and their religious community.[13,52,53] Stigma and minority stress theories, purporting that LGB students experience stress related to their minority sexual orientation, suggest that these youth cope by consuming alcohol.[19,47] The substance use prevention programs available to students, and specifically to sexual minority youth, tend to have a heterocentric focus, which ignores the risk factors specific to LGBT youth.[13]

Interestingly, studies have shown that schools can reduce the drinking disparities among LGBT youth when they have Gay-Straight Alliances (GSAs) on campus and when they protect LGBT students with antibullying policies that include LGBT as a protected group.[47,54–56] In fact, all students, gay and straight, seem to benefit in this way when a GSA is on campus.[47,55,56] Perhaps not surprisingly, an LGBTQ-inclusive curriculum leads to feelings of safety and less victimization among LGBTQ youth.[57] Lower victimization, in turn, likely lowers adolescents' alcohol use. LGBTQ school climate was associated with fewer drinking days at school and fewer heavy episodic drinking days.[47]

BULLYING, VICTIMIZATION, AND DISCRIMINATION

According to several key studies, adolescents who are perceived to be LGBT are at an elevated risk for victimization.[1,3,5,58] A recent, nationwide survey of more than 7800 LGBT students produced the following startling results: 55.5% of respondents felt unsafe at school because of their sexual orientation, 74.1% had experienced verbal harassment, 36.2% had experienced physical harassment, and 49.0% had experienced cyberbullying.[42,57] The high level of bullying becomes a "normalized element" of the lives of LGBT youth.[43,59] Lower grades, absenteeism because of skipping, and less school attachment are the result for many of these young people.[5,42,60,61]

Victimization by cyberbullying is especially pronounced among LGBTQ youth. In one well publicized case from 2010, an 18 year old named Tyler Clementi died by suicide by jumping off of the George Washington Bridge after a college roommate posted a clandestine video of Tyler kissing another man. Studies have concluded that there are higher rates of cyberbullying victims within the LGBTQ population.[62] A 2013 study showed that LGBT youth use the Internet for 45 minutes a day more than their straight peers, and more than twice as many LGBT youth had a close friend they had met online. A total of 42% of the LGBT youth in this study had experienced cyberbullying, compared with just 15% for their straight counterparts. Those experiencing online and in-person bullying reported lower grade-point averages, lower self-esteem, and higher rates of depression.[62,63]

LGBT youth are often reluctant to report bullying to school personnel. In one study, 56.7% of bullied LGBT students "chose not to report the incident to school officials because they felt that interventions were unlikely to occur or that the situation could worsen if records were made of the event." Unfortunately, of those LGBT students who chose to report bullying, 61.6% of them indicated that the school staff did not attempt to address the problem.[43,64] LGBT youth have sometimes believed that school officials and/or the police did not view LGBT bullying as a serious issue, and most participants in one study believed that officials were not doing enough to educate youth about LGBT issues and address the bullying problem.[43,59]

AN ABSENCE OF SAFE HAVENS FOR SOME TRANSITIONAL AGE YOUTH

For many people, the family, school, and house of worship environments represent safe havens where one finds protection from the sometimes harsh realities of the outside world. But this is not always the case with LGBTQ youth. These young people can experience difficulties in all of these settings. In a 2014 study by Higa and colleagues[2] at the University of Washington, 68 LGBTQ youth were recruited to participate in either focus groups or individual interviews to discuss their experiences. "The findings from this study demonstrated a pervasiveness of negative experiences in multiple contexts, and the importance of fostering a positive LGBTQ identity and supportive peer/community networks."[2] A brief summary of this important study's findings follows:

1. In families, for example, some LGBTQ youth described their relationships with parents as distant or strained,[2,65] they feared victimization from family members,[2,66] and there was sometimes a lack of acceptance from socially conservative parents.[2,67] Being kicked out of the house was a real fear among LGBT youth, which is justified given the high rates of homelessness affecting youth in the LGBT community. However, families sometimes choose instead to support their LGBT children, which becomes a positive factor for these young people who have families with a willingness to accept them unconditionally.[2]
2. In schools, LGBT youth bullying and antigay victimization occur at higher rates compared with the straight and cisgender peer group.[58,64] LGBT youth experience verbal and physical harassment, and they note the inaction of school staff, such as teachers and administrators, to intervene on their behalf at these times. There is sometimes resistance from school staff or other students to starting GSAs. "Persons in the school environment who were mentioned most frequently as exhibiting antigay or otherwise nonsupportive behavior were principals, staff, or religious students and teachers." Clearly, there are examples of schools, along with people

working and studying within them, that have created supportive environments for all students, including LGBT youth, and the LGBT youth in these environments have an improved experience.[2]

3. Religion may be a source of distress and contribute to internalized homophobia if religious beliefs are in conflict with one's sexual identity.[2,8] Many LGBT youth cite religion as a negative factor in their lives. They hear negative messages from their faith communities regarding their sexual orientation. They have been told that they are sinners and that they will go to hell for being LGBTQ. Harassment in church communities does occur, and some LGBT youth have been forced out of their religious communities. However, not all LGBT youth have had such negative experiences in church; some even cite religion as a source of strength in their lives. There are religious communities that are openly accepting of LGBTQ people, and the experience for LGBT youth within such an environment is notably different.[2]

4. The larger social environment may affect the well-being of LGBT youth. A recent Oregon study found the risk of attempting suicide for LGB youth was 20% greater in social environments unsupportive of LGBTQ persons compared with LGBTQ-supportive environments.[2,68]

BEST PRACTICES IN SUPPORTING TRANSITIONAL AGE YOUTH: CHANGING THE TRAJECTORY
A Safe Learning Environment

Support by teachers and school staff, when it does exist, has been cited as a protective factor for sexual-minority youth.[43,57] Homophobic bullying seems to be more prevalent in schools where educators remained uninvolved because of being unaware of bullying or ill-equipped to respond appropriately.[43] When LGBT youth feel that there is no adult in the school with whom they can talk about a problem, they are more likely than others to be threatened at school and more likely to make suicide attempts. Staff support of LGBT youth is, conversely, a significant protective factor against suicide attempts.[43,44] Given the high rates of bullying against LGBTQ youth in schools and surrounding environments, schools can choose to become more deliberate in their efforts to prevent LGBTQ victimization by including LGBTQ youth as a protected group in their antibullying campaigns. Adopting policies, training administrators, staff, and teachers, increasing access to and utilization of LGBT-related resources and supports, and bringing LBTQ topics into the curriculum help to promote a safer school climate.[5,45]

An Inclusive Sexuality Curriculum in Schools

Sexuality education has the potential to prevent unhealthy sexual behaviors by delaying the onset of sexual intercourse, reducing pregnancy rates, and reducing rates of human immunodeficiency virus and sexually transmitted infection among youth.[69-71] However, sexuality education in schools tends to be heterocentric, thereby excluding LGB youth from comprehensive sexuality education and lessening the likelihood of positively influencing healthy decision making in this population.[69,72-74] The Gay, Lesbian, and Straight Education Network's 2009 National School Climate Survey indicated that only 17.9% of 7000 LGBTQ students reported their school as having any curricula that contained LGBT-related topics; only 3.8% reported their health curricula acknowledging sexual and/or gender orientation.[61,69]

In one research study in Oregon schools by Gowen and Winges-Yanez,[69] current sexuality education was found to be exclusive to LGBTQ youth. Through silencing (active and passive), adopting a heterocentric perspective, and pathologizing (connecting LGBT with poor outcomes), LGBTQ youth were isolated from "the lessons and conversations within their school-based sexuality education classes." Participants in the study recommended creating sexuality education that would be inclusive of youth of all sexual and gender orientations. The likely outcome of such a change would be the creation of a safer learning environment for LGBT youth.[69]

Informed and Supportive Parents

According to Gonzalez and colleagues,[75] "parenting shapes the development of many adults." With LGBT youth, parents have an opportunity to learn and grow as they are presented with "unique opportunities for personal growth and the development of life skills." Not all parents struggle with a child's coming out, but when they do, opportunities present themselves for positive transformation through a restructuring of views. Some parents look in retrospect at the challenge and recognize that closer familial bonds resulted following their child's coming out.[75] Being raised in a supportive and affirming home environment is one of the goals in promoting the health of LGBT youth.

Health Care Environments

Health care providers and health professions schools have opportunities to establish themselves as sources of support, affirmation, and knowledge for the LGBTQ community. Information regarding sexual identity development can and should be made available to health care professions students, health care providers, patients, and families. To help patients avoid the fear of coming out to one's health care provider, clinics can advertise themselves as LGBTQ-friendly through marketing materials inside and outside the clinic, LGBTQ-friendly intake/questionnaire forms, and the provision of culturally competent health care. Health care providers and health care professions students should take opportunities to educate themselves through self-directed learning and any available conferences or training workshops in their area. One notable, recent AAMC publication entitled, "Implementing curricular and institutional climate changes to improve health care for individuals who are LGBT, gender nonconforming or born with DSD: a resource for medical educators" deserves special mention for health care providers and health professions schools with an interest in learning more.[76]

Gay-Straight Alliances

GSAs are student-directed organizations designed to promote the well-being of LGBTQ students. A growing body of research has demonstrated clear benefits of having GSAs in schools. There is strong evidence showing the association between the presence of GSAs in schools and lower reports of victimization among adolescents. To overcome the occasional politically contentious resistance to having GSAs in schools, it is important to present schools and advocates with convincing data that demonstrate the connection between having GSAs and adolescent well-being.[14]

SUMMARY

Many transitional age youth within the LGBTQ community do well as they mature and enter adulthood. However, a review of this population is necessary because certain health disparities exist, specifically in the areas of mental and sexual health. These disparities are rooted, at least in part, in society's long history of lacking acceptance for the LGBTQ community. With the lack of acceptance comes verbal and physical harassment, bullying, and discrimination. Traditional refuges, such as religious institutions, family, and school, cannot always be relied on for support, leaving these young people to fend for themselves in a sometimes harsh world. Homelessness, resulting from being kicked out of the home, disproportionately affects LGBT youth. Fortunately, there are many people and organizations around the world who are reaching out to the LGBT youth community and offering support. Effective interventions are available and necessary to change the trajectory for LGBT transitional age youth. Overcoming resistance to these changes requires persistence, determination, and a recognition that all young people benefit when no children are harmed. With research providing evidence for best practices along with a groundswell of emerging support from communities, families, schools, LGBTQ allies, and the LGBTQ community, the future is beginning to look brighter for LGBTQ as they transition to young adulthood.

FUTURE DIRECTIONS

Research on sexual minority youth has dealt, in large part, with LGB youth, leaving out transgender individuals. From the few studies available on transgender youth, it is clear that this is an at-risk and vulnerable population, and having more information on the specific risks and protective factors, In addition to the best approaches to care, would greatly improve the ability to optimize and improve their experience.

Most studies related to the mental health of LGBT youth compare rates of mental illness with the larger heterosexual and cisgender youth population. These studies have shown, without exception, that significant mental health disparities do exist, with LGBT youth experiencing mental illness at higher rates than their heterosexual and cisgender counterparts. Now that this disparity has been established, it is worth considering whether there is any variability, based on such factors as race and ethnicity, within the LGBT community itself, without regard to the heterosexual and cisgender youth population. Having such information would enable improved care of LGBT youth across the broad, diverse spectrum of the LGBT population. Furthermore, there is a need for better demographic data, in general, related to the size of the LGBT population. A report by the Institute of Medicine in 2011 discussed this topic, and it is included here as an important reference for review.[77]

The concept of transitional age youth considers development from the teenage years into young adulthood as a key moment in time, rich with possibilities for the direction a person's life can take. A thorough literature review for this article revealed that there are many studies looking at either the mental health of LGBT youth or the mental health of LGBT adults, but there is a dearth of information related to the transition of LGBT youth into adulthood. Understanding resiliency (namely, what allows a person to recover psychologically from hardship) is especially important in the LGBT transitional age group because of the high rates of victimization, homelessness, and discrimination. Taking research one step further and examining the early life course of LGBT youth as they make this transition to adulthood, with attention paid to resiliency, would shed more light on the factors that determine the health outcomes of LGBT transitional age youth.

REFERENCES

1. Centers for Disease Control and Prevention. Health risks among sexual minority youth. 2016. Available at: http://www.cdc.gov/healthyyouth/disparities/smy.htm. Accessed August 12, 2016.
2. Higa D, Hoppe M, Lindhorst T, et al. Negative and positive factors associated with the well-being of lesbian, gay, bisexual, transgender, queer, and questioning (LGBTQ) youth. Youth Soc 2014;46(5):663–87.
3. Centers for Disease Control and Prevention. LGBT youth. 2014. Available at: http://www.cdc.gov/lgbthealth/youth.htm. Accessed August 12, 2016.

4. Williams T, Connolly J, Pepler D, et al. Peer vicitimization, social support, and psychosocial adjustment of sexual minority adolescents. J Youth Adolesc 2005; 34(5):471–82.
5. Hillard P, Love L, Franks H, et al. "They were only joking": efforts to decrease LGBTQ bullying and harassment in Seattle public schools. J Sch Health 2014; 84(1):1–9.
6. Robinson J, Espelage D. Peer victimization and sexual risk differences between lesbian, gay, bisexual, transgender, or questioning and no transgender heterosexual youths in grades 7-12. Am J Public Health 2013;103(10):1810–9.
7. Sanchez N, Rankin S, Callahan E, et al. LGBT trainee and health professional perspectives on academic careers: facilitators and challenges. LGBT Health 2015; 2(4):346–57.
8. Ream G, Savin-Williams R. Reconciling Christianity and positive non-heterosexual identity in adolescence, with implications for psychological well-being. J Gay Lesbian Issues Education 2005;2:19–36.
9. Baams L, Beek T, Hille H, et al. Gender nonconformity, perceived stigmatization, and psychological well-being in Dutch sexual minority youth and young adults: a mediation analysis. Arch Sex Behav 2013;42:765–73.
10. Rieger G, Savin-Williams R. Gender nonconformity, sexual orientation, and psychological well-being. Arch Sex Behav 2012;41:611–21.
11. Birkett M, Newcomb M, Mustanski B. Does it get better? A longitudinal analysis of psychological distress and victimization in lesbian, gay, bisexual, transgender, and questioning youth. J Adolescents Health 2015;56(3):280–5.
12. Heck N. The potential to promote resilience: piloting a minority stress-informed, GSA-based, mental health promotion program for LGBTQ youth. Psychol Sex Orientation Gend Divers 2015;2(3):225–31.
13. Schwinn T, Thom B, Schinke SP, et al. Preventing drug use among sexual-minority youths: findings from a tailored, web-based intervention. J Adolescents Health 2015;56(5):571–3.
14. Marx R, Kettrey H. Gay-Straight alliances are associated with lower levels of school-based victimization of LGBTQ youth: a systematic review and meta-analysis. J Youth Adolescents 2016;45(7):1269–82.
15. De Vries A, McGuire JK, Steensma TD, et al. Young adult psychological outcome after puberty suppression and gender reassignment. Pediatrics 2014;134(4): 696–704.
16. Bos H, Sandfort T, de Bruyn EH, et al. Same-sex attraction, social relationships, psychosocial functioning, and school performance in early adolescence. Developmental Psychol 2008;44:59–68.
17. Pilkington N, D'Augelli A. Victimization of lesbian, gay, and bisexual youth in community settings. J Community Psychol 1995;23:33–55.
18. D'Augelli A, Grossman A, Starks M. Childhood gender atypicality, victimization, and PTSD among lesbian, gay, and bisexual youth. J Interpers Violence 2006; 21(11):1462–82.
19. Meyer I. Prejudice, social stress, and mental health in lesbian, gay, and bisexual populations: conceptual issues and research evidence. Psychol Bull 2003;129: 674–97.
20. Skidmore W, Linsenmeier J, Bailey J. Gender nonconformity and psychological distress in lesbians and gay men. Arch Sex Behav 2006;35:685–97.
21. Toomey R, Ryan C, Diaz RM, et al. Gender-nonconforming lesbian, gay, bisexual, and transgender youth: school victimization and young adult psychosocial adjustment. Developmental Psychol 2010;46:1580–9.

22. Hershberger S, D'Augelli A. The impact of victimization on the mental health and suicidality of lesbian, gay, and bisexual youths. Developmental Psychol 1995;31: 65–74.

23. Bontempo D, D'Augelli A. Effects of at-school victimization and sexual orientation on lesbian, gay, or bisexual youths' health risk behavior. J Adolesc Health 2002; 30:364–74.

24. Meyer I. Minority stress and mental health in gay men. J Health Social Behav 1995;36:38–56.

25. Russell S, Ryan C, Toomey R, et al. Lesbian, gay, bisexual, and transgender adolescent victimization: implications for young adult health and adjustment. J Schol Health 2011;81(5):223–30.

26. Rosario M, Schrimshaw E, Hunter J. Disclosure of sexual orientation and subsequent substance use and abuse among lesbian, gay, and bisexual youths: critical role of disclosure reactions. Psychol Addict Behaviors 2009;23:175–84.

27. Hetrick E, Martin A. Developmental issues and their resolution for gay and lesbian adolescents. J Homosexuality 1987;14:25–43.

28. Frable D, Platt L, Hoey S. Concealable stigmas and positive self-perceptions: feeling better around similar others. J Personal Social Psychol 1998;74:909–22.

29. Lewis R, Millentich R. Minority stress, substance use, and intimate partner violence among sexual minority women. Aggression Violent Behav 2012;17: 247–56.

30. Cox N, Dewaele A, van Houtte M, et al. Stress-related growth, coming out, and internalized homonegativity in lesbian, gay, and bisexual youth. An examination of stress-related growth within the minority stress model. J Homosexuality 2011;58:117–37.

31. Mohr J, Daly C. Sexual minority stress and changes in relationship quality in same-sex couples. J Social Personal Relationships 2008;25:989–1007.

32. Kosciw J, Palmer N, Kull R. Reflecting resiliency: openness about sexual orientation and/or gender identity and its relationship to well-being and educational outcomes for LGBT students. Am J Community Psychol 2015;55:167–78.

33. Centers for Disease Control and Prevention. Sexual identity, sex of sexual contacts, and health-risk behaviors among students in grades 9-12. Youth Risk Behavior Surveillance, selected sites, United States, 2001-2009. MMWR Surveill Summ 2011;60(7):1–133.

34. Friedman M, Marsha M, Guadamuz T, et al. A meta-analysis of disparities in childhood sexual abuse, parental physical abuse, and peer victimization among sexual minority and sexual nonminority individuals. Am J Public Health 2011;101(8): 1481–94.

35. Rice E, Barman-Adhikari A. Homelessness experiences, sexual orientation, and sexual risk taking among high school students in Los Angeles. J Adolescents Health 2013;52(6):773–8.

36. Torres H, Gore-Felton C. Compulsivity, substance abuse, and loneliness: the loneliness and sexual risk model. Sex Addict Compulsivity 2007;14(1):63–75.

37. Rosario M, Hunter J, Maguen S, et al. The coming-out process and its adaptational and health-related associations among gay, lesbian, and bisexual youths: stipulation and exploration of a model. Am J Community Psychol 2001;29(1): 133–60.

38. Martin A, Hetrick E. The stigmatization of the gay and lesbian adolescent. J Homosex 1988;15(1–2):163–83.

39. CDC. HIV surveillance in men who have sex with men (MSM). 2012. Available at: www.cdc.gov/hib/library/slideSets/index.html. Accessed September 1, 2016.

40. Russell S, Joyner K. Adolescent sexual orientation and suicide risk: evidence from a national study. Am J Public Health 2001;91:1276–81.

41. Grossman A, D'Augelli A. Transgender youth and life-threatening behaviors. Suicide life-threatening Behav 2007;37:527–37.

42. D'Augelli A. Developmental implications of victimization of lesbian, gay and bisexual youths. In: Herek G, editor. Stigma and sexual orientation: understanding prejudice against lesbians, gay men, and bisexuals. Thousand Oaks (CA): Sage Publications; 1998. p. 187–210.

43. Kolbert J, Crothers L. Teachers' perceptions of bullying of lesbian, gay, bisexual, transgender, and questioning (LGBTQ) students in a southwestern Pennsylvania sample. Behav Sci 2015;5(2):247–63.

44. Goodenow C, Szalacha L, Westheimer K. School support groups, other school factors, and the safety of sexual minority adolescents. Psychol Schools 2006; 43:573–89.

45. Russell S, Kosciw J, Horn S, et al. Safe schools policy for LGBTQ students. Soc Policy Rep 2010;24(4):1–17.

46. Russell S, Fish J. Mental health in lesbian, gay, bisexual, and transgender (LGBT) youth. Annu Rev Clin Psychol 2016;12:465–87.

47. Coulter R, Birkett ML, Corliss HL, et al. Associations between LGBTQ-affirmative school climate and adolescent drinking behaviors. Drug Alcohol Depend 2016; 161:340–7.

48. Corliss HL, Rosario M, Wypij D, et al. Sexual orientation disparities in longitudinal alcohol use patterns among adolescents: findings from the growing up today study. Arch Pediatri Adolesc Med 2008;162:1071.

49. Marshal MP, Friedman MS, Stall R, et al. Sexual orientation and adolescent substance use: a meta-analysis and methodological review. Addiction 2008;103: 546–56.

50. Talley AE, Hughes TL, Aranda F, et al. Exploring alcohol-use behaviors among heterosexual and sexual minority adolescents: intersections with sex, age, and race/ethnicity. Am J Public Health 2014;104:295–303.

51. Kann L, Olsen E, McManus T, et al. Sexual identity, sex of sexual contacts, and health-risk behaviors among students in grades 9-12—youth risk behavior surveillance, selected sits, United States, 2001-2209. MMWR Surveill Summ 2011; 60:1–133.

52. Goldback J, Tanner-Smith EE, Bagwell M, et al. Minority stress and substance use in sexual minority adolescents: a meta-analysis. Prev Sci 2014;15:350–63.

53. Goffman E. Stigma: notes on the management of spoiled identity. New York: Touchstone; 1963.

54. Heck NC, Livingston NA, Flentje A, et al. Offsetting risks high school gay-straight alliances and lesbian, gay, bisexual and transgender (LGBT) youth. Sch Psychol Q 2011;26:161–74.

55. Konishi C, Saewyc E, Homma Y, et al. Population-level evaluation of school-based interventions to prevent problem substance use among gay, lesbian and bisexual adolescents, in Canada. Prev Med 2013;57:929–33.

56. Poteat V, Sinclair K, DiGiovanni C, et al. Gay-straight alliances are associated with student health: a multischool comparison of LGBTQ and heterosexual youth. J Res Adolesc 2013;23:319–30.

57. Kosciw J, Greytak E, Bartkiewicz M, et al. The 2011 national school climate survey: the experiences of lesbian, gay, bisexual and transgender youth in our Nation's school. New York. New York: GLSEN; 2012.

58. Coker T, Austin SB, Schuster MA, et al. The health and health care of lesbian, gay, and bisexual adolescents. Annu Rev Public Health 2010;31:457–77.

59. Sherriff N, Hamilton W, Wigmore S, et al. "What do you say to them?" Investigating and supporting the needs of lesbian, gay, bisexual, trans, and questioning (LGBTQ) young people. J Commun Psychol 2014;39:939–55.

60. Schwartz D, Gorman A, Nakamoto J, et al. Victimization in the peer group and children's academic functioning. J Educ Psychol 2005;97(3):425–35.

61. Kosciw J, et al. The 2009 National School Climate Survey: the experiences of lesbian, gay, bisexual and transgender youth in our nation's school. 2010. Available at: http://files.eric.ed.gov/fulltext/ED512338.pdf. Accessed January 3, 2017.

62. Wiederhold B. Cyberbullying and LGBTQ youth: a deadly combination. Cyberpsychologly, Behav Social Networking 2014;17(9):569–70.

63. Palmer N, Kosciw J, Greytak E, et al. Out online: the experiences of lesbian, gay, bisexual and transgender youth on the Internet. New York: GLSEN; 2013. http://glsen.org/press/stydy-finds-lgbt-youth-face-greater -harassment-online.

64. Kosciw J, Greytak E, Palmer N, et al. The 2013 National School Climate Survey: the experiences of lesbian, gay, bisexual and transgender youth in our Nation's school. New York: GLSEN; 2014.

65. Floyd F, Stein T, Harter K, et al. Gay, lesbian, and bisexual youths: separation-individuation, parental attitudes, identity consolidation, and well-being. J Youth Adolescence 1999;28:719–39.

66. D'Augelli A. Developmental and contextual factors and mental health among lesbian, gay, and bisexual youths. In: Omoto A, Kurtzman H, editors. Sexual orientation and mental health. Washington, DC: American Psychological Association; 2006. p. 37–53.

67. Newman B, Gerard P. The effects of traditional family values on the coming out process of gay male adolescents. Adolescence 1993;28:213–24.

68. Hatzenbuehler M. The social environment and suicide attempts in lesbian, gay, and bisexual youth. Pediatrics 2011;127:896–903.

69. Gowen L, Winges-Yanez N. Lesbian, gay, bisexual, transgender, queer, and questioning youths' perspectives of inclusive school-based sexuality education. J Sex Res 2014;51(7):788–800.

70. Chin H, Sipe TA, Elder R, et al. The effectiveness of group-based comprehensive risk-reduction and abstinence education interventions to prevent or reduce the risk of adolescent pregnancy, human immunodeficiency virus, and sexually transmitted infections. Am J Prev Med 2012;42(3):272–94.

71. Kirby D. Emerging answers: research findings on programs to reduce teen pregnancy. Washington, DC: National Campaign to Prevent Teen Pregnancy; 2001.

72. Elia J, Eliason M. Discourses of exclusion: sexuality education's silencing of sexual others. J LGBT Youth 2010;7:29–48.

73. Fine M, McClelland S. Sexuality education and desire: still missing after all these years. Harv Educ Rev 2006;76(3):297–338.

74. Linville D, Carlson D. Fashioning sexual selves: examining the care of the self in urban adolescent sexuality and gender discourses. J LGBT Youth 2010;7(3):247–61.

75. Gonzalez K, Rostosky S, Odom RD, et al. The positive aspects of being the parent of an LGBTQ child. Fam Process 2013;52(2):325–37.

76. Hollenback A, Eckstrand K, Dreger A, et al. Implementing curricular and institutional climate changes to improve health care for individuals who are LGBT, gender nonconforming or born with DSD: a resource for medical educators. Washington, DC: Association of American Medical Colleges; 2014.

77. Institute of Medicine (US) Committee on Lesbian. Gay, bisexual, and transgender health issues and research gaps and opportunities. The health of lesbian, gay, bisexual, and transgender people: building a foundation for better understanding. Washington, DC: National Academies Press (US); 2011. Available at: https://www.ncbi.nlm.nih.gov/books/NBK64801/.

Facilitating Transition from High School and Special Education to Adult Life

Focus on Youth with Learning Disorders, Attention-Deficit/Hyperactivity Disorder, and Speech/Language Impairments

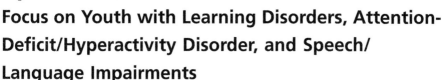

Lee I. Ascherman, MD[a],*, Julia Shaftel, PhD[b]

KEYWORDS

- Postsecondary transition • Learning disorders • ADHD • Communication disorders
- Speech/language disorders • Special education

KEY POINTS

- Comorbidities among learning disorders, speech/language disorders, and attention-deficit/hyperactivity disorder are common throughout the developmental period, resulting in incomplete understanding of the challenges faced by transitional age youth in the absence of thorough evaluation and timely intervention.
- Special education categories and Diagnostic and Statistical Manual of Mental Disorders, 5th Edition diagnoses do not correspond perfectly, causing confusion for transitional age youth, parents, and clinicians.
- Special education law requires schools to follow strict evaluation procedures and timelines before determining eligibility for special education. Parents and clinicians may misinterpret a school's failure to provide services even though a disability has been diagnosed.
- Transition planning procedures during the teen years are required by special education law to help adolescents attain individualized postsecondary goals and increase self-advocacy skills.
- Child and adolescent psychiatrists can play a crucial role in assisting parents and students throughout the postsecondary transition process and into young adult roles.

Disclosure Statement: The authors have nothing to disclose.
[a] Department of Psychiatry and Neurobiology, Division of Child and Adolescent Psychiatry, University of Alabama at Birmingham, 1713 6th Avenue South, Birmingham, AL 35294, USA;
[b] Independent Practice, 5629 Chimney Rocks Circle, Lawrence, KS 66049, USA
* Corresponding author.
E-mail address: lascherman@uabmc.edu

Child Adolesc Psychiatric Clin N Am 26 (2017) 311–327
http://dx.doi.org/10.1016/j.chc.2016.12.009
1056-4993/17/© 2017 Elsevier Inc. All rights reserved.

INTRODUCTION: THE CHALLENGES OF TRANSITION

The chronologic transition from late teen years into the 20s no longer signals the close of adolescence as a developmental stage. Even well-adjusted teens without disability are challenged during this time with the developmental tasks of identity consolidation, separation from family of origin, the exercise of independent functioning, and the establishment of intimacy. Youth whose developmental journey has been complicated by learning disorders, communication disorders, or attention-deficit/hyperactivity disorder (ADHD) face the additional challenges of managing their disability in order to continue development and, ultimately, function at the leading edge of their abilities. Unfortunately, this transition occurs just at the legal and cultural junction when established resources that previously supported such youth may no longer be available. Adult resources must be located, whether higher education or employment is the goal. Those aware of their rights under special education law (Individuals with Disabilities Education Act of 2004 or IDEA)[1] must now become knowledgeable of their rights and resources under disability law (the Americans with Disabilities Act of 1990 or ADA). Simultaneously, the individual is challenged with the difficult recognition that the vulnerabilities that complicated their education may persist, not only in the realm of higher education but also in many other aspects of adult functioning, including employment. Parents are often conflicted about encouraging their child's self-advocacy, knowing their child may resist acknowledging the impact of their disability and/or may be reluctant to assert their needs. For youth in the foster care and juvenile justice systems, the challenges navigating to functional adulthood are formidable. For those with learning disorders, ADHD, or communication disorders, these challenges are compounded by the deleterious impact of their disorder on the skills necessary for this transition and the toll already taken on esteem and confidence.

Child and adolescent psychiatrists (CAPs) are also challenged to help the adolescents they work with when they arrive at this nodal point. Some clinicians may even work in systems that prohibit continuing services to a teen once they reach the age of 18 or 19, shifting care to adult clinicians less attuned to the developmental challenges these youth face. For those teens fortunate enough to continue working with clinicians who know them from childhood, the transition to adult expectations and demands may still not be an easy one.

Clinical planning for this time should begin many years before a child reaches this age. Consideration of whether teens can manage in a higher education setting and whether they want to pursue further education should be discussed far before the completion of high school. Parents, their teen, and the clinician may have very different understandings of the adolescent's abilities, often complicated by the emotional difficulty of accepting persisting vulnerabilities that the teenager did not "grow out of." The clinician may also be a source of hope, assisting teens and their parents to appreciate what might be possible without aiming too low or too high. For those youth choosing a vocational path, planning is critical so that they are guided into a career that is realistic, is of interest to them, and can serve as a means to independence and esteem. Without such advance planning, young adults may find themselves without structure, direction, or resources, making them all the more vulnerable to discouragement, poor self-esteem, and accompanying psychiatric difficulties.

This contribution is designed to highlight the pitfalls and potentials for youth with learning disorders, communication disorders, and/or ADHD as they transition from adolescence to adulthood. Following a brief overview of these disorders, the legal basis for educational and employment rights and the distinctions between educational and disability law is reviewed, noting which laws apply to whom. Subsequently, vocational and educational pathways are discussed, and the importance of advocacy is reviewed.

OVERVIEW OF DISORDERS
Prevalence

Approximately 8.5% of all students aged 6 to 21 were identified with disabilities under IDEA in the fall of 2013, down from 9.1% in 2004.[2] Specific learning disabilities and speech or language impairments are the 2 most common disabilities, accounting for 57% of all special education students. **Table 1** shows the numbers and percentages of students with disabilities in these 2 categories. As explained more fully in later discussion, ADHD is not an IDEA category of disability. When students with ADHD are deemed eligible for special education, they may be identified with specific learning disabilities, emotional disturbance, other health impairment, or another category.

In contrast to the 8.5% of public school students who were identified with disabilities and served under IDEA, 11% of undergraduate college students were identified with disabilities in 2011 to 2012.[3] According to self-report data from the 2015 Fall National College Health Assessment,[4] 8.1% of college students reported having ADHD, 4.8% reported learning disabilities, and 0.9% reported speech/language disabilities.

Learning Disorders

The Diagnostic and Statistical Manual of Mental Disorders, 5th Edition (DSM-5)[5] category of Specific Learning Disorder is roughly synonymous with Specific Learning Disability under IDEA. The definition of Specific Learning Disability arises from the National Advisory Committee on Handicapped Children in 1968 and was adopted by the US Office of Education (later the Department of Education) in 1977:

> a disorder in one or more of the basic psychological processes involved in understanding or in using language, spoken or written, that may manifest itself in an imperfect ability to listen, think, speak, read, write, spell, or to do mathematical calculations, including conditions such as perceptual disabilities, brain injury, minimal brain dysfunction, dyslexia, and developmental aphasia. The term does not include learning problems that are primarily the result of visual, hearing, or motor

Table 1
Number and percent of all students with disabilities, specific learning disabilities, and speech or language impairments served in public schools under Individuals with Disabilities Education Act

Category	Number of All Students (%)	Percent of Students with Disabilities	Percent of Students Aged 12–17	Percent of Students Aged 18–21
All students with disabilities	5.7 million (8.5)	100	10.8	2
Specific learning disabilities	2.3 million (3.5)	39.5	NA	NA
Speech or language impairments	1 million (1.6)	17.9	NA	NA

Abbreviation: NA, not available.

disabilities, of intellectual disabilities, or emotional disturbance, or of environmental, cultural, or economic disadvantage.

Learning disorders are heterogeneous and may exist in one or more academic domains. They may be masked by behavior problems such as task avoidance, the appearance of attentional difficulties, failure to complete homework, conflict with parents, and emotional issues. Learning disorders may go undetected when students (and parents) compensate through extra effort and time. Academic struggles surface or recede as task demands change over time. For example, reading problems often materialize in kindergarten, whereas impairment in math reasoning may not emerge until high school or even college.

Many youth with learning disorders experience consistent frustration in school as they struggle to complete assignments too difficult for independent work. Support in special education often includes tutoring, assistance with homework, tests administered in resource rooms, or an additional teacher or paraprofessional in the regular classroom. By the time these students reach transition age, however, the focus of special education turns to postsecondary educational and vocational planning as well as maintaining sufficient progress in general classes to achieve graduation. Even so, students with learning disabilities graduate at a lower rate than nondisabled students, with 68% graduating in 2011[6] compared with 79% of students overall.[3]

DSM-5 defines specific learning disorder with impairments in reading, written expression, and mathematics. Special education law under IDEA enumerates 8 types of specific learning disability. Unlike IDEA, DSM-5 does not include disorders of oral language under specific learning disorder but has a separate category of language disorder for impairments in receptive and expressive language.

Table 2 shows approximate correspondences between categories used by IDEA and DSM-5. The overlap between IDEA, the federal law paramount within public schools for identification of students requiring special educational services, and DSM-5 definitions is not exact, often resulting in some confusion between categorical definitions.

Table 2
Approximate correspondence between categories of specific learning disability under Individuals with Disabilities Education Act contrasted with types of specific learning disorder and language disorder in Diagnostic and Statistical Manual of Mental Disorders, 5th Edition

Individuals with Disabilities Education Act Specific Learning Disability	Diagnostic and Statistical Manual of Mental Disorders, 5th Edition Specific Learning Disorder
Written Expression	Impairment in written expression: spelling; grammar and punctuation; clear and organized writing
Basic Reading Skills	Impairment in reading: word reading
Reading Fluency Skills	Impairment in reading: reading rate or fluency
Reading Comprehension	Impairment in reading: reading comprehension
Mathematics Calculation	Impairment in mathematics: calculation; rote learning of arithmetic facts
Mathematics Problem Solving	Impairment in mathematics: number sense; math reasoning
Oral Expression	Language Disorder
Listening Comprehension	Language Disorder

Written expression learning disorders

Written expression learning disorders have distinct underlying causes. Spelling, the flip side of word decoding, usually correlates with basic reading problems. Students laboring to produce and sequence letter sounds when reading will likely have the same difficulty when spelling. Motor skills can interfere when students struggle to put words on paper, particularly while composing what to write. Language impairments and limited vocabulary also constrain writing ability. Written language disorders may therefore be comorbid with reading disorders, fine motor coordination problems, or language disorders.

Reading learning disorders

Reading learning disorders occur with vulnerabilities of reading skills at different developmental stages. Phonemic awareness (the ability to manipulate speech sounds to rhyme, blend word sounds, or segment words) develops in the prereading years and is a reliable indicator of risk for later reading problems. Failure to master basic reading skills such as decoding and spelling (matching letters with speech sounds) can indicate weakness in phonemic awareness. Basic reading skills include the growth of sight word vocabulary, essential to reading fluency (rapid, accurate reading of sentences and longer passages). Fluency cannot be attained when students are laboriously sounding out each word. Finally, comprehension as the synthesis of reading skills depends on the attainment of oral language skills, decoding, and fluency. Hence, delay in oral language development is a marker for enormous risk of later reading difficulty.

Mathematics learning disorders

Mathematics learning disorders comprise problems with calculation and reasoning. Calculation includes the fluent retrieval of math facts, analogous to the identification of sight words during reading, along with learning and remembering appropriate procedures to solve problems. Math reasoning includes the application of computation skills to word problems and real-world situations. Reasoning also refers to numeracy (number sense), which is the ability to understand magnitude and number comparison and to estimate and monitor the results of calculations.

Speech and Language Disorders

According to IDEA, "speech or language impairment means a communication disorder, such as stuttering, impaired articulation, a language impairment, or a voice impairment, that adversely affects a child's educational performance." In school and clinical settings, speech/language impairments are usually diagnosed by speech/language pathologists who have specialized knowledge and assessment skills. Identification of speech problems such as stuttering and articulation errors is emphasized in elementary schools. Language impairments often go undiagnosed or misdiagnosed as inattention, noncompliance, or behavior problems.

Mild to moderate language impairments are subtle and difficult to detect. Students with language disorders may struggle with many aspects of academic work, particularly language-heavy tasks such as reading comprehension and writing. These students may appear inattentive or unmotivated when they do not understand task demands or exhibit inappropriate behavior or noncompliance when they cannot express their feelings and needs. Many students with language disorders but without articulation problems are identified with other disabilities and never receive a speech/language evaluation.

Speech and language impairments are represented in DSM-5 by several diagnostic categories, including speech sound disorder (articulation) and childhood-onset fluency disorder (stuttering). Most relevant to the challenges of transitional age youth are language disorder and social (pragmatic) communication disorder.

Language disorder

Language disorder represents delays in communication across modalities, including oral, written, and sign language, that are characterized by limited vocabulary, sentence structure, and discourse, such as the ability to describe thoughts and events. DSM-5 describes the onset of language disorder early in the developmental period, and emerging speech and language development is routinely assessed by health care providers because developmental milestones are well recognized. For this reason, adolescents and transitional age youth are rarely identified with primary language impairments. Furthermore, the symptoms and challenges of early childhood language impairment have by that age morphed into other disabilities, often learning disabilities or emotional and behavior disorders.[7,8]

Social (pragmatic) communication disorder

Social (pragmatic) communication disorder describes verbal and nonverbal communication problems that result in social impairment. Although perhaps most highly suggestive of some autism spectrum disorders or nonverbal learning disabilities, social (pragmatic) communication disorder may be similar to the impaired communication patterns of some students with ADHD.[9]

Attention-Deficit/Hyperactivity Disorder

ADHD is a complex disorder familiar to clinicians comprising difficulty maintaining focus, excessive activity, and impulsivity, with major impact on academic functioning. Students with ADHD frequently have trouble staying in their seats, attending to instruction, following directions, organizing and completing assignments, and preparing for tests. Although CAPs are quite familiar with ADHD, they may not be as aware that attention problems in the school setting may be exacerbated by language or learning difficulties that have not have been fully evaluated or diagnosed. Persistent academic difficulties despite treatment of ADHD may reflect cumulated deficits from past interferences with learning and/or ongoing comorbid learning disorders. Hence, thorough evaluation for learning disorders is indicated when academic difficulties persist.

ADHD exists only in the DSM-5, and therefore, an ADHD diagnosis should be made by a clinician. School personnel often erroneously conflate inattention and overactivity in the classroom that may have multiple determinants with genuine ADHD. When ADHD is accurately diagnosed and has a measurable adverse impact on academic achievement, special education services may be provided. If the student does not have an IDEA diagnosis such as specific learning disability, the most common category for providing services is other health impairment, defined by IDEA as "limited strength, vitality, or alertness."

OUTCOMES FOR YOUTH WITH LEARNING AND LANGUAGE DISORDERS OR ATTENTION-DEFICIT/HYPERACTIVITY DISORDER

Adolescents with learning disabilities engage in risk-taking behaviors more frequently than other youth, including smoking, marijuana use, delinquency, and aggression. Development of self-determination skills and self-advocacy for future plans is recommended to mitigate adolescents' engagement in risky behaviors.[10] Other risk factors for negative adult outcomes include hyperactivity, poor academic performance, discipline problems, suspensions and expulsions, delinquency, and dropping out. Protective factors include high verbal skills, higher intelligence and academic performance, high self-esteem, healthy family functioning, knowledge about one's disability, and graduation from high school.[11,12] One adult outcome of childhood identification with learning disabilities is a higher rate of internalizing disorders.[13]

The reader should note that the term "learning disability" as used in the United Kingdom is equivalent to what would be termed intellectual disability in the United States. In the United States, intellectual disability, defined by significantly below average cognitive functioning, is an exclusionary criterion for specific learning disorder and specific learning disability. Therefore, the source of empirical data must be evaluated before drawing conclusions.

The National Longitudinal Transition Study 2 (NLTS2) followed a nationally representative sample of more than 11,000 students with disabilities, who were ages 13 to 16 at the start of the study in 2000, for several years. NLTS2 documented the secondary school programs, transition experiences, and postsecondary young-adult achievement outcomes of these students. Although these data are descriptive and correlational, they allow contrasts among the performance of youth with different types of disabilities. In some cases, comparisons with nondisabled youth have also been described.

Youth with disabilities were less likely than peers without disabilities to enroll in or complete postsecondary education or to live independently and earned less than nondisabled peers.[14] These outcomes differed by disability category. Youth with learning disabilities or language impairments reported being engaged in education, employment, or training for employment at much higher rates than some other disabilities, such as autism. These youth also had higher rates of independent living 8 years after leaving high school. Youth with learning disabilities reported higher rates of involvement with the criminal justice system than youth with most other types of disabilities.[14] Unfortunately, the literature does not sufficiently follow youth with learning and language disorders into adulthood to determine longer-term effects. Continued follow-up of the NLTS and NLTS-2 cohorts may begin to address these questions because of the established identification of these youth with disorders in childhood.

In the workplace, 60% of young adults with disabilities who had been out of high school for up to 8 years were employed compared with 66% of the general population aged 21 to 25, not a significant difference.[14] Among young adults with disabilities, those with language disorders or learning disabilities were more likely to be employed than those in other disability categories. Employment was highest for those who had obtained a postsecondary degree or certificate, followed by some postsecondary education and high school completion.

Although IDEA refers to "Speech *or* Language Impairment," clinicians often combine these terms in the mental status examination under "Speech *and* Language." Unfortunately, this has contributed to a lack of attentiveness to the distinction between disorders of speech and disorders of language reviewed in later discussion. Clinicians are encouraged to separate these entities, conceptualizing disorders of speech as those related to articulation and fluency, whereas disorders of language relate to receptive, expressive, and pragmatic communication.

Research findings support the distinction in long-term outcomes between disorders of articulation and disorders of language. In a longitudinal, matched-sample study,[15] youth identified only with speech disorders at age 5 did not differ from controls at age 19 on academic measures, with the exception of one subtest. Youth identified with language disorders at age 5 displayed significantly lower performance than speech-only or control subjects on all subtests at age 19. Learning disabilities were significantly more prevalent in the language-impaired group than for control and speech-only subjects, with risk ratios ranging from 4.4 to 11.7. In another study, adolescents with a history of combined language impairments and speech-sound disorders had higher self- and parent-reported rates of psychosocial impairment than did adolescents with speech-sound disorders alone, reading disability, or ADHD.[16] In contrast, comorbid ADHD and reading disability predicted poorer psychosocial outcomes for young adults. Both of these studies were relatively small (N<300), and one measured academic outcomes whereas the other assessed psychosocial outcomes by parent and self-report. The results indicate the long-term impact of language disorders and suggest that additional research on the language capabilities of transitional age youth deserve further investigation.

Language disorders are highly comorbid with learning disorders, particularly in reading.[17–19] In a meta-analysis of studies involving students identified with emotional and behavior disorders, 85% had undiagnosed language deficits.[20] In a smaller study, 65% of students with emotional disturbance and 91% of students with learning disabilities had concurrent language impairments, whereas 61% of students with a language disorder also exhibited a learning disorder in one or more academic areas.[21] In 2 large samples of students followed longitudinally, language impairments significantly predicted later inattention-hyperactivity and other externalizing behavior problems.[7] In a meta-analysis of longitudinal studies, psychological outcomes including internalizing, externalizing, and ADHD symptoms were worse for those identified with language impairment 2 to 12 years previously.[22] Young adults with previously identified language disorders had poorer language, academic, and cognitive performance at age 25 and lower levels of postsecondary educational attainment.[23] In this study, youth with language impairments demonstrated higher levels of behavior problems, which are also related to worse adult outcomes. Employment rates and quality-of-life ratings did not differ between groups with and without language impairment.

In a large national sample of special education students, 65% of students with emotional disturbance and 28% of children with learning disabilities were concurrently diagnosed with ADHD. Special education students with ADHD had poorer long-term academic, social, and personal outcomes than students with emotional disturbance or learning disabilities alone.[24] In a study of families with ADHD sibling pairs, 24% to 31% of children with ADHD also had learning disabilities.[25] Among a representative sample of schoolchildren, 43% of children with ADHD were also learning disabled, whereas 51% of children with learning disabilities also had ADHD.[26] These findings demonstrate the huge comorbidity of ADHD with learning and emotional challenges.

Adult outcomes for youth with ADHD include lower enrollment in 4-year postsecondary institutions and higher rates of unemployment.[27] However, the negative psychiatric and criminal justice consequences of ADHD are better predicted by academic failure and conduct problems than by the diagnosis of ADHD alone.[27,28] This finding suggests that early intervention to mitigate behavioral and academic difficulties is crucial for enhancing young adult performance: "Ensuring that children with ADHD complete school successfully, rather than treating only symptoms, comorbidities, or specific impairments such as disobedience at home, may be critical for improving adult outcomes."[28(p228)]

BRAIN IMAGING AND LEARNING DISORDERS

According to DSM-5, specific learning disorder is a neurodevelopmental disorder resulting from an interaction of genetic, epigenetic, and environmental influences. Because of the failure to locate specific areas of neural dysfunction common to developmental disorders such as ADHD and dyslexia, the concept of atypical brain development (ABD) was proposed as a model.[29] The ABD model recognized variability in brain anomalies among studies, high comorbidity among these disorders, and heterogeneity of the disorders themselves. The concept of ABD argued against attempting to pigeonhole children and youth into narrow diagnostic categories but instead to recognize the overlap among learning difficulties and broadly conceptualize the outcomes of these disorders.

However, as brain imaging techniques have matured, the search for evidence of neurologic dysfunction associated with these tasks has blossomed. Reading tasks were the first to be studied, with investigation into mathematics now underway.

Considerable work has been done to identify the location of dysfunction in dyslexia using functional MRI. Single-word reading has been the subject of brain imaging showing reduced activation in child and adult dyslexic readers in the left temporal, parietal, and fusiform regions, whereas increased activation has sometimes been found in the left inferior frontal and some right hemisphere areas.[30] These differences have also been found in young children before the onset of reading instruction. In addition, studies of event-related potentials have distinguished infants in families with a history of dyslexia and those without such a history as well as in infants who later developed dyslexia.[30]

In a study of reading fluency assessed with silent sentence reading when words were presented singly to control reading rate, dyslexic readers read significantly more slowly than typical readers with disproportionately reduced comprehension as reading rate increased.[31] Although dyslexic readers and typical readers used the same neural pathways for whole-sentence reading (left prefrontal and left superior temporal cortices, anterior cingulate, brainstem, and cerebellum), dyslexic readers showed less activation as a consequence of increased rate than typical readers.

Despite these valuable findings, further research on brain development for adolescents and young adults with learning disorders will be extremely useful. With increased information on the cause of their difficulties and knowledge of comorbidity risks, late adolescents and young adults might be amenable to treatment of associated psychiatric disorders and be willing to look at alternative career choices based on their individual patterns of strengths and weaknesses. Furthermore, given the understanding that brain development and plasticity continue at least into the mid to late 20s, additional brain research may help target remediation efforts during this age range as well as identify interventions that could be implemented even earlier in development for at-risk children.

LEGAL FRAMEWORK
Eligibility for Special Education Under Individuals with Disabilities Education Act

Under IDEA, eligibility for special education is determined by a school-based multidisciplinary team consisting of school administrator, general education teacher, school psychologist, parents, and other school staff as needed, such as a nurse or social worker. This team reviews the process of special education identification, which is strictly prescribed by IDEA. One of the elements of this process is that the team must review and consider, but does not need to accept, the conclusions and recommendations of an external evaluation, such as one containing a DSM-5 diagnosis.

Diagnosis of a learning disability is especially controversial, due in part to revisions in special education law governing states' options for diagnostic methods. The school-based diagnostic process includes a series of general education interventions before referring a child for an evaluation, a process that can be lengthy. This process may mislead parents and clinicians into thinking that the school is neglecting its responsibility when, in fact, it is respecting the right of the child to obtain and benefit from more intensive intervention before an evaluation takes place.

Accommodations Under Section 504

Accommodations under Section 504 of the Rehabilitation Act of 1973 are available to individuals with a physical or mental impairment that substantially limits one or more major life activities, including learning. Students with attention or learning issues that only require classroom accommodations or supports may qualify for this type of assistance. Section 504 plans are developed and administered by general education staff. There is no funding tied to these services and no specialized staff. Typically, these plans identify and put into place accommodations that allow the child to function productively in the general education classroom. Although many children with disabilities are served through IDEA, it is appropriate and sufficient for some students to be served only under Section 504.

The general education program continues to bear responsibility for instruction for all children. If a child has learning difficulties that are not so pronounced as to require special instruction, it is the task of the general education curriculum and staff to provide an appropriate educational program. Regular assessment is carried out in the classroom in all schools in compliance with federal education laws. In this way, the progress of all students should be monitored and instructional interventions should be initiated as needed.

Transition Services Under Individuals with Disabilities Education Act

Since 1990, IDEA has mandated transition services for students in special education in order to improve postsecondary outcomes. Transition services were inserted into IDEA because of the poor outcomes many students with disabilities experienced, such as higher dropout rates, higher rates of unemployment, poorer postsecondary educational attainment, and continued dependence on parents.[14,32,33] Transition services as defined by IDEA are shown in **Box 1**.

Transition services are intended to help the student fulfill individualized postsecondary goals as identified by the members of the student's Individualized Education Program (IEP) team, including the student and his/her parents. Postsecondary goals

---

Box 1
Transition services defined by the Individuals with Disabilities Education Improvement Act of 2004

The term "transition services" means a coordinated set of activities for a child with a disability that:

- Is designed to be within a results-oriented process, that is focused on improving the academic and functional achievement of the child with a disability to facilitate the child's movement from school to postschool activities, including postsecondary education, vocational education, integrated employment (including supported employment), continuing and adult education, adult services, independent living, or community participation

- Is based on the individual child's needs, taking into account the child's strengths, preferences, and interests; and

- Includes instruction, related services, community experiences, the development of employment and other postschool adult-living objectives, and, when appropriate, acquisition of daily living skills and functional vocational evaluation.

Individuals with Disabilities Education Improvement Act, 20 U.S.C. § 1400 602(34) (2004).

outline specific plans for education and employment, plus independent living skills if needed by that student. Annual IEP goals are linked to these postsecondary goals to define a plan of action for the student. Finally, transition services are identified to assist the student with those goals.

Ideally, the student is at the center of this entire process. Students are encouraged to be actively involved in their own transition planning and transition IEP meetings, even to the point of leading those meetings. The student's strengths, needs, preferences, and interests should guide the transition process, not those of parents or other IEP team members. Beginning this process by the time the student turns 16, or earlier if mandated by state law, allows the student and IEP team to develop and implement a robust plan well before the completion of high school. Parents, students, and clinicians are encouraged to become aware of IDEA regulations around transition and to use its requirements to the fullest extent for the benefit of the student with disabilities.

Based on a comparison of NLTS2 data with a similar cohort of youth with disabilities established in the mid-1980s, postsecondary educational participation, employment, and other outcomes improved for the second cohort in all categories of disability following the addition of transition services into IDEA.[32] Evidence-based predictors of improved postschool outcomes, drawn from analysis of correlational studies with NLTS and NLTS2 data, include many elements of strong transition programs, such as career awareness, interagency collaboration, occupational coursework, work experience, self-advocacy and self-determination, and vocational education, among others.[34,35] Predictors of successful employment following high school include attendance at a regular school, work experience in high school, and parental expectations for employment.[36]

The Rehabilitation Act and Americans with Disabilities Act in Postsecondary Education and Employment

Section 504 of the Rehabilitation Act of 1973 requires appropriate supports and accommodations for individuals with disabilities in all institutions that receive federal funds, which includes many if not most colleges and universities. The ADA of 1990 built upon the Rehabilitation Act and extended its protections to public places and services and most businesses, extending the mandate of Section 504 beyond recipients of federal funds. More recently, the ADA Amendments Act of 2008 provided clarification and further regulations intended to restore the mandate of ADA to eliminate discrimination against individuals with disabilities in response to case law that had limited its coverage.

The consistent definition of disability in these 3 acts is "a physical or mental impairment that substantially limits one or more major life activities." ADA describes extremely broad coverage, including protections for individuals who previously experienced a disability or who may be erroneously thought to have a disability. The most visible public accommodations are ADA provisions in architecture and design for individuals with physical limitations, such as wheelchair-accessible bathroom stalls, curb cuts, audible stop lights, and Braille signage in elevators.

Unlike IDEA, which requires specialized instruction and related services delivered by qualified teachers until high school completion, ADA does not provide or require special education in postsecondary settings. 504 Plans established in high school do not automatically carry over to postsecondary education settings. Therefore, students may find that the level of support they received through high school may be suddenly and sharply reduced. Postsecondary students who previously received special education services under IDEA or accommodations under Section 504 may underestimate the impact that specialized instruction and classroom accommodations had on their performance. Although they thought they no longer need supports, they may find that they are again struggling with school work or cannot pass required courses. At this point, students may seek an adult evaluation or may be referred by instructors. It is not unusual to find college-aged youth newly diagnosed with DSM-5 learning disorders or ADHD. When accommodations are implemented, these students may again be able to complete coursework and take tests competitively with their peers. Particularly for college students with learning disorders in mathematics, failure to pass required math courses, even after several attempts, threatens graduation and may prompt a referral as late as the senior year.

In postsecondary education, accommodations such as extended time on tests, taking tests in quiet or private settings, and having tests read aloud are frequently provided for students with learning and attention issues. Other options may include note-takers, recordings of class sessions, and tutoring services. Postsecondary institutions typically work with students on an individual basis to review evaluation results and determine a plan of action describing necessary accommodations that is communicated to instructors.

Some colleges and universities offer specialized programs for students with ADHD and learning disabilities that go above and beyond the requirements of ADA. For example, the Strategic Alternative Learning Techniques program at the University of Arizona offers students with attention problems and learning disorders weekly meetings with learning specialists and seminars on test taking, time management, and reading, among other topics.

Students apply for ADA supports by working with their institution's ADA office. Usually, that office will require the results of a recent evaluation that follows certain guidelines, such as examiner qualifications, permissible or recommended tests and assessments, and contents of the evaluation report, often including DSM-5 diagnosis. Each institution must post guidelines and requirements for the evaluation on their Web site so that evaluators and clinicians can meet those requirements when preparing documentation for their clients.

In vocational settings, individuals with hidden disabilities such as learning disorders, ADHD, and language impairments may display subtle difficulties in remembering and following directions, prioritizing and sequencing tasks, reading and writing, and sustaining attention. As in education, accommodations for these problems must be tailored to individual need. In addition to common workplace accommodations like accessible workstations and modified schedules, employees may obtain screen reading or dictation software, written rather than oral instructions, additional training, and assistance with prioritization and organization of tasks. Accommodations are determined through discussion with the employer (Human Resources staff or Equal Employment Opportunity officer) and with the assistance of agencies such as the Job Accommodation Network, a federal agency within the US Department of Labor, which supports workers with disabilities. Similarly, requests for accommodations in rental apartments are made to the landlord, who must abide by the Fair Housing Act, which, in addition to ADA, prohibits discrimination against individuals with disabilities in the sale or rental of most housing.

Barriers for transitional age youth in vocational and educational settings may include the desire to minimize the impact of their disability as well as reluctance to disclose their disability. For example, only 28% of youth who had been identified with a disability in high school disclosed that disability to their postsecondary institutions.[14] Employees with disabilities may fear that they will not be hired or will lose their jobs if they reveal a disability. Disclosing a disability before job performance suffers activates the umbrella of ADA and can prompt action toward the implementation of appropriate accommodations. In educational settings, disclosing a disability opens the door to a variety of supports that can enhance academic performance. Another significant barrier can be the cost and availability of a clinical or psychoeducational evaluation. ADA offices at educational institutions maintain referral lists that often include low-cost student clinics. Vocational rehabilitation departments can refer adults to private clinicians who conduct affordable evaluations.

THE ROLE OF THE CHILD AND ADOLESCENT PSYCHIATRIST
Education and Vocation

The treatment plan for any child should consider whether there are educational needs related to a disability that interfere with optimal learning. Failure to address these issues enhances vulnerability to academic frustration and failure that leads to consequent psychiatric vulnerabilities. Children with learning disorders, ADHD, and speech/communication disorders carry risks for disruptive behavior disorders, anxiety, depression, and polysubstance abuse.[5,23,27,28] It is not unusual for a parent or guardian to be confused about whether their child carries an academic vulnerability by virtue of being told that their child is not eligible for services. School districts vary considerably on the means by which eligibility is determined, and ultimately, from a school perspective, qualification is binary: one either qualifies or does not. Drawing the line for qualification is ultimately linked to funding resources and limitations. From a clinical perspective, learning disorders, communication disorders, or difficulty with ADHD symptoms are not binary. These disorders fall on a spectrum of severity, and even mild manifestations may interfere with functioning and warrant intervention. The clinician's diagnosis of the disorder, the need for services and accommodation, and the need for advocacy should not be directly determined by a school's negative decision regarding eligibility for services.

By the time youth are in their mid-teen years, discussion of postsecondary school needs and planning should be part of the treatment plan. Students and parents immersed in the challenges of the immediate demands of school are often reluctant to look forward. However, even by early high school, decisions pertaining to whether a child anticipates pursuing postsecondary education are required, especially if the school offers a junction for vocational or academic diplomas. Students and parents often are in need of information about postsecondary educational options, whether they be traditional colleges and universities, colleges or college programs designed for the needs of students with learning and communication disorders, or technical and vocational programs. For those not planning to pursue further education, reasonable employment options, whether the services of Vocational Rehabilitation are requested, also warrant exploration. Vocational Rehabilitation is coordinated on the state level. Its purpose is to minimize disability-related barriers to employment and facilitate access to employment opportunities. Determination of eligibility and priority for vocational rehabilitation services requires confirmation of relevant diagnoses in the assessment phase: a CAP is one private provider who can supply such documentation. Most students and their parents or guardians will not understand how structures offering support and accommodation transition at the time their child leaves the public school setting. Schools receiving federal funds have an obligation to educate individuals with appropriate services and accommodations until the student graduates or reaches the age of 22 years. After this point, the school's obligations to the student cease. At that juncture, special education services and accommodations are no longer provided under the mandate of IDEA. Future protections, supports, and accommodations for the individual fall under the mandate of ADA through the Equal Employment Opportunity Commission, the Fair Housing Act in the Department of Housing and Urban Development, and the Office for Civil Rights in the Department of Education.

Students not pursuing higher education have the immediate challenge of obtaining gainful and meaningful employment; employment that can provide them with a beginning means to a livelihood consistent with interests and abilities and, ideally, one that may lead to further opportunities. Any job may not do. The CAP can be of great assistance to students and parents by encouraging them to consider employment options that are in accord with interests and strengths and to avoid demands that are likely to challenge particular vulnerabilities. An individual with stronger verbal abilities may not be suited for a position that demands mechanical reasoning. An individual with excellent mechanical skills may do better in a setting that uses such talents rather than those that rely on verbal skills. An individual who thrives on predictability may perform better in a position with a redundant job task than an individual who craves novelty. The individual who is restless and distractible will likely have better success in a position that is outdoors and demands activity than one that is indoors, sedentary, and routine. Although vocational guidance can help individuals consider a range of options, a clinician who knows the individual and understands their strengths and vulnerabilities can help greatly by beginning a process that considers "fit" into employment planning.

Advocacy

The importance of advocacy for individuals with learning and communication disorders as well as vulnerabilities linked to ADHD cannot be understated. Parents of younger children need the assistance of the CAP to help them understand their child's strengths and weaknesses, legal rights, and the complexity to the system for accessing services at the same time they are emotionally coming to terms with the realization that their child will not necessarily have a smooth or consistently accomplished academic course. Most parents do not inherently understand what eligibility for services means and does not mean, which services fall under special education law (IDEA), and which services fall under disability law (504 Plans and ADA). Most importantly, they also need guidance on how they can best support their child's emotional and academic growth.

By the teen years, students can be encouraged to begin to advocate for themselves. However, this is often a daunting expectation that conflicts with the developmentally appropriate thrust to deny differences from others and to deny vulnerabilities. Here again, the CAP can be of great help to the parents and student toward understanding the obstacles that interfere with self-advocacy. It is also at this time that discussion of postsecondary pathways can begin.

The school's timetable for planning may not always be consonant with that of parents and students. School officials may present options before a student and/or parent(s) are ready to make such decisions, or may defer such decisions when there is motivation from the student or parents to proceed with planning. In either scenario, the CAP can serve as an invaluable liaison in validating the importance of such planning and processing these decisions. By late adolescence, the CAP can help focus on what may inhibit a student from initiating self-advocacy, addressing family dynamics and/or individual inhibitions linked to shame or denial.

The CAP also has an important role as a strong advocate in the community for the provision of appropriate services and as unobstructed access to them as possible, be they services under IDEA or Vocational Rehabilitation/ADA. In addition, there is a great need for advocacy for adequate school-based vocational programs and encouragement of community employers to invest in employing youth in the community, especially those with learning and communication disorders, as they transition from student to employed adult.

Although federal laws offer the frame for educational and vocational services, the application of these laws in individual communities can vary, especially in the form of unique community-based programs to assist youth in transition. It is essential for CAPs to become knowledgeable of resources and programs in their area to help guide individuals and their parents or guardians, and to advocate for the development of strong and creative services for youth transitioning into adult members of the community. Investment in meeting the needs of adolescents with learning and communication disorders as well as those with ADHD is not only for the benefit of these youth but also for the benefit of their community by virtue of the contributions these individuals have to make and the avoidance of personal and community costs that accompany young adults without structure, esteem, or a sense of productive future.

Toward that end, protective factors must be developed and enhanced during the transition period. Family support for the challenges faced by transitional age youth, such as poor school attendance or inadequate vocational planning, can be bolstered by close cooperation among parents, teens, and the clinician along with increased reliance on school and community resources. Resilience factors, such as maximum development of academic abilities to enhance career selection, early exploration of community employment opportunities, development of self-determination and self-advocacy skills, effective school-home communication, and healthy family relationships, can all be reinforced through strong alliance.

REFERENCES

1. Individuals with Disabilities Education Improvement Act, 20 U.S.C. § 1400 (2004). Available at: IDEA.ed.gov.
2. Office of Special Education and Rehabilitative Services, US Department of Education. 37th Annual Report to Congress on the Implementation of the Individuals with Disabilities Education Act, 2015. Available at: http://www2.ed.gov/about/reports/annual/osep/2015/parts-b-c/index.html. Accessed January 4, 2017.
3. National Center for Education Statistics. Fast facts: students with disabilities. Available at: http://nces.ed.gov/fastfacts/display.asp?id=60. Accessed January 4, 2017.
4. American College Health Association. American College Health Association–National College Health Assessment II: reference group executive summary fall 2015. Hanover (MD): American College Health Association; 2016. Available at: http://www.acha-ncha.org/docs/NCHA-II%20FALL%202015%20REFERENCE%20GROUP%20EXECUTIVE%20SUMMARY.pdf. Accessed January 4, 2017.
5. American Psychiatric Association. Diagnostic and statistical manual of mental disorders, fifth edition. Arlington (VA): American Psychiatric Association; 2013.
6. National Center for Learning Disabilities. Diplomas at risk: a critical look at the graduation rate of students with learning disabilities. 2013. Available at: http://ncld.convio.net/site/PageNavigator/Understood/Active/Understood_AD13_Diplomas_061814.html. Accessed January 4, 2017.
7. Petersen IT, Bates JE, D'Onofrio BM, et al. Language ability predicts the development of behavior problems in children. J Abnorm Psychol 2013;122(2):542–57.
8. Sun L, Wallach GP. Language disorders are learning disabilities: challenges on the divergent and diverse paths to language learning disability. Topics in Language Disorders 2014;34(1):25–38.

9. Ketelaars MP, Cuperus J, Jansonius K, et al. Pragmatic language impairment and associated behavioural problems. Int J Lang Commun Disord 2010;45(2): 204–14.

10. McNamara JK, Willoughby T. A longitudinal study of risk-taking behavior in adolescents with learning disabilities. Learn Disabil Res Pract 2010;25(1):11–24.

11. Morrison GM, Cosden MA. Risk, resilience, and adjustment of individuals with learning disabilities. Learn Disabil Q 1997;20(1):43–60. Available at: http://www.jstor.org.www2.lib.ku.edu/stable/1511092. Accessed January 4, 2017.

12. Murray C. Risk factors, protective factors, vulnerability, and resilience: a framework for understanding and supporting the adult transitions of youth with high-incidence disabilities. Remedial Spec Educ 2003;24(1):16–26.

13. Klassen RM, Tze VM, Hannok W. Internalizing problems of adults with learning disabilities: a meta-analysis. J Learn Disabil 2013;46(4):317–27.

14. Newman L, Wagner M, Knokey A-M, et al. The post-high school outcomes of young adults with disabilities up to 8 years after high school. A report from the National Longitudinal Transition Study-2 (NLTS2) (NCSER 2011-3005). Menlo Park (CA): SRI International; 2011. Available at: https://ies.ed.gov/ncser/pubs/20113005/pdf/20113005.pdf. Accessed January 4, 2017.

15. Young AR, Beitchman JH, Johnson C, et al. Young adult academic outcomes in a longitudinal sample of early identified language impaired and control children. J Child Psychol Psychiatry 2002;43(5):635–45.

16. Lewis BA, Patton E, Freebarn L, et al. Psychosocial co-morbidities in adolescents and adults with histories of communication disorders. J Commun Disord 2016;61: 60–70.

17. McArthur GM, Hogben JH, Edwards VT, et al. On the "specifics" of specific reading disability and specific language impairment. J Child Psychol Psychiatry 2000;41(7):869–74.

18. Nash HM, Hulme C, Gooch D, et al. Preschool language profiles of children at family risk of dyslexia: continuities with specific language impairment. J Child Psychol Psychiatry 2013;54(9):958–68.

19. Sices L, Taylor HG, Freebairn L, et al. Relationship between speech-sound disorders and early literacy skills in preschool-age children: impact of comorbid language impairment. J Dev Behav Pediatr 2007;28(6):438–47.

20. Hollo A, Wehby JH, Oliver RM. Unidentified language deficits in children with emotional and behavioral disorders: a meta-analysis. Except Child 2014;80(2): 169–86.

21. Benner G, Mattison R, Nelson J, et al. Types of language disorders in students classified as ED: prevalence and association with learning disabilities and psychopathology. Education & Treatment Of Children [serial online] 2009;32(4): 631–53.

22. Yew SG, O'Kearney R. Emotional and behavioural outcomes later in childhood and adolescence for children with specific language impairments: meta-analyses of controlled prospective studies. J Child Psychol Psychiatry 2013; 54(5):516–24.

23. Johnson CJ, Beitchman JH, Brownlie BE. Twenty-year follow-up of children with and without speech-language impairments: family, educational, occupational, and quality of life outcomes. Am J Speech Lang Pathol 2010;19(1): 51–65.

24. Wei X, Yu JW, Shaver D. Longitudinal effects of ADHD in children with learning disabilities or emotional disturbances. Except Child 2014;80(2):205–19.

25. Del'Homme M, Kim TS, Loo SK, et al. Familial association and frequency of learning disabilities in ADHD sibling pair families. J Abnorm Child Psychol 2007;35(1):55–62.
26. Smith TJ, Adams G. The effect of comorbid AD/HD and learning disabilities on parent-reported behavioral and academic outcomes of children. Learn Disabil Q 2006;29(2):101–12.
27. Kuriyan AB, Pelham WE, Molina BS, et al. Young adult educational and vocational outcomes of children diagnosed with ADHD. J Abnorm Child Psychol 2013;41(1): 27–41.
28. Owens EB, Hinshaw SP. Childhood conduct problems and young adult outcomes among women with childhood attention-deficit/hyperactivity disorder (ADHD). J Abnorm Psychol 2016;125(2):220.
29. Gilger JW, Kaplan BJ. Atypical brain development: a conceptual framework for understanding developmental learning disabilities. Dev Neuropsychol 2001; 20(2):465–81.
30. Norton ES, Beach SD, Gabrieli JDE. Neurobiology of dyslexia. Curr Opin Neurobiol 2015;30:73–8.
31. Christodoulou JA, Del Tufo SN, Lymberis J, et al. Brain bases of reading fluency in typical reading and impaired fluency in dyslexia. PLoS One 2014;9(7):e100552.
32. Newman L, Wagner M, Cameto R, et al. Comparisons across time of the outcomes of youth with disabilities up to 4 years after high school. A report of findings from the National Longitudinal Transition study (NLTS) and the National Longitudinal Transition Study-2 (NLTS2). NCSER 2010-3008 2010;163. Available at: http://www.nlts2. org/reports/2010_09/nlts2_report_2010_09_complete.pdf. Accessed January 4, 2017.
33. Office of Disability Employment Policy. Economic picture of the disability community project: Key points on disability and occupational projections tables. n.d. Available at: https://www.dol.gov/odep/topics/disabilityemploymentstatistics. htm. Accessed January 4, 2017.
34. Mazzotti VL, Rowe DA, Sinclair J, et al. Predictors of post-school success: a systematic review of NLTS2 secondary analyses. Career Dev Transit Except Individ 2015;1–20. http://dx.doi.org/10.1177/2165143415588047. Accessed January 4, 2017.
35. Mazzotti VL, West DW, Mustian AL. Secondary transition evidence-based practices and predictors: implications for policymakers. J Disabil Policy Stud 2014; 25(1):5–18.
36. Wehman P, Sima AP, Ketchum J, et al. Predictors of successful transition from school to employment for youth with disabilities. J Occup Rehabil 2015;25(2): 323–34.

Autism Spectrum Disorders

Challenges and Opportunities for Transition to Adulthood

Gerrit I. van Schalkwyk, MB,ChB, Fred R. Volkmar, MD*

KEYWORDS

- Autism • Autism spectrum disorder • College mental health • Young adults
- Adults with disabilities

KEY POINTS

- Owing to good outcomes, individuals with autism spectrum disorder (ASD) are increasingly transitioning to adulthood with diverse goals regarding their education, vocation, and degree of independent living.
- These individuals may experience substantial challenges during this period owing to the decreased availability of supports, particularly regarding their educational goals.
- Although programs exist to support these individuals, they are, for the most part, limited and without significant evidence.
- Providers need to have both an understanding of the challenges for transition age youth with ASD and an awareness of their unique needs in clinical settings.

INTRODUCTION

The transition to adulthood presents a broad range of challenges and opportunities to individuals with ASD. The nature of the transition experience depends on the levels of functioning of the individual and includes goals as diverse as entry in to the labor force,[1] attending college,[2] and achieving a degree of independent living.[3] A significant increase in the provision of supports to children and adolescents with ASD has broadened the scope of potential opportunities[2] and also provided new impetus for services that support the optimal transition of youth into adulthood.[4] The diversity of individual capacities, resource availability, and family and individual preference significantly complicate the task of providing support during the transitional period, requiring that services be pitched at a range of levels and operate in several contexts. During childhood, school systems frequently serve to organize and provide the necessary

Disclosures: The authors have no relevant disclosures.
Child Study Center, Yale University School of Medicine, New Haven, CT, USA
* Corresponding author. Child Study Center, Yale University, 230 South Frontage Road, New Haven, CT 06510.
E-mail address: fred.volkmar@yale.edu

Child Adolesc Psychiatric Clin N Am 26 (2017) 329–339
http://dx.doi.org/10.1016/j.chc.2016.12.013   **childpsych.theclinics.com**

supports to optimize learning outcomes for individuals with ASD—by contrast, colleges and other postsecondary educational programs do not have a federal mandate to act in this capacity.[5] Furthermore, many individuals with ASD may not be able to, or may choose not to, access postsecondary education programs at all. This underscores the need for both research and service development that extend across multiple settings.

Existing research has raised awareness of the diversity of outcomes for individuals with ASD entering adulthood.[6] Furthermore, some more recent work has explored employment outcomes,[7] and the small body of research pertaining to social, behavioral, and cognitive outcomes has been the subject of systematic review.[8] Emerging understanding is that overall, adaptive functioning may improve in adulthood but that there are risks for deterioration across other domains.[8] Psychiatric comorbidity has been found more common in adults with ASD,[9,10] although these findings are from small samples, and there is significant complexity in appropriately framing comorbidity within an ASD population.[11-13] Even less research involves evaluation of specific programs to support these individuals. Although the literature increasingly contains helpful recommendations for specific contexts, there is a limited understanding of the overall needs of this population and how they can be met most effectively. From a neuroscience perspective, although some work has identified the ongoing presence of cognitive deficits in specific domains, such as theory of mind, understanding of brain development into adulthood for individuals with ASD is extremely limited.[14] Adding a final layer of complexity, preliminary research has identified the inadequacy of training in ASD and developmental disabilities in child and adolescent psychiatry residents[15]—although there are no data available, it is reasonable to assume that training is even less adequate for adult psychiatry residents, who frequently are tasked with the care of these individuals.

This article describes the unique challenges faced by transitional age youth with ASD. It focuses on both less and more cognitively able young adults and highlights existing research and approaches to psychosocial support. Specific legal issues that are pertinent during this period are discussed further and tentative best practice recommendations for clinicians working with these individuals are offered. Finally, the most critical areas for future research are highlighted, which will improve understanding and capacity to deliver effective supports.

CHALLENGES FOR INDIVIDUALS WITH AUTISM SPECTRUM DISORDER ENTERING COMMUNITIES AND WORKPLACES

As for all young adults making the transition from high school to adulthood, there are several challenges for individuals with ASD—in particular, the less cognitively able. With earlier diagnosis and intervention, more students are functioning at higher levels; unfortunately, some students remain in need of substantial supports.[4] For these students, support from state departments of developmental disabilities are usually available; depending on the state/jurisdiction, eligibility may be arbitrary, often centering around full-scale IQ rather than individual needs. This is particularly unfortunate given that individuals with relatively normal full-scale IQ but significant deficits in certain domains—such as adaptive functioning—may be particularly responsive to a range of supports. In addition to cognitive disability, difficulties in adaptive skills pose real obstacles for daily functioning.[16] As Howlin[4] notes, it is important to underscore that what adults with ASD might prefer in terms of living arrangements may differ from societal or parental expectations. Societal ideals might emphasize independent living, whereas for some a sense of privacy and safety may be more important.[4]

A range of programs have been developed for adults needing employment sup-ports,[17] with preliminary evidence suggesting that vocational support programs may increase the likelihood of sustained employment.[18] Unfortunately, however, employ-ment options remain limited.[19] Individuals with ASD are more frequently denied voca-tional rehabilitation services for being considered too severely disabled.[20] Even for individuals without intellectual disability, results of one study have found that fewer than half access community employment, with a majority spending time in workshops or adult day care settings.[1] As is the case for most individuals, there is some sugges-tion that having a good vocational placement is associated with better behavioral adaptations in ASD.[21] There is a need for more information on this topic, with better integration of the entire package of services beginning as part of the high school tran-sitional planning process. To the authors' knowledge, there are no formal data describing this process, but clinical experience suggests that individualized educa-tional plans rarely pay sufficient attention to concrete attempts at preparing students for the next phase. It is important to respect student interest while also being realistic. Planning should include a consideration of strengths and weaknesses as well as a realistic assessment of adaptive skills.

In the US, major federal supports include Supplemental Security Income and Social Security Disability Insurance. These programs are of special benefit to those adults who cannot engage in substantive employment. Services provided by these programs may include home-based interventions (such as home health aides, visiting nurses, and behaviorists) as well as funding for residential placement. There are few data to guide understanding of the optimal approach for more severely affected individuals, and the decision needs to take into account the capacities and preferences of the fam-ily and individual. Preliminary research notes that the decision to have an adult with ASD coreside versus live out of living may have complex impacts on both the individ-ual and family—specifically, mothers of adults with ASD consider the former of great-est benefit to the family and the latter to be of greatest benefit to the individual.[22] Longitudinal studies examining the comparative biopsychosocial outcomes of individ-uals in both settings are a critical priority.

Other issues arise with health insurance coverage, because after age 26 (with the passage of the Affordable Care Act), individuals can no longer remain on their parents' insurance plans and often receive state-supported programs. Although providing a certain basic coverage, access to specialist care can be limited. Finding medical care providers knowledgeable in the care of individuals with ASD is a challenge. The risk for some mental health problems, notably mood and anxiety disorders, is increased in the more cognitively able individuals with ASD and the same is probably true for the more cognitively challenged although research is limited. For individuals with little or no spoken language, these problems are complex and sometimes overlap with medical issues, for example, undiagnosed pain leads to behavior problems. In such an instance, it is the pain that is most profitably treated. The few data available suggest that although knowledge remains limited, pharmacologic interventions are common, with antipsy-chotics most frequently used and polypharmacy an increasing concern.[23,24]

It must be emphasized that some good resources and practice guidelines are avail-able.[16,25] Knowledge has mostly been limited, however, to outcome studies of young adults, with little information available on the aging population. For example, it is not known if the risk for epilepsy is increased in adults as it is in children and adoles-cents[26]; similarly, information on suicidality and suicide rates is almost nonexistent,[27] as is information on aging in general.[28] Many of the interventions used, with some ex-ceptions in the area of psychopharmacology, are based on generalization of experi-ence from younger populations.

CHALLENGES FOR COLLEGE STUDENTS WITH AUTISM SPECTRUM DISORDER

As is the case for all students, individuals with ASD may experience challenges when attending college across a range of dimensions, including social, academic, and psychological functioning. The difficulties encountered during the transition to college are related to (1) an abrupt change in the primary environment, (2) a shift from parental responsibility to students being responsible for their own success, and (3) changing legal mandates.[5] Whereas schools are required to do whatever is necessary to ensure the best possible education, colleges are required only to provide "reasonable accommodations" to students with unique needs.[5] This leaves considerable responsibility with students, who need to assertively request any supports that they think are necessary to achieve success. Furthermore, the process of preparing a student with ASD for college involves a long, collaborative process between the student, parents, school, college, and health care team and should include prolonged consideration of the appropriate college setting and the necessary skills that need to be learned prior to a student graduating high school. Even when this is done adequately, students may continue to require supports once making this transition.

Mental Health Issues

Mental health concerns are highly prevalent among college students.[29] Students with ASD seem at risk for the same disorders that affect other students, with case reports describing symptoms of depression,[30] attention-deficit/hyperactivity disorder (ADHD),[12] and anxiety.[31] Although there are no larger epidemiologic studies in this population, high rates of psychiatric comorbidity have been reported for high-functioning adults with ASD in general.[32] The etiology of these comorbid difficulties may include despair about capacity to function effectively in the more complex social environments that characterize college campuses[33] as well as increased demands on executive function that unmask ongoing difficulties with attention and planning.[12] Social anxiety may become increasingly prominent as a recognition of the importance of social engagement is paired with an increased awareness of social limitations.[34] Clinicians and support services at universities may not be optimally equipped to recognize these difficulties in students with ASD, who may have idiosyncratic presentations and treatment needs (discussed later).

Social Issues and Sexuality

The college environment provides uniquely challenging social demands. Whereas the high school environment provides a relative degree of consistency in terms of physical space and expectations, college campuses may involve widely varying classroom sizes, different approaches from lecturers, and rapid shifts between contexts with different social rules—this is particularly the case for students living on residential college campuses. In the authors' clinical experience, students have been encountered who were mailing their dirty clothes back home on a weekly basis to avoid the complex social rules that governed the dormitory laundry room. These realities are consistent with findings of high loneliness rates among college students with ASD.[35] The literature includes a range of practical recommendations to support the social functioning of students with ASD, including social skills training[36] and the identification of peer or staff mentors.[37]

Sexuality is an issue that warrants specific attention. Previous investigators have highlighted the risk for college students with ASD to be taken advantage of sexually,[2] a salient concern as awareness grows regarding the rates of sexual misconduct on college campuses. Furthermore, individuals with ASD seem to more frequently express gender-related concerns[38,39] and may continue in their efforts to clarify their own gender roles during college. Clinicians can likely be most helpful to students by providing them with concrete support in exploring their own gender identity as they navigate new social contexts.[40]

Challenges related to both social engagement and sexuality should be recognized as well for their potential positive implications. The success of students with ASD in making it to college suggests improving support services during young childhood, and the motivation of these students to be positively engaged with peers may contribute to positive outcome. Despite earlier assumptions to the contrary, recent literature indicates that most adolescents and young adults with ASD do have significant interest in pursuing appropriate sexual relationships.[41] The need then is for a better understanding of how to support individuals in achieving these goals.

Adaptive Skills

The college environment may place new demands on an individual's capacity for independent function. Academically skilled students with ASD may nevertheless need preparation to successfully navigate tasks like setting up complex time tables, developing effective routines, doing laundry, shopping, and obtaining food.[5] Offices for disability services are variably helpful in this regard, and it is important that students work on developing these capacities in the years preceding the college transition.[37] This need is underscored by data showing that decreased capacity for independent functioning seems to be a significant barrier to students with ASD engaging in postsecondary education.[42] Students may also experience difficulty in academic performance, despite average or above-average intelligence. The need for significant planning, balancing different academic priorities, and being increasingly self-directed with regard to academic work may present a challenge even for students who have been academically successful in high school.[12] In this sphere, some support may be possible, with disability offices frequently available to help teach students strategies for planning their college studies effectively—however, more extensive accommodations (such as waivers of certain course requirements) are unlikely to be available.[5] College transition programs exist at many colleges, and some have been found helpful for individuals with disabilities by providing early insight into the nature of the college experience and jump-starting the formation of relationships[43]—these programs may vary in their usefulness for individuals with ASD specifically.

LEGAL ISSUES

Legal issues can arise in various circumstances. There is a marked increase in risk for adults with ASD to become caught up in the criminal justice system.[44] This can arise in myriad ways, for example, being a victim, witnessing criminal activity, being involved in bullying (as a victim or, at times, as a participant), making true but highly inappropriate comments, searching for information online, and so forth. For the less cognitively able individual, inappropriate behavior, for example, an outburst at a store or mall, can get the police involved. Such individuals may also be ready targets for criminal activity or bullying; having ASD probably at least doubles the risk for bullying above the base rate and additional problems only further increase this risk.[45] For the more cognitively able, issues like inappropriate sexual requests or activities can lead to legal difficulties. On occasion, individuals with ASD, in particularly those with Asperger syndrome, may become fixated on a particular friend or possible romantic partner and engage in what may be seen as stalking.[46] The limited available literature suggests that although individuals with Asperger syndrome are more likely to come into contact with the criminal justice system, they are no more likely to face conviction.[47,48] The response of law enforcement to these individuals at multiple levels of the criminal justice process may play an important role in mediating this increased involvement.[40] Furthermore, given issues with social judgment, individuals may also engage unwittingly in criminal activity, for example, an adolescent with Asperger syndrome who is approached at the airport and asked by a stranger if he would do a favor by carrying a package to his elderly mother who would be waiting at the airport at the end of the flight—the package containing cocaine!

Other issues arise relative to the need some adults have for more intense supervision and support. For such individual's guardianship by parents, siblings or others may be appropriate. Issues of estate planning and provision of special trusts can also arise and parents may need informed legal help to insure that assets are passed in some way to the person.[49] States vary in their approach to this problem. Some of the most complicated issues arise for individuals with IQs above the intellectually deficient range, who may need some help but do not qualify for full guardianship.[50]

BEST PRACTICES AND THE ROLE OF MENTAL HEALTH PROFESSIONALS

As discussed previously, the capacity to make broad recommendations for supporting transition age youth with ASD is limited by the heterogeneity of their needs; the multiple contexts in which these individuals may be living, working, and learning; and the limited evidence base. Nevertheless, several practical recommendations are appropriate based on emerging understanding. Most obviously, efforts at raising awareness are indicated, and these should involve individuals with ASD, family members, teachers at school, and relevant staff in postsecondary education or work settings. In particular, there is an immediate need for the transition process to be codified in the individualized education plan of students with ASD several years prior to completion of high school.[5,30,37] Mental health professionals, disability services staff, and other relevant staff on college campuses need to have a robust understanding of the potential needs of students with ASD and have some form of programming that is available to support their needs.[51] Peer support interventions are increasingly popular and seem a promising way to support these individuals.[2,52]

Mental health professionals need a higher level of understanding as to the potential difficulties that may arise for individuals with ASD, including psychiatric comorbidities. Frequently, psychiatrists in college mental health services (as well as those seeing young adults in community settings) are adult psychiatrists, with comparatively limited experience in developmental disabilities. There is a need for these psychiatrists to familiarize themselves with the available literature around psychopharmacology for adults with ASD[12]—these are well reviewed by Doyle and colleagues[53] and summarized in **Table 1**. When college students have concerns that are appropriate for psychotherapy, counselors should at least be aware of relevant considerations that may influence the therapy process.[36,54] Specifically, therapists need to be comfortable with providing a more directive approach and are tasked with helping translate the social world for their patients. Strictly analytical therapies are generally believed contraindicated and in general therapists may find themselves relying less on subtleties of communication. Where appropriate, social skills–based interventions should be made available to students hoping to improve their capacity for positive peer interaction. The evidence for these interventions comes from studies of group-based interventions,[55,56] although in practice it may only be feasible for this

Table 1
Pharmacotherapy for comorbid symptoms and diagnoses in adults with autism spectrum disorder

	Available Evidence	Practical Recommendation
ADHD	Case reports in adults of methylphenidate[12] and atomoxetine[57]	Stimulants first line but less likely to be effective and greater risk for poor tolerance
Behavioral symptoms	Risperidone and haloperidol shown effective in a RCT.[58,59] Haloperidol discontinued due to side effects in 7/33 subjects.[59] Case series for other antipsychotics, including aripiprazole.[60] Limited study of SSRIs, TCAs, and mood stabilizers.	Atypical antipsychotics risperidone and aripiprazole likely first-line choice. Haloperidol an option if significant weight gain occurs on these agents, although rates of dystonia and other side effects are concerning.
Depression	Case series of fluoxetine[61]	Trial of SSRI; monitor from improved communication and decreased irritability as a sign of response.
Anxiety	Case reports of fluvoxamine[62] and fluoxetine[63] in OCD	SSRI trial may be appropriate; note increased risk for activation.

Abbreviations: OCD, obsessive-compulsive disorder; RCT, randomized controlled trial; SSRI, selective serotonin reuptake inhibitor; TCA, tricyclic antidepressant.

Data from Doyle C, McDougle C, Stigler K. Pharmacotherapy of behavioral symptoms and psychiatric comorbidities in adolescents and adults with autism spectrum disorders. Adolescents and adults with autism spectrum disorders. New York: 2014. p. 161–91.

work to be done on an individual basis given the logistic challenges of coordinating groups of students.

SUMMARY AND FURTHER RESEARCH

Available research suggests that positive outcomes are increasingly common for transition age youth with ASD. This progress has created an enormous need for both services and research into how these individuals can be best supported. Both recommendations and research in this area are complicated by the diverse trajectories that are possible for individuals with ASD. Future work should seek to better define the most common desires and needs of youth with ASD and their families as they transition from high school into young adulthood. A starting point for developing better evidenced-based interventions is to collect good data on existing efforts at supporting this population—for example, outcome data in peer support programs on college campuses. Clinicians need to be actively engaged in publishing and presenting case reports on their experiences supporting youth with ASD, to increase the availability of common sense recommendations and identify specific areas where further discussion and research are required. Relatedly, effective education needs to be implemented for employers, colleges, and law enforcement regarding the idiosyncratic working, learning, and coping styles of individuals with ASD. Pharmacologic research should be focused on studying the efficacy and tolerability of the existing armamentarium of medications that are currently used in younger individuals and on an off-label basis in adults. The dramatic need for additional research should be recognized and addressed, but at the same time clinicians and families need to advocate for increased availability of resources at all levels that are informed by available evidence and that include mechanisms for measuring change. The needs of transition age youth with ASD are significant and cannot be delayed in anticipation of a more complete scientific understanding.

REFERENCES

1. Taylor JL, Seltzer MM. Employment and post-secondary educational activities for young adults with autism spectrum disorders during the transition to adulthood. J Autism Dev Disord 2011;41(5):566–74.
2. Vanbergeijk E, Klin A, Volkmar F. Supporting more able students on the autism spectrum: college and beyond. J Autism Dev Disord 2008;38(7):1359–70.
3. Marriage S, Wolverton A, Marriage K. Autism spectrum disorder grown up: a chart review of adult functioning. J Can Acad Child Adolesc Psychiatry 2009; 18(4):322–8.
4. Howlin P. Outcome in adult life for more able individuals with autism or asperger syndrome. Autism 2000;4(1):63–83.
5. Thierfeld Brown J, Wolf LE, King L, et al. The parent's guide to college for students on the autism spectrum. Shawnee Mission (KS): AAPC Publishing; 2012.
6. Levy A, Perry A. Outcomes in adolescents and adults with autism: a review of the literature. Res Autism Spectr Disord 2011;5(4):1271–82.
7. Cimera RE, Cowan RJ. The costs of services and employment outcomes achieved by adults with autism in the US. Autism 2009;13(3):285–302.
8. Magiati I, Tay XW, Howlin P. Cognitive, language, social and behavioural outcomes in adults with autism spectrum disorders: a systematic review of longitudinal follow-up studies in adulthood. Clin Psychol Rev 2014;34(1):78–86.
9. Joshi G, Wozniak J, Petty C, et al. Psychiatric comorbidity and functioning in a clinically referred population of adults with autism spectrum disorders: a comparative study. J Autism Dev Disord 2013;43(6):1314–25.
10. Lugnegård T, Hallerbäck MU, Gillberg C. Psychiatric comorbidity in young adults with a clinical diagnosis of Asperger syndrome. Res Dev Disabil 2011;32(5): 1910–7.
11. Dossetor D. "All that glitters is not gold": misdiagnosis of psychosis in pervasive developmental disorders—a case series. Clin Child Psychol Psychiatry 2007; 12(4):537–48.
12. van Schalkwyk GI, Beyer C, Martin A, et al. College students with autism spectrum disorders: a growing role for adult psychiatrists. J Am Coll Health 2016; 64(7):575–9.
13. Van Schalkwyk GI, Peluso F, Qayyum Z, et al. Varieties of misdiagnosis in ASD: an illustrative case series. J Autism Dev Disord 2015;45(4):911–8.
14. Baron-Cohen S, Wheelwright S, Hill J, et al. The "reading the mind in the eyes" test revised version: a study with normal adults, and adults with asperger syndrome or high-functioning autism. J Child Psychol Psychiatry 2001;42(2):241–51.
15. Marrus N, Veenstra-VanderWeele J, Hellings JA, et al. Training of child and adolescent psychiatry fellows in autism and intellectual disability. Autism 2014; 18(4):471–5.
16. Shea V, Mesibov GB. Adolescents and adults with autism. In: Volkmar FR, Rogers SJ, Paul R, et al, editors. Handbook of autism and pervasive developmental disorders. Hoboken (NJ): Wiley; 2014. p. 288–311.
17. Gerhadt PF, Cicero F, Mayville E, et al. Employment and related services for adults with ASD. In: Volkmar FR, Rogers SJ, Paul R, et al, editors. Handbook of autism and pervasive developmental disorders. Hoboken (NJ): Wiley; 2014.
18. Hillier A, Campbell H, Mastriani K, et al. Two-year evaluation of a vocational support program for adults on the autism spectrum. Career Dev Transit Except Individ 2007;30(1):35–47.

19. Nicholas DB, Attridge M, Zwaigenbaum L, et al. Vocational support approaches in autism spectrum disorder: a synthesis review of the literature. Autism 2015; 19(2):235–45.

20. Lawer L, Brusilovskiy E, Salzer MS, et al. Use of vocational rehabilitative services among adults with autism. J Autism Dev Disord 2009;39(3):487–94.

21. Taylor JL, Smith LE, Mailick MR. Engagement in vocational activities promotes behavioral development for adults with autism spectrum disorders. J Autism Dev Disord 2014;44(6):1447–60.

22. Krauss MW, Seltzer MM, Jacobson HT. Adults with autism living at home or in non-family settings: positive and negative aspects of residential status. J Intellect Disabil Res 2005;49(2):111–24.

23. Khanna R, Jariwala K, West-Strum D. Use and cost of psychotropic drugs among recipients with autism in a state Medicaid fee-for-service programme. J Intellect Disabil Res 2013;57(2):161–71.

24. Schubart JR, Camacho F, Leslie D. Psychotropic medication trends among children and adolescents with autism spectrum disorder in the Medicaid program. Autism 2014;18(6):631–7.

25. Volkmar F, Reichow B, McPartland J. Adolescents and adults with autism spectrum disorders. New York: Springer; 2014.

26. Volkmar FR, Nelson DS. Seizure disorders in autism. J Am Acad Child Adolesc Psychiatry 1990;29(1):127–9.

27. Paquette-Smith M, Weiss J, Lunsky Y. History of suicide attempts in adults with Asperger syndrome. Crisis 2014;35(4):273–7.

28. Piven J, Rabins P, Autism-in-Older Adults Working Group. Autism spectrum disorders in older adults: toward defining a research agenda. J Am Geriatr Soc 2011;59(11):2151–5.

29. Zivin K, Eisenberg D, Gollust SE, et al. Persistence of mental health problems and needs in a college student population. J Affect Disord 2009;117(3):180–5.

30. Connor DJ. Actively navigating the transition into college: narratives of students with learning disabilities. Int J Qual Stud Educ 2012;25(8):1005–36.

31. MacLeod A, Green S. Beyond the books: case study of a collaborative and holistic support model for university students with Asperger syndrome. Studies in Higher Education 2009;34(6):631–46.

32. Hofvander B, Delorme R, Chaste P, et al. Psychiatric and psychosocial problems in adults with normal-intelligence autism spectrum disorders. BMC Psychiatry 2009;9:35.

33. Pinder-Amaker S. Identifying the unmet needs of college students on the autism spectrum. Harv Rev Psychiatry 2014;22(2):125–37.

34. Bauminger N, Shulman C, Agam G. Peer interaction and loneliness in high-functioning children with autism. J Autism Dev Disord 2003;33(5):489–507.

35. Jobe LE, Williams White S. Loneliness, social relationships, and a broader autism phenotype in college students. Pers Individ Dif 2007;42(8):1479–89.

36. Van Schalkwyk GI, Volkmar FR. Autism spectrum disorders: in theory and practice. Psychoanal Study Child 2015;69:219–41.

37. Adreon D, Durocher JS. Evaluating the college transition needs of individuals with high-functioning autism spectrum disorders. Interv Sch Clin 2007;42(5):271–9.

38. de Vries ALC, Doreleijers TA, Steensma TD, et al. Psychiatric comorbidity in gender dysphoric adolescents. J Child Psychol Psychiatry 2011;52(11):1195–202.

39. Jacobs LA, Rachlin K, Erickson-schroth L, et al. Gender dysphoria and co-occurring autism spectrum disorders: review, case examples, and treatment considerations. LGBT Health 2014;1(4):277–82.

40. van Schalkwyk GI, Klingensmith K, Volkmar FR. Gender identity and autism spectrum disorders. Yale J Biol Med 2015;88(1):81–3.

41. Fernandes LC, Gillberg CI, Cederlund M, et al. Aspects of sexuality in adolescents and adults diagnosed with autism spectrum disorders in childhood. J Autism Dev Disord 2016;46(9):3155–65.

42. Shattuck PT, Narendorf SC, Cooper B, et al. Postsecondary education and employment among youth with an autism spectrum disorder. Pediatrics 2012; 129(6):1042–9.

43. Rothman T, Maldonado JM, Rothman H. Building self-confidence and future career success through a pre-college transition program for individuals with disabilities. J Vocat Rehabil 2008;28(2):73–83.

44. Woodbury-Smith M. Unlawful behaviors in adolescents and adults with autism spectrum disorders. Adolescents and adults with autism spectrum disorders. New York: Springer; 2014. p. 269–81.

45. Zeedyk SM, Rodriguez G, Tipton LA, et al. Bullying of youth with autism spectrum disorder, intellectual disability, or typical development: victim and parent perspectives. Res Autism Spectr Disord 2014;8(9):1173–83.

46. Stokes M, Newton N, Kaur A. Stalking, and social and romantic functioning among adolescents and adults with autism spectrum disorder. J Autism Dev Disord 2007;37(10):1969–86.

47. Browning A, Caulfield L. The prevalence and treatment of people with Asperger's syndrome in the criminal justice system. Criminol Crim Justice 2011; 11(2):165–80.

48. Hippler K, Viding E, Klicpera C, et al. No increase in criminal convictions in Hans Asperger's original cohort. J Autism Dev Disord 2010;40(6):774–80.

49. Volkmar FR, Wiesner LA. A practical guide to autism. Hoboken (NJ): Wiley; 2009.

50. Zablotsky B, Bradshaw CP, Anderson CM, et al. Risk factors for bullying among children with autism spectrum disorders. Autism 2014;18(4):419–27.

51. Wolf L, Brown J, Kukiela Bork G, et al. Students with Asperger syndrome: a guide for college personell. Shawnee Mission (KS): AAPC Publishing; 2009.

52. Rao PA, Beidel DC, Murray MJ. Social skills interventions for children with Asperger's syndrome or high-functioning autism: a review and recommendations. J Autism Dev Disord 2008;38(2):353–61.

53. Doyle C, McDougle C, Stigler K. Pharmacotherapy of behavioral symptoms and psychiatric comorbidities in adolescents and adults with autism spectrum disorders. Adolescents and adults with autism spectrum disorders. New York: Springer; 2014. p. 161–91.

54. Volkmar FR. Asperger's disorder: implications for psychoanalysis. Psychoanal Inq 2011;31(3):334–44.

55. Gantman A, Kapp SK, Orenski K, et al. Social skills training for young adults with high-functioning autism spectrum disorders: a randomized controlled pilot study. J Autism Dev Disord 2012;42(6):1094–103.

56. Howlin P, Yates P. The potential effectiveness of social skills groups for adults with autism. Autism 1999;3(3):299–307.

57. Niederhofer H, Damodharan SK, Joji R, et al. Atomoxetine treating patients with Autistic disorder. Autism 2006;10(6):647–9.

58. McDougle CJ, Holmes JP, Carlson DC, et al. A double-blind, placebo-controlled study of risperidone in adults with autistic disorder and other pervasive developmental disorders. Arch Gen Psychiatry 1998;55(7):633–41.
59. Remington G, Sloman L, Konstantareas M, et al. Clomipramine versus haloperidol in the treatment of autistic disorder: a double-blind, placebo-controlled, crossover study. J Clin Psychopharmacol 2001;21(4):440–4.
60. Shastri M, Alla L, Sabaratnam M. Aripiprazole use in individuals with intellectual disability and psychotic or behavioural disorders: a case series. J Psychopharmacol 2006;20(6):863–7.
61. Ghaziuddin M, Tsai L, Ghaziuddin N. Fluoxetine in autism with depression. J Am Acad Child Adolesc Psychiatry 1991;30(3):508–9.
62. McDougle CJ, Price LH, Goodman WK. Fluvoxamine treatment of coincident autistic disorder and obsessive-compulsive disorder: a case report. J Autism Dev Disord 1990;20(4):537–43.
63. Koshes RJ. Use of fluoxetine for obsessive-compulsive behavior in adults with autism. Am J Psychiatry 1997;154(4):578.

Schizophrenia and Psychosis

Diagnosis, Current Research Trends, and Model Treatment Approaches with Implications for Transitional Age Youth

Vivien Chan, MD[a,b,c],*

KEYWORDS

- Schizophrenia • Psychotic disorders • Therapeutics • Education • Adolescence

KEY POINTS

- Current best-practice models of schizophrenia treatment are multidisciplinary, recovery oriented, and include medications, with psychosocial interventions involving as many of the patient's supports as possible.
- Psychosocial interventions with families may be helpful to improve outcomes for youth at high risk for psychosis, but these interventions still require significant validation.
- There are imprecisions in the definitions of psychosis and first episode, especially in the ultrahigh-risk/clinical-high-risk literature.
- The emerging adult period is a critical stage in which the developmental trajectory can be significantly altered but can also be a time of higher treatment responsiveness toward stable remission.

INTRODUCTION

At first glance, a diagnosis of schizophrenia seems distinct, and the clinical signs have long been described by Kraepelin and Bleuler.[1] Frequently with onset coincident with the developmental age of emerging adulthood, particularly in young men, its annual incidence is up to 0.70/1000/y consistently worldwide.[2,3] There is a well-known bimodal peak of onset during ages 15 to 24 years, which is slightly

Disclosure: Dr V. Chan has common stock holdings in AbbVie, Inc, Abbott Laboratories, Bristol-Myers Squibb Co, Eli Lilly & Co., and Johnson & Johnson.

[a] 501 Student Health, Student Health Center, University of California Irvine, Irvine, CA 92697-5200, USA; [b] Behavioral Health Services, Children, Youth & Prevention Division, Center for Resiliency Wellness & Education (First Episode Psychosis), Orange County Health Care Agency, 729 W Town & Country Road, Building E, Orange, CA 92868, USA; [c] Department of Psychiatry & Human Behavior, UCI Health, Orange, CA 92868, USA

* 501 Student Health, Student Health Center, University of California Irvine, Irvine, CA 92697-5200.
E-mail address: vchan1@uci.edu

Child Adolesc Psychiatric Clin N Am 26 (2017) 341–366
http://dx.doi.org/10.1016/j.chc.2016.12.014
1056-4993/17/© 2017 The Author. Published by Elsevier Inc. This is an open access article under the CC BY-NC-ND license (http://creativecommons.org/licenses/by-nc-nd/4.0/).

childpsych.theclinics.com

weighted toward men, and weighted toward women at 55 to 64 years.[3,4] The disorder affects men and women, with a higher lifetime risk in men.[4]

Having genetic familial clustering, schizophrenia carries a standard mortality ratio of 2.6, usually from suicide or cardiovascular risk.[5] Although familial clustering is important (eg, 22q11.2 deletion), sporadic cases of schizophrenia occur more often, possibly due to associated decreased fertility and fecundity.[6,7] The reasons for this decrease are unclear, but clinicians should still discuss family planning, social, sexual and romantic relationships, particularly in the late adolescent and young adult population. Familial risks of schizophrenia are outlined in **Table 1**.[3,8,9]

The course of schizophrenia, from acute to stabilization and recovery phase, varies widely from total incapacity to remission.[10] Rapid initiation of antipsychotic pharmacologic treatment is indicated; when the first episode of schizophrenia is treated, it has a better prognosis and requires a lower antipsychotic dosage than a long duration of untreated psychosis (DUP).[10] The 5 years following the first episode, often called the critical period forecasting illness progression, usually includes relapse.[10,11] Beyond this initial critical period and through the following decade, schizophrenia tends to plateau and not devolve to a progressively deteriorating condition.[11] This is useful psychoeducation for young adult patients in order to instill hope, encourage compliance, and work toward recovery. Some favorable prognostic indicators of schizophrenia are listed in **Box 1**.[10]

Readers are invited to contemplate how the disorder and treatments described can affect traditional adolescent and young adult milestones: for example, self-reliance and affiliation with peers; sense of identity; empathy; affect regulation and impulse control; development of sexuality and intimate relationships; ethical and moral development; and negotiating familial relationships. Additional milestones include expanded capacity for abstract thought, creative pursuits, and academic and/or occupational productivity. The model program NAVIGATE described in this article addresses the treatment of schizophrenia that follows system-of-care values and principles and emphasizes individual placement and supported employment.[10,12] This publication has also produced a 2013 edition dedicated to psychosis in youth, referenced throughout this article.[13]

MAKING THE DIAGNOSIS: CURRENT CRITERIA
Schizophrenia

Using the Diagnostic and Statistical Manual of Mental Disorders (DSM), Fifth Revision, schizophrenia is identified by signs of disordered thinking manifest in disorganized

Table 1 Familial risks in schizophrenia	
General Population Prevalence (12 mo)	1% (1 in 100)
Lifetime Development Risk (%)	0.7 (0.3–2)
Family History First-degree Relative (%)	9–18
Family History Second-degree Relative (%)	3–6
Family History Third-degree Relative (%)	2–3
Nontwin Sibling Risk (%)	8 (9–18)
Twin Risk: Monozygotic (%)	47–48 (41–65)
Twin Risk: Dizygotic (%)	12 (0–28)
Child with 1 Parent with Schizophrenia (%)	12–14 (2–35)
Child of 2 Parents with Schizophrenia (%)	40–46 (40–60)

Data from Refs.[3,9,10]

> **Box 1**
> **Favorable prognostic indicators of schizophrenia**
>
> - Shorter DUP (with antipsychotic medication)
> - Fewer negative symptoms
> - Predominantly only delusions and hallucinations as positive symptoms
> - Higher baseline premorbid functioning (eg, social function, intelligence quotient)
> - Onset associated with acute precipitating stressor
> - No co-occurring psychiatric disorders (including substance use disorders)
> - Absent family history of schizophrenia
> - Present family history of mood disorder
> - Living in a nonurban area; in a developing country
>
> *From* Lehman AF, Lieberman JA, Dixon LB, et al. Practice guideline for treatment of patients with schizophrenia, second edition. Am J Psychiatry 2004;161(Suppl 2):1–56; with permission.

behaviors and speech, along with prominent reductions in emotional expression and decrease in self-motivated useful activities, which, together, markedly impair functioning from an individual's baseline.[14] The "checklist" criteria of DSM-5 only require 2 or more symptoms, so that having only hallucinations and delusions that impair functioning are sufficient for diagnosis, although most clinicians recognize that disorganized behaviors and negative symptoms often also occur. The major diagnostic criteria have been similar since 1980, but, in DSM-5, the former subtypes of schizophrenia have been removed, and catatonia has been restructured.[14,15] Early-onset schizophrenia (EOS), defined as occurring before age 18 years, and childhood-onset schizophrenia (COS) before age 13 years are not separate conditions in DSM-5.[16] The conditions share key diagnostic symptoms with adult-onset schizophrenia (AOS) but their prognoses and comorbidities differ. It remains unclear why earlier onset disorder often has more severe symptoms.

The core symptoms of schizophrenia disrupt development when the disorder occurs in the young adult population. Traditional positive symptoms alter the patient's sense of reality. Negative symptoms result in decreased daily activities, such as self-care, persistence in structured activity, and socialization. Negative symptoms, together with cognitive and executive functioning symptoms, impede academic and occupational progression. Some patients can acknowledge their symptoms as distressing and perceive illness, whereas others do not recognize in themselves any form of disorder displaying a lack of insight. A therapeutic alliance allows concerned clinicians to explore these areas and to relate them back to functional recovery and achieving developmental milestones. Ultimately, reentry into a career has been shown to cause less stress than unemployment; clinicians should actively promote ongoing recovery, including help navigating the educational system.[17–19]

DSM-5 encourages practitioners to rank the dimensional severity of psychosis, a word that is often imprecisely used as an equivalent for schizophrenia, by using the WHODAS 2.0 (World Health Organization Disability Assessment Schedule)[14] found in its appendix. The removal of the multiaxial diagnostic system with Global Assessment of Functioning (GAF) score has widened the imprecision in assessing symptom criteria, clinical significance, and functional impairments.[14,20,21] Much of the high-risk-to-psychosis research criteria, discussed later, relied on the GAF or the associated SOFAS (Social and Occupational Functioning Assessment Scale). There is no current standardized clinical method to validate impairment; the self-reported WHODAS 2.0, can be vulnerable when patients are "not motivated to be accurate".[21] For such a critical part of making a diagnosis, evaluating treatment efficacy, and measuring recovery, this is a significant gap in the current understanding of schizophrenia and perhaps mental illness.

Early-onset Schizophrenia

A systematic literature review on EOS noted that DUP was longer in EOS (17 months ± 1 year) compared with AOS.[22] Most patients in the literature review had a schizophrenia spectrum primary diagnosis, but comorbidities such as posttraumatic stress disorder (PTSD), attention-deficit/hyperactivity disorder (ADHD), disruptive behaviors, and conduct disorders each occurred in about one-third of the subjects. Pervasive developmental disorder spectrum was comorbid in about 12.5% of cases. Mean illness age was 15.6 years, with mean illness onset at 14.5 years. Better premorbid functioning predicted better outcome.[22]

The review cited needing time to discern the overlap between mood disorders with psychosis and primary psychotic disorders given common errors of diagnosing schizophrenia instead of mood disorders.[22] Also, distinguishing psychosis from autism spectrum disorders (ASDs), obsessive-compulsive disorder, generalized anxiety disorders, and social anxiety disorders can be difficult.[22] Misdiagnosis leads to mistreatment and incorrect prognoses. In this digital era, in which adolescents (and others) turn to the Internet as a reliable source of information, a recent study found that 15% of a popular video-sharing Web site contained inaccurate content on schizophrenia.[23]

Two clinical presentations of emerging adulthood schizophrenia are described in **Box 2**.

Childhood-onset Schizophrenia

Driver and colleagues[16] recently reviewed the rare but highly disabling condition, COS. They warn about overly focusing on psychosis when it occurs, neglecting comorbidities. This approach can lead to undertreatment and can perpetuate schizophrenia diagnosis–related myths and stigma that may follow throughout the developmental trajectory. COS also seems to have a strong relationship with ASD, being comorbid in up to 50% of cases.[24,25] Note that this strong correlation occurs in COS but is not yet noted in EOS, AOS, or schizophrenia spectrum disorders.[25]

Schizophrenia Spectrum Disorders

The remaining schizophrenia spectrum disorders are well described in DSM-5.[14] Although schizoaffective disorder is included, it is reviewed separately. One study prospectively followed for at least 2 years 114 patients with a mean age of 30 years who were hospitalized for non-affective psychosis.[26] In this group, DUP, slightly less than 2 years, was longest for the diagnosis of schizophrenia.[26] More than half the patients underwent a later diagnostic change, which would be expected for the time-transitional diagnoses.[26] The most prevalent diagnoses were unspecified psychosis, schizophreniform disorder, and brief psychotic disorder.[26] Of those diagnosed with schizophrenia, 37% had a diagnosis change to schizoaffective disorder.[26] Three-quarters had 8 weeks or more of remission/recovery, whereas 24% did not.[26] Such wide-ranging diagnostic shifts in a first-episode adult population suggest even more elusive diagnoses with a younger population whose typical development is marked by constant change.

Box 2
Clinical presentations of emerging adulthood schizophrenia

Clinical vignette: adult-onset schizophrenia

A 22-year-old married woman was referred to mental health services after multiple trips to the emergency department (13 times in the past 9 months) for repeated concerns that her stomach was not where it should be, and who believed that metal was embedded in her bones as a conspiracy by others in the neighborhood. She had halting and disjointed speech, covered her mouth with her hand when she spoke, fearfully cowered in her chair, and made regular fleeting glances out of the sides of her eyes to no particular object. According to collateral sources, she had deteriorated from being an active, engaged family and community member to being someone who no longer could prepare meals, was isolated in her room, repeatedly reading religious texts in book form or online. When asked, she denied that she heard any auditory hallucinations and denied other hallucinations. She did not believe that she had any illness other than a bodily one that she thought multiple health care providers had failed to detect.

Clinical vignette: early-onset schizophrenia

A 15-year-old boy was referred to psychiatric services for behaving bizarrely in the classroom for the past year. These behaviors included irritability, appearing to speak to himself, and getting out of his chair to pace aimlessly in the aisle. He had a history of language disorders and/or specific learning disorders since elementary school, which sometimes was attributed by the school to being an English second-language learner. After the transition to middle school, he associated with behaviorally disordered peers and showed truancy and cannabis-use behaviors. In the 6 months preceding presentation, his family stated that he was afraid to sleep alone. He was disheveled, neglecting his hygiene, and his academic productivity precipitously decreased in the past year. His mother believed he had not used cannabis in the past few months' because he no longer socialized with anyone. In the office, he showed thought blocking, avoided all eye contact, and stated that he heard auditory voice hallucinations, which he thought were bad spirits.

CHALLENGING DIFFERENTIAL DIAGNOSES AND CO-OCCURRING CONDITIONS
Schizoaffective Disorder

Schizoaffective disorder remains in the psychotic diagnostic grouping, while DSM-5 notes, "there is growing evidence that schizoaffective disorder is not a distinct nosologic category."[14,27] A recent review and meta-analysis concluded that the diagnosis has poor stability compared with the stability of a schizophrenia diagnosis.[28] Schizoaffective disorder is often used to indicate a milder subgroup of schizophrenia or a more severe subcategory of mood disordered patients and has low diagnostic reliability.[28,29]

Childhood Trauma

PTSD is not part of the schizophrenia spectrum of conditions. In children, trauma, especially sexual, and maltreatment have been associated with psychotic symptoms.[30–33] A dose of 3 childhood traumas can be predictive of developing hallucinations.[30]

Substance Use Disorders

There is little expert guidance on managing co-occurring substance disorders.[34] A sufficient sustained period of abstinence from substances needed to rule out substance etiology is often arbitrarily determined, with a 2-month period suggested in DSM-IV Text Revision (TR) and no time period mentioned in DSM-5.[14,20] With the adolescent and young adult population, this can be a period of steep increase in the use of illicit drugs.[35] In particular with cannabis and methamphetamine, it can be difficult to apportion the contributions of psychotic symptoms from substance use. Cannabis is known to be residual in the body, with long-term effects considered after 20 days of use.[36] For substances like methamphetamines, psychotic symptoms can persist well past stopping drug use.[37,38] Psychosis-specific research also tends to exclude both groups for study.[39,40] When obvious psychotic symptoms do arise, the general approach is to attempt to stabilize with antipsychotic medication. It remains unclear how effective stabilization is with concurrent substance use. Although many studies exist that comment on the relationship between cannabis, cognitive functioning, psychotic symptoms, and mortality, work remains to be done to show clinical application.[41–44] Nicotine, prenatally, is implicated in higher schizophrenia risk but is also described in animal studies as attenuating negative and cognitive symptoms.[45,46] Patients with schizophrenia may develop tobacco use disorder, attempting to alleviate symptoms, which should be discussed with all patient age groups. Alcohol is frequently used, often in binge form, in this population and no studies provide guidance on the concomitant ingestion of antipsychotic medications and alcohol.[47]

Attention-deficit/Hyperactivity Disorder

To further complicate matters, symptoms of ADHD are often found in retrospective reviews of patients with psychosis histories.[48,49] Knowledge gaps of ADHD and psychosis are well reviewed in an article by Levy and colleagues.[50] Having hallucinations can be an infrequent side effect with stimulant medication use.[51]

Autism Spectrum Disorders

There are shared aspects of odd thinking, rigid behaviors, and impaired socialization in schizophrenia and ASD.[24] Both disorders are described as having Theory of Mind (ToM) impairments of mentalization and introspection (ie, impairments in patients' ability to understand intentions and beliefs of others and drawing on context-specific autobiographical memory to decide their own mental state).[52] These skills typically improve with age from 2 years old through adolescence.[53] Less mature adolescents and adults may have difficulty observing and reporting on their inner states and appropriately attributing others' thoughts, intentions, and beliefs. These concepts may complicate a clinical interview for the purposes of exploring psychotic symptoms. Several groups have examined these concepts by using psychological tests, such as paranoia scales, delusional inventories, and Strange Stories tests.[54–56] Although patients with schizophrenia tend to perform worse on these tests compared with patients with ASD and normal controls, there are still significant gaps in separating out ToM features in this population and in typical adolescence.

A REVIEW OF THE POSTMODERN ERA IN SCHIZOPHRENIA RESEARCH

In 1992, the National Institutes of Health convened a workgroup to discuss the National Institute of Mental Health's (NIMH) 1988 schizophrenia research goal of examining patients in their first episodes of psychosis.[57] Much of the previous research was conducted on chronic, refractory cases, and more information on treatment-innocent or new-onset cases was sorely needed. Researchers also developed standardized assessments, including the Measurement and Treatment Research to Improve Cognition in Schizophrenia (MATRICS) Consensus Cognitive Battery (**Table 2**).[58–61] Several first-episode psychosis programs also emerged, designed to intervene within the critical period of schizophrenia and to reduce DUP.[62] These intensive interventions have

Table 2	
MATRICS Consensus Cognitive Battery tests	
Measured Domain	**MCCB Component Tests**
Processing speed	Trail Making Test Part A
	Brief Assessment of Cognition in Schizophrenia Symbol Coding Test
	Category Fluency Test, animal naming
Verbal learning	Hopkins Verbal Learning Test
Working memory	Wechsler Memory Scale Spatial Span
	University of Maryland Letter Number span
Reasoning and problem solving	Neuropsychological Assessment Battery: Mazes
Visual learning	Brief Visuospatial Memory Test: Revised
Social cognition	Mayer-Salovey Caruso Emotional Intelligence Test Managing Emotions Branch
Attention/vigilance	Continuous Performance Test: Identical Pairs

Abbreviation: MCCB, MATRICS Consensus Cognitive Battery.
Data from McCleery A, Ventura J, Kern RS, et al. Cognitive functioning in first-episode schizophrenia: MATRICS Cognitive Consensus Battery (MCCB) profile of impairment. Schizophr Res 2014;157:33–9.

been shown to be promising in reducing hospitalizations and in improving social outcomes. The model NAVIGATE program, created in response to the NIMH's Recovery After an Initial Schizophrenia Episode (RAISE) initiative,[63,64] is discussed later.

A review of recent literature specifically focused on child and adolescent perionset first episodes of psychosis, prodrome, or clinical-high-risk/ultrahigh-risk states also reveals that the investigational community may be using the vocabulary of first episode and psychosis at variance, requiring careful reading and cautious application of definitions, findings, and outcomes. There is much in the literature that is promising about trying to capture (pre)development of schizophrenia, but it still requires replication and validation.

In 2008, a group met to review 10 consensus statements about schizophrenia management and to grade them by expert review and survey results.[65] These consensus statements and challenges, many of which still remain unanswered, are summarized in **Table 3** and are used to launch discussion of prodrome.

Statement 1

Studies have started to examine milder psychotic experiences and risk factors for emerging psychosis. These groups tend to call themselves first-episode psychosis programs, which can lead unwary readers to confuse the findings with first-episode schizophrenia programs. The point of conversion from a high-risk state to a more seriously pathologic state can be unclear because of varying definitions. Most groups focus on prospectively trying to examine the prodromal stage, which remains defined as a retrospective event of a period of time. One review remarked that prodrome is an imprecise shorthand for at-risk populations.[66] However, these laudable efforts offer hope to families, teenagers, and preteens with low-risk interventions during this early time with the wish to avert schizophrenia.[80]

Prodrome can be defined as a period of nonpsychotic symptoms but with emotional disturbance and decrease in functioning, or, as described in DSM-5, mild or subthreshold hallucinations and more prominent negative symptoms before the development of schizophrenia.[10,14] Researchers have attempted to define, identify, and measure a set of clinical high risk (CHR)/ultrahigh risk (UHR) for psychosis criteria.[81]

Table 3
Summary of 2008 Schizophrenia Summit's 10 consensus statements

Statement Number	Section Author	Statement	Discussion/Directions
1	Perkins	Identification of the earliest prodromal phase of schizophrenia is feasible	Clinical definition of psychosis is not standard; need to refine at-risk criteria; need to examine mood disorders with psychotic features; current studies limited by examining clinical populations but not the general population
2	Benes	Schizophrenia is a neurodegenerative disease resulting in brain changes that parallel symptom progression and functional decline	Decrease in gray matter occurs, but it is unclear whether the loss reflects neurodegeneration in step with symptoms *Imaging studies do not yet well demarcate neurodegeneration in step with symptoms, especially given that COS sibling and CHR/UHR imaging studies have also found significant changes[67,68]
3	Keshavan	Cognitive Impairment, especially executive dysfunction and memory loss, is a key diagnostic component of schizophrenia	Neurocognitive impairment is a core component of the illness, but it is not seen robustly in all patients. It can also be found in nonpsychotic relatives and in other conditions *Cognitive impairment is not exclusive to this diagnosis, requiring more specificity as a diagnostic area. Some of the UHR/CHR studies show that verbal learning on the MATRICS can be impaired up to 4 y past a first episode.[69] Using the battery in healthy adolescents shows general improvement in domains over time, associated with normal development.[70] In practice, clinicians may consider tools like the UPSA (University of Calfornia, San Diego, Performance-Based Skills Assessment), which tests making phone calls, paying bills, as well as other methods summarized in the referenced article[71]
4	Braff	Genetic factors are the best-established causal determinants of schizophrenia	Although true, replicable and clinically translatable findings are yet to occur *Many studies have identified genomic regions and susceptibility loci to further examine[6,7,72,73]
5	Weinberger	Neuroimaging is a tool for elucidating biological and genetic mechanisms of illness and treatment response	It is an essential research tool, but it is not yet clinically useful *Brain imaging schizophrenia studies point to cortical thinning, prefrontal gray matter volume loss, increased lateral ventricle size, smaller amygdala size, and smaller hippocampal size.[74–79] Andreasen et al[76] note that antipsychotic medications, while offering the best relapse prevention, can also incur generalized brain tissue loss (compared with more focalized frontotemporal loss of the illness)

(*continued on next page*)

Table 3
(continued)

Statement Number	Section Author	Statement	Discussion/Directions
6	Nasrallah	Atypical antipsychotic drugs are neuroprotective in patients diagnosed with schizophrenia	Treatment with medication is important, but whether it is neuroprotective remains to be seen. Also, the definition of neuroprotective needs to be clarified
7	Weiden	Treatment in the prodromal phase of schizophrenia improves patient outcomes	Early intervention is indicated as soon as psychosis occurs, but the term prodrome is ambiguous. Antipsychotic pharmacologic interventions in prodrome are not clearly helpful but psychosocial interventions may be
8	Kane and Correll	Patients with treatment-resistant schizophrenia require combination antipsychotic treatment	Even though this may be done clinically, there is little evidence to support this practice. Also, definitions of treatment resistance remain unclear
9	Gur	Improvement in cognitive function is an essential treatment target in patients with schizophrenia	There was agreement on this statement, but pharmacologic interventions are not shown to significantly improve cognitive function. Second-generation antipsychotics were associated with some improvement, but not first-generation medications. However, cognitive function is not generally measured in trials
10	Green	Managing substance abuse is a key target of treatment	Everyone agrees, but substance-induced psychosis complicates the picture. Excluding substance use disorders from studies would limit findings. The panel had consensus that ultrahigh-risk individuals should be encouraged not to use cannabis. Assessing readiness for change, implementing contingency management, and considering medications to decrease cravings need to be investigated further

Updates to some statements are marked by asterisks (*).
Abbreviations: CHR, clinical high risk; UHR, ultrahigh risk.
Data from Nasrallah HA, Keshavan MS, Benes FM, et al. Proceedings and data from the Schizophrenia Summit: a critical appraisal to improve the management of schizophrenia. J Clin Psychiatry 2009;70(Suppl 1):4–46.

Many writings, including a review article in 2010, have summarized the state of research findings.[82] The regularly published CHR/UHR researchers include subgroups of the transnational European Prediction of Psychosis Study (EPOS); Australian Orygen/ PACE (Personal Assessment and Crisis Evaluation) clinic; and a consortium of separate programs collaborating as the NAPLS (North American Prodrome Longitudinal Study).[83–86] The groups have identified 3 vulnerable populations to study, although the distribution of subjects has fallen largely into 1 category: attenuated psychotic symptoms (a proposed DSM-5 syndrome, recently published in a case presentation).[14,87] The risk criteria are compared in **Table 4**.[83–85] **Table 4** also references assessment instruments used and/or developed by these groups to standardize CHR/UHR criteria: the PANSS (Positive and Negative Syndrome Scale for Schizophrenia),

Table 4 Comparisons of risk criteria for psychosis development			
Criteria	Europe	Australia	North America
Attenuated positive symptoms	Using the SIPS, occurring several times a week for at least 1 wk within past year: unusual thought content/delusions; suspiciousness/persecutory ideas; grandiosity; hallucinations; disorganized communications; odd behavior or appearance	Using the CAARMS, at least several times a week for ≥1 wk and ≤5 y within the past year: ideas of reference; odd beliefs or magical thinking; perceptual disturbance; paranoid ideation; odd thinking and speech; odd behavior and appearance	Using the SIPS, occurring at least once a week in the past month, 1 or more, begun or worsened in the past year: unusual thought content; suspiciousness; grandiose ideas; perceptual abnormalities; disorganized communication
Brief limited intermittent psychotic symptoms	Using the PANSS, having 1 of hallucinations, delusions, or formal thought disorder that resolves spontaneously in 7 d and separated by 1 wk of occurrence	Using the CAARMS, transient symptoms lasting ≤1 wk but spontaneously resolving, ≥1 of ideas of reference, magical thinking, perceptual disturbance, paranoid ideation, and odd thinking or speech	Using the SIPS, any 1 of unusual thought content, suspiciousness, grandiosity, perceptual abnormalities, and disorganized communication; reaching a psychotic intensity within past 3 mo but not seriously disorganizing or dangerous; symptom does not last for more than average 1 h/d 4 d/wk over 1 mo
Familial risk + reduced functioning	A 30% reduction on the GAF for at least 1 mo to 1 y and a first-degree or second-degree relative with a history of psychotic disorder; having a schizotypal personality disorder	Schizotypal personality disorder in the identified individual or a first-degree relative with a psychotic disorder; past year decline in functioning maintained for 1 mo and <5 y (30% reduction in GAF)	First-degree relative with psychosis or patient with schizotypal personality disorder; 30% reduction in GAF compared with past year sustained over the past month

Abbreviations: CAARMS, Comprehensive Assessment of At-Risk Mental States; PANSS, Positive and Negative Syndrome Scale for Schizophrenia; SIPS, Structured Interview for Prodromal States.
   Data from Refs.[83–85]

CAARMS (Comprehensive Assessment of At-Risk Mental States), and SIPS (Structured Interview for Prodromal States).[88–92] These groups then prospectively followed subjects aged 12 to 35 years who had met CHR/UHR criteria. The NAPLS-2 described its predictive algorithm as having an 80% positive predictive value and 40% sensitivity.[86] It generated a psychosis risk calculator (**Box 3**).[93] When this constellation of factors occurs, clinicians should consider more careful monitoring and deliver the psychosocial interventions for CHR/UHR states until a clear diagnosis emerges.

Because the structured assessments used in research have training and administrative costs, several groups developed a 2-step process: screening, then structured interview.[94–96] Some examples of screeners and how to access them are listed in **Box 4**.[97–99] Depending on the study, researchers assert that these screeners are valid, whereas others assert that they are not.[100] Readers are encouraged to examine the UHR/CHR criteria and to recognize the broad scope of the screeners as well as the potential for perpetuating ambiguity against precise terminology.

Psychotic-like or psychotic symptoms in the general population

There are people in the general population who have psychotic-like experiences (PLEs), such as subclinical hallucinations and delusions, but who are not distressed by them.[101] Some investigators carefully excluded imaginary friends, immature responses, ghosts, hypnagogic and hypnopompic hallucinations, and eidetic images, especially when surveying children and adolescents.[102–104] The frequency of PLEs depends on the study, with a range from 0.6% to 84%.[105] Most studies report a lifetime prevalence of 6% to 8% in children and adolescents and up to 28% in adults.[106–108] In one study with a 17.5% sample prevalence of PLEs, only 2.1% of subjects had a diagnosis of nonaffective psychosis.[109] In two European studies, PLEs decreased with time; for example, 2 years and 20 years later.[110,111] As in adults, most PLEs that do not cause distress in children have been transient.[112] **Table 5** lists these common thoughts and their frequencies, showing the high rate in an emerging adult population.[111] The long, 92-item form of the Prodromal Questionnaire was administered to college undergraduate students; 43% of students met the cutoff for screening intervention, which decreased to 25% when clinically screened, and only 2% of college students reported distress from their PLEs.[113] An Australian study surveyed 875 high school students and categorized 4 types of psychotic-like experience: bizarre experiences, perceptual abnormalities, persecutory ideas, and magical thinking, with magical thinking having poor clinical predictive value.[114] In a European sample of 103 healthy individuals with auditory verbal hallucinations, 71% heard no negative

---

Box 3
Six factors in the psychosis risk calculator model

- Baseline age
- Unusual thought content and suspiciousness
- Family history of a psychiatric disorder
- Verbal learning (on Hopkins Verbal Learning Test)
- Processing speed performance (on Brief Assessment of Cognition in Schizophrenia Symbol Coding Test)
- Decline in social functioning

Data from Carrion RE, Cornblatt BA, Burton CZ, et al. Personalized prediction of psychosis: external validation of the NAPLS-2 psychosis risk calculator with the EDIPPP project. Am J Psychiatry 2016;173(10):989–6.

Box 4
High-risk potential for psychosis screeners

42-item CAPE (Community Assessment of Psychic Experience) http://cape42.homestead.com/files/CAPE-42.htm

YPARQ-B (Youth Psychosis at Risk Questionnaire-brief): proprietary https://www.orygen.org.au/Campus/Expert-Network/Resources/Paid/Manuals/Pace-Manual

General information at: http://oyh.org.au/, accessed September 1, 2016

Yale-PRIME (Prevention through Risk Identification, Management, and Education) screen http://www.schizophrenia.com/sztest/primetest.pdf

PQ-B (Prodromal Questionnaire-brief) http://www.mentalhealthamerica.net/mental-health-screen/psychosis-screen, Accessed Sept 1, 2016

content and 25% heard negative and positive content.[115] Having negative emotional content (distress) was predictive of clinical conversion.[110] **Fig. 1** shows the frequency of PLEs in a UK population study.[101] None of the investigators explained PLEs further and described psychosis as a nonspecific marker, with a greater need to determine distress and impairment disruption.[105,107]

One UHR research group wrote reflections on how the current focus on risk neglects clinical phenomena.[116] Current research does not explore features of consciousness, such as people's ability to describe and reflect on themselves, or the complexities of subjective experience (like a sense of self, sense of bodily experience, inner speech, stream of thoughts).[116] Few articles discuss misdescription or malingering of pediatric PLEs.[117] This is a major gap in the current state of understanding of developing psychosis and this emphasizes the importance of having clear nosology.

Statement 7

Leaving aside the imprecise vocabulary, the CHR/UHR programs have delivered interventions[65] with some trends emerging. An average of 30% of CHR/UHR patients (range, 12%–54%) converted to psychosis.[82,86,118–120] Most conversions occurred in the first 2 years, but some occurred almost 10 to 15 years later.[84,121] Note that conversion to psychosis is variably defined. Several of the CHR/UHR programs define conversion to psychosis as having positive symptoms that occur several times a week for more than 1 week.[84,86] One study includes severe disorganization or dangerous behavior as conversion.[86] Others refer to diagnoses in the schizophrenia spectrum category.[116]

Table 5
Twenty-year study of general population psychotic experiences

Endorsement	At Age 20–21 y (%)	At Age 40–41 y (%)
Someone else can control your thoughts	38.3	15.2
Others being aware of your thoughts	18.5	4.7
Having thoughts that are not your own	22.6	7
Auditory hallucinations	3.2	0.1
Feeling lonely even when with people	33.8	29.4
Not feeling close to another person	21.5	22.9
Having ideas that others do not share	58	32
Feeling that people take advantage of you	32	33.9
Feeling that you are watched by others	42.8	33.3
Feeling that most people cannot be trusted	37.1	29.2

Data from Rössler W, Rieche-Rössler A, Angst J, et al. Psychotic experiences in the general population: a 20-year prospective community study. Schizophr Res 2007;92:1–14.

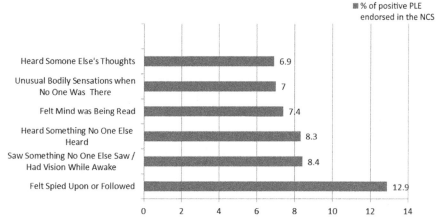

Fig. 1. Percentage of positive PLE endorsed in the US National Comorbidity Survey. (*Data from* Shevlin M, Murphy J, Dorahy M, et al. The distribution of positive psychosis-like symptoms in the population: a latent class analysis of the National Comorbidity Survey. Schizophr Res 2007;89:101–9.)

The 70% (on average) of subjects who did not convert to a primary psychotic condition in the UHR/CHR studies were functionally impaired on the GAF/SOFAS compared with normal controls, and although they did not have psychosis, they may not have been false-positives.[121–123] Nonconverters had other diagnosable problems; for example, in the United Kingdom, more than 70% of the CHR population had at least 1 DSM-IV TR diagnosis at baseline, as shown in **Fig. 2.**[124]

To date, there is little to no evidence to deliver antipsychotic pharmacologic interventions in this stage of possible disorder, which is a different approach to care

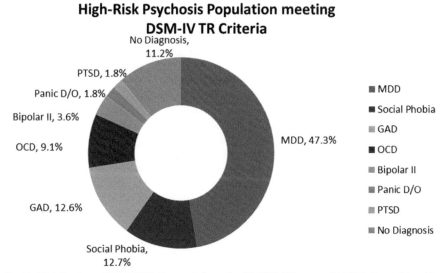

Fig. 2. Distribution of DSM-IV TR diagnosis from the CAMEO UK group. CAMEO, Cambridgeshire and Petersborough Assessing Managing and Enhancing Outcomes; D/O, disorder; GAD, generalized anxiety disorder; MDD, major depressive disorder; OCD, obsessive compulsive disorder. (*Data from* Morcillo C, Stochl J, Russo D, et al. First-rank symptoms and premorbid adjustment in young individuals at increased risk of developing psychosis. Psychopathology 2015;48:120–6.)

than shortening DUP with medications.[125] A 12 week trial of omega-3 fatty acids claimed to reduce conversion to psychosis and to improve functional outcomes; a current US study is ongoing for 740 mg of eicosapentaenoic acid and 400 mg of docosa-hexaenoic acid per day (https://clinicaltrials.gov/ct2/show/NCT01429454).[126,127]

The psychosocial interventions delivered to help-seeking patients included community outreach and education about psychosis in targeted dissemination through specialized family-aided assertive community treatment teams to deliver proprietary curricular-based psychoeducation, multifamily groups, and other individual interventions, with available resources linked in the Miklowitz and colleagues[128] study.[128–131] Another review suggested that family interventions need to be provided for a duration of at least 6 to 9 months to sustain significant improvement.[132] Proponents of family psychoeducation have amassed data supporting their efficacy.[133]

Other studies delivered cognitive behavior therapy (CBT) aimed specifically at early psychosis (CBTp).[134,135] Some groups offered cognitive remediation, usually through computer-based tasks.[136] Another combines cognitive training with aerobic exercise.[137] Outcome measures vary across studies, with the same ambiguity of defining psychosis and conversion.[82,91] Although studies show risk reductions or improvement in select cognitive domains, a meta-analysis concluded that all interventions require experimental replication and that diminished effects as time progresses indicate that interventions are not likely to give immunity.[122]

CBTp has been the most studied and most recommended individual psychotherapeutic intervention for this UHR/CHR period. Its proponents proclaim its efficacy (particularly compared with supportive or psychodynamic therapies), but a few studies have remarked on the low quality of evidence.[119,138] A Delphi study about components specific to CBTp found that many of its elements shared foundations with general robust therapeutic relationships, like distress reduction; eliciting hope; planning for maintenance; homework as a standing agenda; and designing therapeutic goals to be SMART (specific, measurable, achievable, realistic, and time-limited).[139–141] Other studies reported that the basic cognitive schemas, like jumping to conclusions, were not exclusive to psychosis.[142,143] Despite problems regarding specificity and delivery, it is important to recognize that UHR/CHR individuals may benefit from cognitive-based approaches. Killackey and colleagues[17] reviewed the disruption of employment skills caused by symptoms but also reported on clinician biases and attitudes about psychosis vocational recovery. The investigators identified that intensive psychosocial interventions may be helpful, particularly those focused on supportive education and employment, but the key components of other CHR/UHR interventions are yet to be proved, manualized, and replicated on a large scale.

The consensus statements do not address psychosocial interventions in the treatment of schizophrenia. A recent meta-analysis compared psychological interventions (befriending, CBT, cognitive remediation, psychoeducation, social skills training, and supportive counseling for psychosis) and is contemporary since the National Institute for Health and Care Excellence (NICE) guidelines.[144] Different psychosocial interventions each modified different symptoms or aspects of treatment (eg, CBT, positive symptoms; social skills, negative symptoms; cognitive remediation, all symptoms; psychoeducation, treatment adherence).[144] Investigators cautioned that differences were small, and the significance of some findings changed when all analyses were applied.[144]

Statement 6

The consensus statement and discussion on this is self-explanatory.[65]

Recommendations for treating schizophrenia have been widely disseminated and are available in many resources.[10,138,145–148] For the purposes of this article, pertinent information on psychopharmacologic options is summarized in tabular form to assist clinicians in delivering medication treatments. Primary-action dopamine receptor blockade medications that are currently available in the United States are listed in **Table 6**.[149,150] **Table 6** also lists when oral medications are additionally available as oral dissolvable tablets, intramuscular injections, or long-acting injectables (LAIs). A meta-analysis also reviewed adding antidepressants primarily to address negative symptoms which is a recommended intervention in the United States but not in other countries.[151] With a 5% lifetime risk of suicide associated with schizophrenia, suicide prevention includes "identification of those at risk, treating comorbid depression and substance misuse as well as providing the best available treatment for psychotic symptoms.[152] The NAVIGATE model includes LAIs as a second medication progression.[153] **Table 7** lists second-generation and third-generation antipsychotic medications and their nonpsychotic indications. Nicotine, often smoked concurrently with antipsychotic medications, and caffeine can affect drug blood levels based on cytochrome interactions. These interactions are described in **Table 8** and should be regularly discussed with patients.[46,154]

RECOMMENDED BEST PRACTICE: MODEL NAVIGATE PROGRAM

Participants, aged 15 to 40 years, who had less than a 6 months' duration of antipsychotic treatment and who met criteria for schizophrenia spectrum disorder were randomized into usual care or the NAVIGATE model.[63,64,153,155,156] Results were not stratified by age within the participant group. Designed to be replicated in nonacademic settings, its 4 components (personalized medication management assisted by a Web-based decision tool, family psychoeducation, resilience-focused individual therapy, and supported employment and education; implementation manuals are available at http://www.nimh. nih.gov/health/topics/schizophrenia/raise/coordinated-specialty-care-for-first-episode-psychosis-resources.shtml) were found to be effective by patient measures of being less

Table 6
List of antipsychotic medications available in the United States and pediatric approval

First-generation Approved (#12)	Second-generation Approved (#11)
Chlorpromazine (IM), >1 y[a]	Asenapine, >10 y[a]
Droperidol (IM), >2 y[a]	Clozapine
Fluphenazine (IM, LAI)	Iloperidone
Haloperidol (IM, LAI), >3 y[a]	Lurasidone
Loxapine, >12 y[a]	Olanzapine (ODT, IM, LAI), >13 y[a]
Molindone, >12 y[a]	Paliperidone (LAI), >12 y[a]
Perphenazine, >12 y[a]	Quetiapine (oral extended release), >10 y[a]
Pimozide, >2 y[a]	Risperidone (ODT, LAI), >10 y[a]
Prochlorperazine[a]	Ziprasidone (IM)
Thiothixene, >12 y[a]	Third generation
Thioridazine, >2 y[a]	Aripiprazole (oral, ODT, IM, LAI), >13 y[a]
Trifluoperazine, >6 y[a]	Brexpiprazole
Combination	Cariprazine
Perphenazine + amitriptyline	Olanzapine + fluoxetine

Abbreviations: IM, intramuscular; LAI, long-acting injectable; ODT, oral dissolvable tablets.
[a] Approved for use in the pediatric age group.
Adapted from Agency for Healthcare Research and Quality. First and second generation antipsychotics in children and young adults – comparative effectiveness review update. 2015. Available at: https://effectivehealthcare.ahrq.gov/ehc/products/615/2149/antipsychotics-children-update-protocol-151204.pdf. Accessed September 4, 2015.

Table 7
Second-generation and third-generation antipsychotic medication

Medication/Indication	Aripiprazole	Asenapine	Brexpiprazole	Cariprazine	Clozapine	Olanzapine	Quetiapine	Risperidone	Ziprasidone
Schizophrenia (adolescent)	X	—	—	—	—	X	X	X	—
Bipolar I mixed/manic monotherapy	X	X	—	X	—	X	X	X	X
Bipolar I mixed/manic adjunctive	—	—	—	—	—	—	X	—	X
Bipolar depressed	—	—	—	—	—	—	X	—	—
MDD adjunct	X	—	X	—	—	—	X	—	—
Resistant MDD	—	—	—	—	—	X	—	—	—
Autism irritability	X	—	—	—	—	—	—	X	—
Agitation 2° mania or psychosis	X	—	—	—	—	X	—	—	X
Suicide Risk Reduction	—	—	—	—	X	—	—	—	—

Adapted from Agency for Healthcare Research and Quality. First and second generation antipsychotics in children and young adults – comparative effectiveness review update. 2015. Available at: https://effectivehealthcare.ahrq.gov/ehc/products/615/2149/antipsychotics-children-update-protocol-151204.pdf. Accessed September 4, 2015.

Table 8
Possible effect of nicotine and caffeine on antipsychotic drug levels (P450)

Antipsychotic Medication	Nicotine	Caffeine
Clozapine	Decreases drug levels	Increases drug levels
Olanzapine	Decreases drug levels	Possibly increases
Haloperidol	Possibly decreases	Unknown
Phenothiazines	Decreases drug levels	Unknown
Risperidone	None reported	None reported
Ziprasidone	None reported	None reported
Quetiapine	None reported	None reported
Aripiprazole	None reported	None reported

Data from Pinniti N, Mago R, Leon JD. Coffee, cigarettes, and meds: what are the metabolic effects? Psychiatric Times 2005. Available at: http://www.psychiatrictimes.com/articles/coffee-cigarettes-and-meds-what-are-metabolic-effects/page/0/1. Accessed August 28, 2016.

symptomatic in PANSS scores; more likely to remain in treatment; enjoying better quality of life; and participating more in work/school than usual care.[89,155] The overarching theme is a shared decision-making strategy using as much appropriate collateral information as possible. Collaboration is the key to NAVIGATE, which should be an alliance strategy in all forms of treatment and especially with an adolescent–young adult cohort. Its guided medication model reviews framing the discussion and key points to consider about medication treatment; progressive management options, including those of metabolic side effects; and addressing adherence/nonadherence. The family education program manual discusses tailoring family work to individual needs, encourages engagement along motivational interviewing to elicit change behaviors, and outlines 8 basic topics for family education. It encourages inclusion of any key supports in this process. The individual resiliency training manual outlines 14 modules, 7 of which are considered required. The remaining modules are customized based on collaborative decision making. The supported employment and education (SEE) manual templates discussion for work and academic recovery led by an SEE specialist. It reviews an assessment phase that inventories employment, school, and career history and preferences. The next phase, job search or school enrollment, is self-explanatory, with a final phase of follow-along supports to promote and maintain success. It also gives guidance on disability benefits programs.

NAVIGATE reported a difference in effect sizes separated at DUP less than or equal to 74 weeks for change in treatment with greater mental disorder improvement and quality of life; the goal remains to move DUP to less than 3 months.[64] The RAISE model aligns well with a recovery-oriented model, often found in public and community mental health sectors.[18] Within the recovery model, a goal is to provide not just acute interventions but continuous assistance toward resilience and community reintegration (ie, wraparound services). This complete model exemplified by NAVIGATE diverges from usual care, which often includes medication but not explicit self-management skills. The ideal is to provide a 1-stop integrated system of care that facilitates recovery for co-occurring conditions and offers wraparound services.[18]

Based on this research and the ongoing federal dollar investment into the RAISE coordinated specialty care model, with existing examples of state partnerships, these programs are expected to proliferate.[155,157] Note that the aim of RAISE addresses recovery after schizophrenia, and the programs are designed for diagnoses within the wider schizophrenia spectrum of conditions, including schizoaffective disorder.

SUMMARY

Although the treatment of schizophrenia remains anchored in medication management, evidence supports system-of-care psychosocial interventions and psychoeducation in a team-support model that is familiar to child and adolescent psychiatrists. Necessary research is occurring with first-episode patient populations, but critical readers of the literature need to be aware that definitions of prodrome, first-episode, and psychosis high-risk investigation are not standardized. Also, a portion of the general population of adults, adolescents, and children report symptoms that are often ascribed to psychosis but do not report any experience of distress. This omission suggests that an emphasis on what are typically identified as delusions and hallucinations as disease markers may be misleading. Further, there are few recommendations coming from large-scale evidence for the intersection of mood, substance abuse, and other comorbidities with schizophrenia. Clinicians are encouraged to render evidence-based practices facilitating social and occupational recovery while seeking to understand the subjective experience of patients. This effort includes explicitly addressing developmentally appropriate daily life skills, verbal and nonverbal communications, interpersonal relationships, purposeful careers, and meaningful recreation. Promising practices in the treatment of schizophrenia are still forthcoming.

REFERENCES

1. Ciompi L. The natural history of schizophrenia in the long term. Br J Psychiatry 1980;136:413–20.
2. Arnett J. Emerging adulthood: a theory of development from the late teens through the twenties. Am Psychol 2000;55(5):469–80.
3. Messias E, Chen C, Eaton W. Epidemiology of schizophrenia: review of findings and myths. Psychiatr Clin North Am 2007;30(3):323–38.
4. Welham J, Thomas R, McGrath J. Age-at-first-registration for affective psychosis and schizophrenia. Schizophr Bull 2004;30(4):849–53.
5. Saha S, Chant D, McGrath J, et al. A systematic review of mortality in schizophrenia: is the differential mortality gap worsening over time? Arch Gen Psychiatry 2007;64(10):1123–31.
6. Yang J, Visscher P, Wray N. Sporadic cases are the norm for complex disease. Eur J Hum Genet 2010;18:1039–43.
7. Roos B, Roos JL, Levy S, et al. Strong association of de novo copy number mutations with sporadic schizophrenia. Nat Genet. 2008;40(7):880–5.
8. Available at: http://www.nimh.nih.gov/health/statistics/prevalence/schizophrenia.shtml. Accessed August 18, 2016.
9. Tandon R, Keshavan M, Nasrallah H. Schizophrenia, "Just the Facts" what we know in 2008. 2. Epidemiology and etiology. Schizophr Res 2008;102:1–18.
10. Lehman AF, Lieberman JA, Dixon LB, et al, American Psychiatric Association. Practice guideline for treatment of patients with schizophrenia, second edition. Am J Psychiatry 2004;161(Suppl 2):1–56.
11. Emsley R, Bonginkosi C, Asmal L, et al. The nature of relapse in schizophrenia. BMC Psychiatry 2013;13:50.
12. Available at: http://www.tapartnership.org/SOC/SOCvalues.php. Accessed September 1, 2016.
13. Dvir Y, Frazier J. Psychotic disorders in youth. Child Adolesc Psychiatr Clin N Am 2013;22.
14. American Psychiatric Association. Diagnostic and statistical manual of mental disorders. 5th edition. Arlington (VA): American Psychiatric Association; 2013.

15. Phillips J. Diagnosing schizophrenia from DSM II to DSM-5: A Quiz. Psychiatric Times. July 2011. Available at: http://www.psychiatrictimes.com/schizophrenia/diagnosing-schizophrenia-dsm-ii-dsm-5-quiz. Accessed August 28, 2016.

16. Driver D, Gogtay N, Rapoport J. Childhood onset schizophrenia and early onset schizophrenia spectrum disorders. Child Adolesc Psychiatr Clin N Am 2013;22: 539–55.

17. Killackey E, Alvarez-Jiminez M, Allott K, et al. Community rehabilitation and psychosocial interventions for psychotic disorders in youth. Child Adolesc Psychiatr Clin N Am 2013;22:745–58.

18. Cavanaugh D, Goldman S, Friesen B, et al. Designing a recovery-oriented care model for adolescents and transition age youth with substance use or co-occurring mental health disorders: Substance Abuse and Mental Health Services Administration Center for Substance Abuse Treatment and Center for Mental Health Services; 2009. Report from CSAT/CMHS/SAMHSA Consultative Session. November 13–14, 2008. Available at: https://gucchdtacenter.georgetown.edu/resources/Recovery_Report_Adolescents%20-%20FINAL.pdf. Accessed January 18, 2017.

19. Chan V. Special needs: scholastic disability accommodations from K-12 and transitions to higher education. Curr Psychiatry Rep 2016;18(2):21.

20. American Psychiatric Association. American Psychiatric Association: Diagnostic and statistical manual of mental disorders, 4th text revision edition. Washington, DC: American Psychaitric Association; 2000.

21. Gold L. DSM-5 and the assessment of functioning: The World Health Organization Disability Assessment Schedule 2.0 (WHODAS 2.0). J Am Acad Psychiatry Law 2014;42:173–81.

22. Stentebjerg-Olesen M, Pagsberg A, Fink-Jensen A, et al. Clinical characteristics and predictors of outcome of schizophrenia-spectrum psychosis in children and adolescents: a systematic review. J Child Adolesc Psychopharmacol 2016; 26(5):410–27.

23. Nour M, Nour M, Tsatalou O, et al. Schizophrenia on YouTube. Psychiatr Serv 2016. http://dx.doi.org/10.1176/appo.ps.201500541.

24. Rapoport J, Chavez A, Greenstein D, et al. Autism-spectrum disorders and childhood onset schizophrenia: clinical and biological contributions to a relationship revisited. J Am Acad Child Adolesc Psychiatry 2009;48(1):10–8.

25. Cochran D, Dvir Y, Frazier J. "Autism-plus" spectrum disorders: intersection with psychosis and the schizophrenia spectrum. Child Adolesc Psychiatr Clin N Am 2013;22:609–27.

26. Tohen M, Khalasa H, Salvatore P, et al. The McLean-Harvard first-episode project: early course in 114 cases of first-episode nonaffective psychoses. J Clin Psychiatry 2016;77(6):781–8.

27. Kotov R, Leong S, Mojtaba I, et al. Boundaries of schizoaffective disorder revisiting Kraepelin. JAMA Psychiatry 2013;70(12):1276–86.

28. Murru A, Pacchiarotti I, Nivoli A, et al. What we know and what we don't know about the treatment of schizoaffective disorder. J Euroneuro 2011;21:680–90.

29. Rink L, Pagel T, Franklin J, et al. Characteristics and heterogeneity of schizoaffective disorder compared with unipolar depression and schizophrenia - a systematic literature review and meta-analysis. J Affect Disord 2016;191(8):8–14.

30. Shevlin M, Dorahy M, Adamson G. Childhood traumas and hallucinations: an analysis of the National Comorbidity Study. J Psychiatr Res 2007;41:222–8.

31. Daalman K, Diedren K, Derks E, et al. Childhood trauma and auditory verbal hallucinations. Psychol Med 2012;42:2475–84.

32. Holshausen K, Bowie C, Harkness K. The relation of childhood maltreatment to psychotic symptoms in adolescents and young adults with depression. J Clin Child Adolesc Psychol 2016;45(3):241–7.

33. Dvir Y, Denietolis B, Frazier J. Childhood trauma and psychosis. Child Adolesc Psychiatr Clin N Am 2013;22:629–43.

34. Gorke DKS. Substance abuse and psychosis. Child Adolesc Psychiatr Clin N Am 2013;22:643–54.

35. Young S, Corley R, Stallings M, et al. Substance use, abuse and dependence in adolescence: prevalence, symptom profiles and correlates. Drug Alcohol Depend 2002;68:309–22.

36. Crean R, Crane N, Mason B. An evidence based review of acute and long-term effects of cannabis use on executive cognitive functions. J Addict Med 2011; 5(1):1–8.

37. Lin S, Wang L, Chen Y, et al. Differences in clinical features of methamphetamines users with persistent psychosis and patients with schizophrenia. Psychopathology 2016;49:108–15.

38. Grant KM, LeVan T, Wells S, et al. Methamphetamine-associated psychosis. J Neuroimmune Pharmacol 2012;7:113–39.

39. Rounsville B. DSM-V research agenda: substance abuse/psychosis comorbidity. Schizophr Bull 2007;33(4):947–52.

40. Litt M, Kadden R, Petry N. Behavioral treatment for marijuana dependence: randomized trial of contingency management and self-efficacy enhancement. Addict Behav 2013;38(3):1764–75.

41. Manrique-Garcia E, Ponce de Leon A, Dalman C, et al. Cannabis, psychosis, and mortality: a cohort study of 50,373 Swedish men. Am J Psychiatry 2016; 173:790–8.

42. Kelley M, Wan C, Broussard B, et al. Marijuana use in the immediate 5-year premorbid period is associated with increased risk of onset of schizophrenia and related psychotic disorders. Schizophr Res 2016;171:62–7.

43. Bechtold J, Hipwell A, Lewis D, et al. Concurrent and sustained cumulative effects of adolescent marijuana use on subclinical psychotic symptoms. Am J Psychiatry 2016;173(8):781–9.

44. Henquet C, Krabbendam I, Spauwen J, et al. Prospective cohort study of cannabis use, predisposition for psychosis, and psychotic symptoms in young people. BMJ 2005;330(7481):11.

45. Niemelä S, Sourander A, Surcel H, et al. Prenatal nicotine exposure and risk of schizophrenia among offspring in a national birth cohort. Am J Psychiatry 2016; 173:799–806.

46. Levin E, Rezvani A. Nicotinic interactions with antipsychotic drugs, models of schizophrenia and impacts on cognitive function. Biochem Pharmacol 2007; 74(8):1182–91.

47. Available at: http://www.samhsa.gov/specific-populations/age-gender-based. Accessed September 1, 2016.

48. Peralta V, de Jalón E, Camps M, et al. The meaning of childhood attention-deficit hyperactivity symptoms in patients with a first-episode of schizophrenia-spectrum psychosis. Schizophr Res 2011;126:28–35.

49. Donev DR, Greenstein D, Davidson A, et al. Comorbidity of schizophrenia and adult attention-deficit hyperactivity disorder. World J Biol Psychiatry 2011; 12(Suppl 1):52–6.

50. Levy E, Traicu A, Iyer S, et al. Psychotic disorders comorbid with attention-deficit hyperactivity disorder: an important knowledge gap. Can J Psychiatry 2015; 60(3):s48–52.

51. Mosholder A, Gelperin K, Hammad T, et al. Hallucinations and other psychotic symptoms associated with use of attention-deficit/hyperactivity disorder drugs in children. Pediatrics 2009;123:611–6.

52. Abell F, Hare D. An experimental investigation of the phenomenology of delusional beliefs in people with Asperger syndrome. Autism 2005;9(5):515–31.

53. Bosco F, Gabbatore I, Tirassa M. A broad assessment of theory of mind in adolescence: the complexity of mindreading. Conscious Cogn 2014;24:84–97.

54. Craig J, Hatton C, Craig F, et al. Persecutory beliefs, attributes and theory of mind: comparison of patients with paranoid delusions, Asperger's syndrome and healthy controls. Schizophr Res 2004;69:29–33.

55. Cederlof M, Petterson E, Sarislan A, et al. The association between childhood autistic traits and adolescent psychotic experiences is explained by general neuropsychiatric problems. Am J Med Genet B 2015;171B:153–9.

56. Happe F. An advanced test of theory of mind: understanding of story characters' thoughts and feelings by able autistic, mentally handicapped and normal children and adults. J Autism Dev Disord 1994;24(2):129–54.

57. Kirch D, Keith S, Matthews S. Research on first-episode psychosis: report on a national institute of health workshop. Schizophr Bull 1992;18(2):179–84.

58. Marder S. The NIMH-MATRICS project for developing cognition-enhancing agents for schizophrenia. Dialogues Clin Neurosci 2006;8:109–13.

59. Available at: http://www.mhs.com/product.aspx?gr=cli&prod=mccb&id=overview. Accessed September 1, 2016.

60. McCleery A, Ventua J, Kern R, et al. Cognitive functioning in first-episode schizophrenia: MATRICS Consensus Cognitive Battery (MCCB) profile of impairment. Schizophr Res 2014;157:33–9.

61. Green M, Harris J, Nuechterlein K. The MATRICS Consensus Cognitive Battery: what we know 6 years later [commentary]. Am J Psychiatry 2014;171(11): 1151–4.

62. Srihari V, Tek C, Kucukgoncu S, et al. First-episode services for psychotic disorders in the U.S. public sector: a pragmatic randomized controlled trial. Psychiatr Serv 2015;66:705–12.

63. Muser K, Penn D, Addington J, et al. The NAVIGATE program for first-episode psychosis: rationale, overview and description of psychosocial components. Psychiatr Serv 2015;66:680–90.

64. Kane J, Robinson D, Schooler N, et al. Comprehensive versus usual community care for first-episode psychosis: 2-year outcomes from the NIMH RAISE early treatment program. Am J Psychiatry 2016;173(4):362–72.

65. Nasrallah H, Keshavan M, Benes F, et al. Proceedings and data from the Schizophrenia Summit: a critical appraisal to improve the management of schizophrenia. J Clin Psychiatry 2009;70(Suppl 1):4–46.

66. Woodberry K, Shapiro D, Bryant B, et al. Progress and future directions in research on psychosis prodrome: a review for clinicians. Harv Rev Psychiatry 2016;24(2):87–103.

67. Velakoulis D, Wood S, Wong M, et al. Hippocampal and amygdala volumes according to psychosis stage and diagnosis a magnetic resonance imaging study of chronic schizophrenia, first-episode psychosis, and ultra-high-risk individuals. Arch Gen Psychiatry 2006;63(2):139–49.

68. Watsky R, Ludov K, Pollar D, et al. Severity of cortical thinning correlates with schizophrenia spectrum symptoms. J Am Acad Child Adolesc Psychiatry 2016;55(20):130–6.
69. Kenney J, Anderson-Schmidt H, Scanlon C, et al. Cognitive course in first-episode psychosis and clinical correlates: a 4 year longitudinal study using the MATRICS Consensus Cognitive Battery. Schizophr Res 2015;169:101–8.
70. Stone W, Msholam-Gately R, Giuliano A, et al. Healthy adolescent performance on the MATRICS Consensus Cognitive Battery (MCCB): developmental data from two samples of volunteers. Schizophr Res 2016;172:106–13.
71. Harvey P, Velligan D, Bellack A. Performance-based measures of functional skills: usefulness in clinical treatment studies. Schizophr Bull 2007;33(5): 1138–48.
72. Cariaga-Martinez A, Saiz-Ruiz J, Alelú-Paz R. From linkage studies to epigenetics: what we know and what we need to know in the neurobiology of schizophrenia. Front Neurosci 2016;10:202.
73. Asarnow R, Forsyth J. Genetics of childhood-onset schizophrenia. Child Adolesc Psychiatr Clin N Am 2013;22:675–87.
74. Brent B, Thermenos H, Keshavan M, et al. Gray matter alteration in schizophrenia high-risk youth and early-onset schizophrenia a review of structural MRI findings. Child Adolesc Psychiatr Clin N Am 2013;22:689–714.
75. Thompson P, Vidal C, Giedd J, et al. Mapping adolescent brain change reveals dynamic wave of accelerated gray mater loss in very early-onset schizophrenia. Proc Natl Acad Sci U S A 2001;98(20):11650–5.
76. Andreasen N, Liu D, Ziebell S, et al. Relapse duration, treatment intensity, and brain tissue loss in schizophrenia: a prospective longitudinal MRI study. Am J Psychiatry 2013;170:609–15.
77. Kempton M, Stahl D, Williams S, et al. Progressive lateral ventricular enlargement in schizophrenia: a meta-analysis of longitudinal MRI studies. Schizophr Res 2010;120(1–3):54–62.
78. Nelson M, Saykin A, Flashmam L, et al. Hippocampal volume reduction in schizophrenia as assessed by magnetic resonance imaging: a meta-analytic study. Arch Gen Psychiatry 1998;55(5):433–40.
79. Chung Y, Cannon D. Brain imaging during the transition from psychosis prodrome to schizophrenia. J Nerv Ment Dis 2015;203:336–41.
80. Seidman L, Nordentoft M. New targets for prevention of schizophrenia: is it time for interventions in the premorbid phase? Schizophr Bull 2015;41(4):795–800.
81. Miller T, McGlashan T, Woods S, et al. Symptom assessment in schizophrenic prodromal states. Psychiatr Q 1999;70(4):273–87.
82. McFarlane W. Prevention of the first episode of psychosis. Psychiatr Clin North Am 2011;34:95–107.
83. Klosterkötter J, Ruhrmann S, Schultze-Lutter F, et al. The European Prediction of Psychosis Study (EPOS): integrating early recognition and intervention in Europe. World Psychiatry 2005;4(3):161–8.
84. Nelson B, Yuen H, Wood S, et al. Long-term follow up of a group at ultra high risk ("prodromal") for psychosis: the PACE 400 Study. JAMA Psychiatry 2013;70(8): 793–802.
85. Addington J, Cadenhead K, Cannon T, et al. North American prodrome longitudinal study: a collaborative multisite approach to prodromal schizophrenia research. Schizophr Bull 2007;33(3):665–72.
86. Addington J, Liu L, Buchy L, et al. North American Prodrome Longitudinal Study (NAPLS 2): the prodromal symptoms. J Nerv Ment Dis 2005;203:328–35.

87. Cadenhead K, Mirzakhanian H. A case of attenuated psychosis syndrome: a broad differential diagnosis requires broad-spectrum treatment. Am J Psychiatry 2016;173(4):321–9.

88. Available at: http://www.rcpsych.ac.uk/pdf/Brief%20CAARMS%20with%20SO FAS%202016.pdf. Accessed May 30, 2016.

89. Wunderink L, Nienhuis F, Systema S, et al. Predictive validity of proposed remission criteria in first-episode schizophrenic patients responding to antipsychotics. Schizophr Bull 2007;33(3):792–6.

90. Yung A, Yuen H, McGorry P, et al. Mapping the onset of psychosis: the comprehensive assessment of at-risk mental states. Aust N Z J Psychiatry 2005;39: 964–71.

91. Miller T, McGlashan T, Rosen J, et al. Prodromal assessment with the structured interview for prodromal syndromes and the scale of prodromal symptoms: predictive validity, interrater reliability, and training to reliability. Schizophr Bull 2003; 29(4):703–15.

92. Miller TJ, McGlashan TH, Rosen JL, et al. Prospective diagnosis of the initial prodrome for schizophrenia based on the structured interview for prodromal syndromes: preliminary evidence of interrater reliability and predictive value. Am J Psychiatry 2002;159:863–5.

93. Carrión R, Cornblatt B, Burton C, et al. Personalized prediction of psychosis: external validation of the NAPLS-2 psychosis risk calculator with the EDIPPP Project. Am J Psychiatry 2016;173(10):989–96.

94. Available at: http://cape42.homestead.com/files/CAPE-42.htm. Accessed September 1, 2016.

95. Available at: http://www.schizophrenia.com/sztest/primetest.pdf. Accessed September 1, 2016.

96. Loewy R, Pearson R, Vinogradov S, et al. Psychosis risk screening with the prodromal questionnaire - brief version (PQ-B). Schizophr Res 2011;129:42–6.

97. Kline E, Thompson E, Demro C, et al. Longitudinal validation of psychosis risk screening tools. Schizophr Res 2015;165:116–22.

98. Ising H, Veling W, Loewy R, et al. The validity of the 16-item version of the Prodromal Questionnaire (PQ-16) to screen for ultra high risk of developing psychosis in the general help-seeking population. Schizophr Bull 2012;38(6):1288–96.

99. Mossaheb N, Becker J, Schaefer M, et al. The Community Assessment of Psychic Experience (CAPE) questionnaire as a screening-instrument in the detection of individuals at ultra-high risk for psychosis. Schizophr Res 2012;141: 210–4.

100. Addington J, Stowkowy J, Weiser M. Screening tools for clinical high risk for psychosis. Early Interv Psychiatry 2015;9:345–56.

101. Shevlin M, Murphy J, Dorahy M, et al. The distribution of positive psychosis-like symptoms in the population: a latent class analysis of the National Comorbidity Survey. Schizophr Res 2007;89:101–9.

102. Schreier H. Hallucinations in nonpsychotic children: more common than we think? J Am Acad Child Adolesc Psychiatry 1999;38(5):623–5.

103. McGee R, Poulton SWR. Hallucinations in nonpsychotic children [Letter to the Editor]. J Am Acad Child Adolesc Psychiatry 2000;19(1):12–3.

104. Jadri R, Bartels-Velthuis A, Debbane M, et al. From phenomenology to neurophysiological understanding of hallucinations in children and adolescents. Schizophr Bull 2014;40(S4):S221–32.

105. Johns L, Kompus K, Connell M, et al. Auditory verbal hallucinations in persons with and without a need for care. Schizophr Bull 2014;40(S4):S255–64.

106. de Leede-Smith S, Barkus E. A comprehensive review of auditory verbal hallu-cinations: lifetime prevalence, correlates and mechanisms in healthy and clinical individuals. Front Hum Neurosci 2013;7(367):1–25.

107. McGrath J, Saha S, Al-Hamzawi A, et al. The bidirectional association between psychotic experiences and DSM-IV mental disorders. Am J Psychiatry 2016; 173(10):997–1006.

108. Scott J, Martin G, Bor W, et al. The prevalence and correlates of hallucinations in Australian adolescents: results from a national survey. Schizophr Res 2008;107: 179–85.

109. van Os J, Hannssen M, Bijl R, et al. Straus (1969) revisited: a psychosis contin-uum in the general population? Schizophr Res 2000;459:11–20.

110. Hanssen M, Bak M, Bijl M, et al. The incidence and outcome of subclinical psy-chotic experiences in the general population. Br J Clin Psychol 2005;44:181–91.

111. Rössler W, Rieche-Rössler A, Angst J, et al. Psychotic experiences in the gen-eral population: a twenty-year prospective community study. Schizophr Res 2007;92:1–14.

112. Bartels-Velthuis A, Wigman J, Jenner J, et al. Course of auditory vocal halluci-nations in childhood: 11-year follow up study. Acta Psychiatr Scand 2016;134: 6–15.

113. Loewy R, Johnson J, Cannon T. Self-report of attenuated psychotic experiences in a college population. Schizophr Res 2007;93(1–3):144–51.

114. Yung A, Nelson B, Baker K, et al. Psychotic-like experiences in a community sample of adolescents: implications for the continuum model of psychosis and prediction of schizophrenia. Aust N Z J Psychiatry 2009;43:118–28.

115. Sommer I, Daalman K, Rietkerk T, et al. Healthy individuals with auditory verbal hallucinations: who are they? Psychiatric assessments of a selected sample of 103 subjects. Schizophr Bull 2010;36(3):633–41.

116. Nelson B, Yung A, Bechdolf A, et al. The phenomenological critique and self-disturbance: implications for ultra-high risk ("prodrome") research. Schizophr Bull 2007;34(2):381–92.

117. Sikich L, et al. Diagnosis and evaluation of hallucinations and other psychotic symptoms in children and adolescents. Child Adolesc Psychiatric Clin N Am 2013;22:655–73.

118. Yung A, Phillips LJ, Yuen H, et al. Risk factors for psychosis in an ultra high risk group: psychopathology and clinical features. Schizophr Res 2004;67:131–42.

119. Stafford M, Jackson H, Mayo-Wilson E, et al. Early interventions to prevent psy-chosis: systematic review and meta-analysis. BMJ 2013;346:1–13.

120. Fusar-Poli P, Bonoldi I, Yung A, et al. Predicting psychosis: meta-analysis of transition outcomes. Arch Genpsychiatry 2012;69(3):220–9.

121. Fusar-Poli P, Borgward S, Bechdolf A, et al. The psychosis high-risk state: a comprehensive state-of-the-art review. JAMA Psychiatry 2013;70(1):107–20.

122. van der Gaag M, Smit F, Bechdolt A, et al. Preventing a first episode of psycho-sis: meta-analysis of randomized controlled prevention trials for 12 month and longer-term follow ups. Schizophr Res 2013;149:56–62.

123. Addington J, Cornblatt B, Cadenhead K, et al. At clinical high risk for psychosis: outcome for nonconverters. Am J Psychiatry 2011;168:800–5.

124. Morcillo C, Stochl J, Russo D, et al. First-rank symptoms and premorbid adjust-ment in young individuals at increased risk of developing psychosis. Psychopa-thology 2015;48:120–6.

125. McGlashan T, Zipursky R, Perkins D, et al. The PRIME North American random-ized double-blind clinical trial of olanzapine versus placebo in patients at risk of

being prodromally symptomatic for psychosis. I. Study rationale and design. Schizophr Res 2003;61:7–18.

126. Amminger G, Schafer M, Papageorgiiou K, et al. Long-chain omega-3 fatty acids for indicated prevention of psychotic disorders: a randomized, placebo-controlled trial. Arch Gen Psychiatry 2010;67(2):146–54.

127. Amminger G, Schäfer M, Schlögelhofer M, et al. Longer-term outcome in the prevention of psychotic disorders by the Vienna omega-3 study. Nat Commun 2015;6:7934.

128. Miklowitz D, O'Brien M, Schlosser D, et al. Family-focused treatment for adolescents and young adults at high risk for psychosis: results of a randomized trial. J Am Acad Child Adolesc Psychiatry 2014;53(8):848–58.

129. McFarlane W, Levin B, Travis L, et al. Clinical and functional outcomes after 2 years in the early detection and intervention for the prevention of psychosis multisite effectiveness trial. Schizophr Bull 2015;41(1):30–43.

130. Calvo A, Moreno M, Ruiz-Sancho A, et al. Intervention for adolescents with early onset psychosis and their families: a randomized controlled trial. J Am Acad Child Adolesc Psychiatry 2015;53(6):688–96.

131. Calvo A, Moreno M, Ruiz-Sancho A, et al. Psychoeducation group intervention for adolescents with psychosis and their families: a two year follow-up. J Am Acad Child Adolesc Psychiatry 2015;54(12):984–90.

132. Sadath A, Muralidhar D, Vrambally S, et al. Family intervention in first-episode psychosis: a qualitative systematic review. Sage Open 2015. http://dx.doi.org/10.117/2158244015613108.

133. McFarlane W. Family interventions for schizophrenia and the psychoses: a review. Fam Process 2016;55:460–82.

134. Ising H, Lokkerbo J, Rietdijk J, et al. Four-year cost-effectiveness of cognitive behavior therapy for preventing first episode psychosis: the Dutch Early Detection Intervention Evaluation (EDIE-NL) Trial. Schizophr Bull 2016. http://dx.doi.org/10.1093/schbul/sbw084.

135. van der Gaag M, Nieman D, Rietdjik J, et al. Cognitive behavioral therapy for subjects at ultrahigh risk for developing psychosis: a randomized controlled clinical trial. Schizophr Bull 2012;38(6):1180–8.

136. Lewandowksi K. Cognitive remediation for the treatment of cognitive dysfunction in the early course of psychosis. Harv Rev Psychiatry 2016;24(2):164–72.

137. Nuechterlein H, Ventura J, McEwen S, et al. Enhancing cognitive training through aerobic exercise after a first schizophrenia episode: theoretical conception and pilot study. Schizophr Bull 2016;42(s1):s42–52.

138. National Institute for Health and Care Excellence. Psychosis and schizophrenia in children and young people: recognition and management 2013. Clinical guideline; Available at: nice.org.uk/guidance/cg155nice.org.uk/guidance/cg155.

139. Morrison A, Barratt S. What are the components of CBT for psychosis? A Delphi study. Front Psychol 2010;36(1):136–42.

140. Hagen R, Turkington D, Berge R, et al, editors. CBT for psychosis: a symptom-based approach. The International Society for the Psychological Treatments of the Schizophrenias and Other Psychoses. Routledge; 2011.

141. Norcross J, editor. Psychotherapy relationships that work. 2nd edition. Oxford University Press; 2011.

142. Thomas N. What's really wrong with cognitive behavior therapy for psychosis? Front Psychol 2015. http://dx.doi.org/10.3389/psyg.2015.00232.

143. Tai S, Turkington D. The evolution of cognitive behavior therapy for schizophrenia: current practice and recent developments. Schizophr Bull 2009; 35(5):865–73.
144. Turner D, van der Gaag M, Karyotaki E, et al. Psycholgocial interventions for psychosis: a meta-analysis of comparative outcome studies. Am J Psychiatry 2014;171:525–8.
145. Kulpers E, Yesufu-Udenchuku A, Taylor C, et al. Management of psychosis and schizophrenia in adults: summary of updated NICE guidance. BMJ 2014;348. http://dx.doi.org/10.1136/bmj.g1173.
146. McClellan J, Stock S. Practice parameter for the assessment and treatment of children and adolescents with schizophrenia. J Am Acad Child Adolesc Psychiatry 2013;52(9):976–90.
147. Buchanan R, Kreyenbuhl J, Kelly D, et al. The 2009 schizophrenia PORT psychopharmacological treatment recommendations and summary statements. Schizophr Bull 2010;36(1):71–93.
148. Dixon L, Dickerson F, Bellack A, et al. The 2009 schizophrenia PORT psychosocial treatment recommendations and summary statements. Schizophr Bull 2010; 36(1):47–80.
149. Christian R, Saavedra L, Gaynes B, et al. Future research needs for first- and second- generation antipsychotics for children and young adults. Rockville (MD): Agency for Healthcare Research and Quality; 2012 (Prepared by the RTI-UNC Evidence-based Practice Center under Contract No. 290 2007 10056 I); Future Research Needs Paper No. 13.
150. Maglione M, Ruelez Maher A, Hu J, et al. Off-label use of atypical antipsychotics: an update. (prepared by the Southern California Evidence-based Practice Center under contract no. HHSA290-2007-10062-1). Rockville (MD): Agency for Healthcare Research and Quality; 2011. Comparative Effectiveness Review No. 43.
151. Helfer B, Samara M, Huhn M, et al. Efficacy and safety of antidepressants added to antipsychotics for schizophrenia: a systematic review and meta-analysis. Am J Psychiatry 2016 Sep 1;173(9):876–86.
152. Hor K, Taylor M. Suicide and schizophrenia: a systematic review of rates and risk factors. J Psychopharm 2010;(11 S4):81–90.
153. Kreyenbuhl J, Medoff D, McEvoy J, et al. The RAISE connection program: psychopharmacological treatment of people with a first episode of schizophrenia. Psychiatr Serv Adv 2015;67(12):1300–6.
154. Pinniti N, Mago R, Leon JD. Coffee, cigarettes, and meds: what are the metabolic effects? Psychiatr Times 2005. Available at: http://www.psychiatrictimes.com/articles/coffee-cigarettes-and-meds-what-are-metabolic-effects/page/0/1. Accessed August 28, 2016.
155. Rosenheck R, Leslie D, Sint K, et al. Cost effectiveness of comprehensive, integrated care for first episode psychosis in the NIMH RAISE early treatment program. Schizophr Bull 2016;42(4):896–906.
156. Marino L, Nossel I, Choi J, et al. The RAISE connection program for early psychosis: secondary outcomes and mediators and moderators of improvement. J Nerv Ment Dis 2015;203:365–71.
157. Essock S, Goldman H, Hogan M, et al. State partnerships for first-episode psychosis Services. Psychiatr Serv 2015;66:671–3.

Model Programs

Transition to Adult Health Care Services for Young Adults with Chronic Medical Illness and Psychiatric Comorbidity

Margaret McManus, MHS*, Patience White, MD, MA

KEYWORDS

- Transition to adult care • Adolescent • Young adult • Chronic conditions

KEY POINTS

- Youth with chronic medical illness are at increased risk of psychiatric illness, and those with chronic psychiatric illness are at elevated risk of medical illness.
- Most youth with chronic medical and psychiatric conditions are not receiving needed transition support from pediatric to adult medical and behavioral health care.
- Medical professional recommendations call for transition preparation to begin early in adolescence and continue through young adulthood.
- A nationally recognized transition approach, called the *Six Core Elements of Health Care Transition*, offers a tested model for broad application in pediatric and adult medical and behavioral health care.
- Practical lessons learned are offered for implementing the *Six Core Elements* and measuring transition process and impacts.

INTRODUCTION

Advances in pediatric care have resulted in dramatic increases in the number of children and adolescents with chronic conditions.[1,2] The increasing prevalence of childhood chronic conditions has important implications for transition to adult care because well over 90% of this population will survive into adulthood.[1] In fact, an estimated one million adolescents with chronic conditions turn 18 annually and need transition support as they move from pediatric to adult health care.[3]

Obtaining a precise estimate of transition-aged youth with chronic medical illness and psychiatric comorbidity is currently impossible because national survey datasets

Disclosure Statement: The authors have nothing to disclose.
Got Transition, The National Alliance to Advance Adolescent Health, 1615 M Street Northwest, Suite 290, Washington, DC 20036, USA
* Corresponding author.
E-mail address: mmcmanus@thenationalalliance.org

identify youth with special health care needs (YSHCN) based on either (1) the presence of an ongoing physical, mental, behavioral and/or other health condition that results in elevated need for services and/or an activity limitation; or (2) a listing of selected chronic conditions. In the first instance, YSHCN are defined broadly and combined to include all types of chronic conditions. In the second instance, youth with selected chronic conditions are defined to include only a subset of the total childhood population with chronic conditions. Furthermore, the limited published literature on childhood comorbidities is often disease specific, dated, or based on small study samples.

Despite these limits, evidence clearly supports that children with chronic medical illness are at increased risk of impaired psychological adjustment or psychiatric illness, and those with chronic psychiatric illness are at elevated risk of medical illness.[4–8] Considerable variation in rates of comorbidity is found by type of medical condition, with neurodevelopmental and sensory conditions having the highest rates of psychiatric illness.[7,8] Increased risk of comorbidity is also associated with the severity or the number of chronic medical conditions.[4] In a seminal study on adult medical and psychiatric disorders published in 2011, called the Synthesis Project, the authors found that exposure to adverse childhood experiences, chronic stress, poverty, and poor educational attainment were risk factors for comorbidity.[9]

In this article, national data on lack of transition preparation among YSHCN, including those with emotional, behavioral, and developmental conditions, are presented along with transition barriers identified by consumers and providers. These transition gaps are followed by a summary of US transition goals and US and UK health professional recommendations for transition. In addition, an in-depth examination of the nationally recognized transition approach, the *Six Core Elements of Health Care Transition*, is discussed along with a summary of practice-based lessons learned. Finally, the article concludes with a discussion of transition measurement and evaluation.

GAPS IN RECEIPT OF TRANSITION SUPPORT AND CONSUMER AND PROVIDER BARRIERS

Transition gaps are pervasive for all YSHCN, including those with medical and psychiatric comorbidities. National survey data reveal that an estimated 25% of youth between 12 and 17 have a special health care need.[10] Research shows that most of these YSHCN have not received needed transition preparation. According to the 2009/2010 National Survey of Children with Special Health Care Needs, 60% of YSHCN failed to receive needed transition support.[11] This survey, conducted by the National Center for Health Statistics, uses a nationally representative sample of parents or legal guardians with children less than the age of 18 years who have special health needs, identified by a 5-item screener.[12] A total of 17,114 parent respondents who have YSHCN ages 12 through 17 answered 4 transition questions in this survey, from which a composite score was obtained.[10] Parents or guardians were asked about discussions that YSHCN have had with health care providers (HCPs) about changing to an adult HCP, taking increased responsibility for self-care, changing health care needs, and maintaining health insurance coverage.

As shown in **Table 1**, certain health characteristics were associated with a lack of transition preparation: (1) having an emotional, behavioral, or developmental condition (EBD), and (2) having a condition that limits activities. As many as 71% of youth with EBD, with or without one or more comorbid medical conditions, did not receive needed transition preparation compared with 54% of youth with medical conditions without associated comorbid EBD conditions. Also, of note, the extent to which HCPs encourage self-care responsibility differed sharply depending on whether the

Table 1
Proportion of youth with special health care needs *not* meeting transition goal and individual component measures: United States, 2009/2010

Health Characteristics	Overall Proportion of YSHCN Not Meeting Transition Goal	HCP Not Discussed Shift to Adult Provider	HCP Not Discussed Changing Health Needs	HCP Not Usually/ Always Encouraged Youth to Take Self-Care Responsibility	No One Discussed Maintaining Health Insurance as Adult
All YSHCN, %	60	56	41	22	65
Youth with EBD, behavioral, or developmental conditions					
EBD ± other SN	71	61	49	32	71
Other SN without EBD	54	53	37	17	61
Youth with activity impacts					
Always, usually, great deal affected	75	62	47	37	70
Somewhat, moderately affected	61	55	41	19	66
Never affected	48	51	36	14	58

Abbreviations: EBD, emotional, behavioral, developmental conditions; HCP, health care professionals; SN, special needs (in the table this refers to chronic medical conditions with SN); YSCHN, youth with special health care needs.

YSHCN had an EBD condition or whether the youth's condition significantly impacted activities. Other factors associated with lack of transition preparation included male gender, non-white race, Hispanic ethnicity, family income less than 400% of poverty, not having a medical home, and being uninsured or publicly insured.

Barriers associated with poor transition performance are widespread and are commonly reported by youth with specific chronic medical or psychiatric illnesses and their parents.[13–19] Provider barriers, which appear to mirror several of the consumer barriers, reflect distinct concerns among pediatric and adult clinicians.[20–30] **Box 1** summarizes these barriers.

Box 1
Barriers associated with lack of transition support

Barriers Cited by Consumers

- Difficulty letting go of long-standing relationships with pediatric medical and behavioral health providers
- Reticence among parents and caregivers of relinquishing care and decision-making responsibilities
- Limited engagement of youth and young adults in planning for transition
- Lack of information about the transition process and available adult providers
- Lack of explicit and continuous attention to young adults' needs for decision-making supports
- Lack of coordination and communication among all pediatric and adult providers, including across disciplines
- Stigma associated with seeking mental health care
- Low utilization of medical and behavioral care during adolescent and young adult period
- Changes in and more rigid eligibility criteria for adult services, insurance, and disability assistance

Barriers Cited by Pediatric Providers

- Difficulty identifying available adult clinicians
- Fragmentation between pediatric and adult systems
- Difficulty breaking bond with patients and parents
- Concern that adult clinicians may not be sufficiently trained in the care of young adults with childhood-onset, complex, medical or psychiatric conditions
- Lack of time and staff
- Reimbursement issues

Barriers Cited by Adult Providers

- Practices are full
- Inadequate exchange of medical and psychiatric information from and communication with pediatric provider
- Lack of experience with complex conditions and with the developmental stage of young adults
- System infrastructure inadequacies
  - Lack of access to adult medical specialty and mental health clinicians
  - Inadequate care coordination support
  - Lack of information about and availability of community resources, including public program services

---

UNITED STATES PUBLIC HEALTH TRANSITION GOALS

Transition from pediatric to adult care is a national public health priority. Healthy People 2020 calls for the United States to increase the proportion of YSHCN whose HCPs have discussed transition planning from pediatric to adult health care.[31] In addition, the federal Maternal and Child Health Bureau (MCHB) recently selected transition to adult health care for all youth as 1 of its 15 national priorities.[32] In response to MCHB's national priorities, 32 states have selected transition as their priority for the next 5 years.[33]

UNITED STATES PROFESSIONAL SOCIETY RECOMMENDATIONS
AAP/AAFP/ACP Clinical Report on Health Care Transition

In 2011, the American Academy of Pediatrics (AAP), the American Academy of Family Physicians (AAFP), and the American College of Physicians (ACP) published their joint statement defining a recommended process for transition for all youth.[34] The authors acknowledged the lack of progress made in transition over the past decade and called for a specific health care transition planning algorithm, starting early in adolescence and continuing into young adulthood. The Clinical Report calls for all clinicians/practices to have a written transition policy, which is shared with the youth and caregiver, describing the practice's approach to an adult model of care and the recommended age for transfer. Transition preparation and planning should start at age 14 with an assessment of self-care skills and development of a care plan to support youth independence and preparation for adult care. Before the age of 18, legal documentation of supported decision-making or guardianship should be put in place, if determined to be necessary by youth, caregiver, or provider. This preparation is critical because, at age 18, youth start to receive an adult model of care, requiring privacy and confidentiality considerations, even if they are still being seen by pediatric medical and behavioral health clinicians. Between the ages of 18 and 21, most young adults transfer to an adult clinician. Continued transition support from adult clinicians is necessary following the transfer, and pediatric consultation support should be made available to adult clinicians as a resource, if needed, during the post-transfer period.

United Kingdom's Guideline for Transition from Child to Adult Services

The UK's National Institute for Health and Care Excellence (NICE) released its transition guideline in February 2016 for clinicians in child and adult health, mental health, and social care services.[35] It is similar to the AAP/AAFP/ACP Clinical Report and the Six Core Elements, described in later discussion. NICE recommends that transition planning begin at ages 13 or 14 and, for those close to the point of transfer, planning should begin immediately. Annual transition planning meetings are recommended with the young person, family, and HCPs involving a "named worker" responsible for coordinating health, education, employment, community inclusion, and independent living and housing supports. NICE recommends that the young person meet the new adult provider before leaving children's services and that a transfer folder be prepared with information about the youth's health condition, education, and social care needs; preferences about parent involvement; emergency care plans; and strengths and future goals. After transfer to an adult provider, the NICE guideline calls for active outreach and follow-up to ensure young adult engagement and continuity of adult providers at least for the first 2 appointments. Importantly, a supporting infrastructure is recommended with senior leadership accountability for implementing transition strategies, supporting consumers, providing community education, and identifying and addressing gaps.

THE *SIX CORE ELEMENTS* OF HEALTH CARE TRANSITION

Following the release of the 2011 Clinical Report, the national resource center, Got Transition, published the *Six Core Elements*.[36] This transition approach is aligned with the Clinical Report and can be used by both medical and behavioral health providers. This approach incorporates the key activities associated with transition: preparation, transfer of care, and integration into adult care and can be applied by providers caring for youth with medical, psychiatric, and intellectual/developmental conditions as well as for youth without chronic conditions. The intervention can be delivered in pediatric and adult primary care, medical specialty, and behavioral health settings and incorporated into large systems of care, managed care organizations, care coordination programs, and public health and mental health programs.

The *Six Core Elements* define the basic components of health care transition support with linked sample tools and measurement resources. The results of transition learning collaboratives in several states, an examination of transition innovations in the United States and abroad, and reviews by more than 100 pediatric and adult health professionals and consumers informed the approach. **Fig. 1** displays the *Six Core Elements* timeline for transitioning youth to an adult provider. Three *Six Core Elements* packages, with sample tools, are available for (1) transitioning youth to an adult provider, (2) transitioning youth to an adult approach to care without changing providers, and (3) integrating young adults into adult health care. A description of the content of each core element is shown in **Box 2**, from the Got Transition package for pediatric, family medicine, and med-peds providers, "Transitioning Youth to Adult Health Care," available at www.gottransition.org.

Recently, several subspecialty societies of the ACP have customized some of the *Six Core Elements* for youth with selected chronic medical illnesses.[37] With the ACP, the Society of Adolescent Health and Medicine and the Society of General Internal Medicine customized the transition readiness assessment tool and medical summary for youth with intellectual/developmental disabilities and for youth with physical disabilities.[37]

Several transition readiness/self-care assessments/patient activation instruments have been developed and can be used as part of the *Six Core Elements* approach. Some of these tools, such as the Transition Readiness Assessment Questionnaire, have been validated and are summarized in the resources section on www.

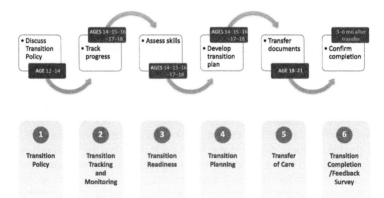

Fig. 1. *Six Core Elements* of Health Care Transition: timeline example for a youth transferring to an adult provider.

Box 2
Content of the *Six Core Elements* for "youth transitioning to adult care"

1. Transition policy
   - Develop a transition policy/statement with input from youth and families that describes the practice's approach to transition, including privacy and consent information.
   - Educate all staff about the practice's approach to transition, the policy/statement, the *Six Core Elements* approach, and distinct roles of the youth, family, and pediatric and adult health care team in the transition process, taking into account cultural preferences.
   - Post policy and share/discuss with youth and families, beginning at age 12 to 14, and regularly review as part of ongoing care.

2. Transition tracking and monitoring
   - Establish criteria and process for identifying transitioning youth and enter their data into a registry.
   - Use individual flow sheet or registry to track youth's transition progress with the *Six Core Elements*.
   - Incorporate *Six Core Elements* into clinical care process, using EHR if possible.

3. Transition readiness
   - Conduct regular transition readiness assessments, beginning at age 14, to identify and discuss with youth and parent/caregiver their needs and goals in self-care.
   - Jointly develop goals and prioritized actions with youth and parent/caregiver and document regularly in a plan of care.

4. Transition planning
   - Develop and regularly update the plan of care, including readiness assessment findings, goals and prioritized actions, medical summary and emergency care plan, and, if needed, a condition fact sheet and legal documents.
   - Prepare youth and parent/caregiver for adult approach to care at age 18, including legal changes in decision-making and privacy and consent, self-advocacy, and access to information.
   - Determine need for decision-making supports for youth with intellectual challenges and make referrals to legal resources.
   - Plan with youth and parent/caregiver for optimal timing of transfer. If both primary and subspecialty care are involved, discuss optimal timing for each.
   - Obtain consent from youth/guardian for release of medical information.
   - Assist youth in identifying an adult provider and communicate with selected provider about pending transfer of care.
   - Provide linkages to insurance resources, self-care management information, and culturally appropriate community supports.

5. Transfer of care
   - Confirm date of first adult provider appointment.
   - Transfer young adult when his/her condition is stable.
   - Complete transfer package, including final transition readiness assessment, plan of care with transition goals and pending actions, medical summary and emergency care plan, and, if needed, legal documents, condition fact sheet, and additional provider records.
   - Prepare letter with transfer package, send to adult practice, and confirm adult practice's receipt of transfer package.
   - Confirm with adult provider the pediatric provider's responsibility for care until young adult is seen in adult setting.

6. Transfer completion
   - Contact young adult and parent/caregiver 3 to 6 months after last pediatric visit to confirm transfer of responsibilities to adult practice and elicit feedback on experience with transition process.
   - Communicate with adult practice confirming completion of transfer and offer consultation assistance, as needed.
   - Build ongoing and collaborative partnerships with adult primary and specialty care providers.

gottransition.org.[38] In addition, Martel and colleagues[39] have developed a readiness checklist for youth going to college with behavioral health issues.

LESSONS LEARNED: PRIMARY CARE, SPECIALTY MEDICAL CARE, AND MANAGED CARE

To test the use of the *Six Core Elements* approach, health care transition learning collaboratives were conducted between 2011 and 2013 in Washington DC, Colorado, Massachusetts, New Hampshire, and Wisconsin. These collaboratives used the evidence-based quality improvement methodology from the National Initiative for Children's Healthcare Quality and pioneered by the Institute for Healthcare Improvement.[40] Findings demonstrated that the *Six Core Elements* approach and tools were feasible to use in both primary and subspecialty clinical settings and resulted in measurable improvements in the transition process and in the development of collaborative arrangements between pediatric and adult providers.[41]

This transition approach has also been incorporated into a Washington, DC Medicaid-managed care plan for YSHCN receiving Supplemental Security Income.[42] Youth and young adults participating in this Medicaid pilot study had developmental/intellectual, behavioral health, and complex medical conditions. Got Transition staff worked closely with the managed care leadership to customize the *Six Core Elements* tools and identify what core elements were the responsibility of the Medicaid plan's care managers and what were the responsibility of the pediatric and adult primary care clinicians. Results showed that the Medicaid-managed care plan demonstrated improvement in incorporating the *Six Core Elements* using Got Transition's process measurement tool and consumer feedback survey.

To further demonstrate the application of this approach in a subspecialty medical setting, Got Transition staff collaborated with the University of Rochester's pediatric and adult divisions to successfully incorporate the *Six Core Elements* into their diabetes, cystic fibrosis, and sickle cell disease programs. Got Transition staff also collaborated with several large integrated delivery systems, such as Kaiser of Northern California, Cleveland Clinics, and the Henry Ford Health Systems. These systems summarized their recommendation in a tip sheet for other practices/systems starting a health care transition quality improvement process.[43]

Box 3 summarizes the lessons learned from all of the above-mentioned practice settings. Got Transition staff are currently partnering with DC's Department of Behavioral Health to customize the *Six Core Elements* tools for their transition-aged youth, ages 16 to 25, to pilot the approach with 2 child and adult public mental health clinics as part of DC's Substance Abuse and Mental Health Services Administration–funded transition initiative. The transition policy has been modified to explain the specific type of transition support that will be provided by the mental health clinic, the age for transfer to adult mental health services, and information about privacy and consent. The transition readiness assessment has been customized to include questions about behavioral health needs, understanding stressors, knowing what to do in cases of a crisis, and so forth. This quality improvement effort will be summarized in a subsequent publication.

For practices or systems planning to implement the *Six Core Elements* approach and customize specific sample tools, it is important to recognize that older youth will need to go through an accelerated transition planning process compared with those who are in their early adolescent years, where there is more time for planning. The longer youth/families and clinicians/systems wait to initiate this process, the greater the challenges. Often, many older adolescents become disconnected from care, making transition planning assistance and transfer support very difficult. Compressing all of the core elements into 1 or 2 visits is not recommended. Importantly,

---

Box 3
Summary of transition lessons learned in primary, specialty, and managed care settings

Team Effort

- Leadership (eg, senior providers in a practice, clinic, or behavioral/medical system) must be engaged.
- Fitting transition into a larger strategic plan for the practice/system makes the leadership more likely to support it.
- Involvement of both pediatric and adult provider leaders from the beginning is essential.
- Transition is a team-based effort with consumer and clinic staff (social workers, front desk staff) involvement. It cannot be accomplished by a transition specialist or care manager alone.

Key Processes

- Starting with a pilot to test the processes is necessary before broad implementation and always apply quality improvement methods.
- It is important in the transition readiness assessment tool to separate the ongoing behavioral and medical aspects of the care from the transition self-care and health care skills needed for transition.
- Waiting until age 18 or older to start the transition process is much more difficult than starting at a younger age.
- Practice change to make transition improvements takes time. Transition implementation takes more than writing a policy, doing a readiness assessment, or putting tools into the electronic medical record.

Evidence

- Defining the processes, outcomes, and evaluation strategies up front is critical so everyone is on board and knows what success looks like.
- Adaptation and implementation of the *Six Core Elements* in primary, specialty, and managed care settings is feasible.
- Patients and families appreciate participating in a structured, ongoing process.
- Health care providers find transition improvement is rewarding and sustainable.

---

though, clinicians and systems can choose what core elements are best suited for their patients and their available resources. Using a quality improvement process, there can be flexibility regarding the level of assistance individual youth is provided to gain the needed self-care and health care navigation skills.

Many youths with medical illness and psychiatric comorbidity have several providers—primary care, medical specialty, and mental health. Having a coordinated plan on how to stage the transfer of care process for each provider is important so the youth does not get lost in the process or overwhelmed with too many transitions at once. When multiple providers are involved, the overall transition process should be collaborative in nature and may be best initiated and led by the clinicians managing the major health issue (either psychiatric or medical) or by the primary care provider that is coordinating all of the care.

MEASUREMENT AND EVALUATION OF HEALTH CARE TRANSITION INTERVENTIONS

Despite the fact that transition from pediatric to adult-focused health care is a topic that affects all youth, especially those with chronic medical and behavioral health conditions, research in this field is very limited. Transition evaluation studies that include preintervention and postintervention data, intervention and nonintervention comparisons, or randomized clinical trials are for the most part limited to youth with selected medical conditions such as diabetes; very few rigorously evaluated studies have evaluated transition interventions for youth with mental health conditions, with intellectual/developmental disabilities, and with comorbid medical and behavioral conditions (Gabriel P, McManus M, Rogers K, et al. The outcome evidence for structured pediatric to adult health care transition interventions: a systematic review. Submitted for publication). Most evaluation studies have small sample sizes and are based in non-US countries with different health care delivery systems. Furthermore, transition studies seldom adhere to any conceptual or professional framework, and measures used to evaluate transition outcomes vary considerably.[44] The Institute of Medicine's (IOM's) report, *Investing in the Health and Well-Being of Young Adults*, called attention to this research gap, stating that "there has been minimal systematic implementation and evaluation of institutional change to address concerns about the increasing numbers of pediatric patients with chronic conditions who are now living into adulthood."[45] The IOM report articulated several recommendations for improving the state of health care transition research, as shown in **Box 4**.

As researchers and clinicians consider ways to better measure transition process and impact, it is important to focus special attention on youth and young adults with medical illness and psychiatric comorbidities because they fare so poorly in terms of receipt of transition support. The conceptual design of such new research should take into consideration that multiple systems of care are often involved, including, at the very least, medical and behavioral health systems. Moreover, the intervention components to be evaluated should encompass (1) *transition planning or preparation* preferably between ages 12 and 17, (2) *transfer of care* preferably between 18 and 21, and (3) *integration into adult care* preferably between 18 and 25. All too often transition interventions are inadequately described in published evaluation studies, making the association between outcomes and associated transition interventions difficult to ascertain. Using 1 of the 2 transition measurement tools in the *Six Core Elements*[46] offers a way to create more uniformity in describing the specific components of a transition quality improvement intervention.

The triple aim framework of population health, consumer experience of care, and utilization and costs of care has been widely used to measure impacts of various interventions and holds promise for transition interventions as well.[44] With respect to population health impacts, measures that could be considered for youth with chronic

---

Box 4
Institute of Medicine recommendations for improving the state of health care transition research

- Development of quality performance measures on the transition process by the Agency for Healthcare Quality and Research and the Maternal and Child Health Bureau

- Funding of transition innovation models by the Centers for Medicare and Medicaid Services

- Inclusion of transition performance as part of reporting frameworks by the National Committee on Quality Assurance and the National Quality Forum

- Collection of relevant transition data elements as part of meaningful use criteria

- Provision of pay-for-performance initiatives and other provider assessments based on transition metrics

medical conditions with or without psychiatric health conditions pertain to adherence to medications or functional status improvements or attainment of self-care skills. With respect to experience of care, measures that could be considered to pertain to assessments of consumer engagement (using, for example, the Patient Activation Measure) and consumer experience (using, for example, the *Six Core Elements'* Transition Feedback Survey). With respect to utilization and costs of care, measures that can be considered include (1) length of time between the last child medical or mental health visit and the initial adult medical or mental health visit, (2) proportion of transferred patients arriving in adult medical or mental health care with up-to-date health records and a plan of care, (3) utilization of adult medical or mental health ambulatory services, (4) use of emergency room and hospital services, and (5) associated costs of care.

SUMMARY

Transition support for youth and young adults with chronic medical illness and psychiatric comorbidity is not widely available in the United States. National public health goals and health professional guidance are available to support future medical and behavioral health clinicians and health efforts. The *Six Core Elements* offers a comprehensive approach available to both medical and behavioral clinicians that has been successfully implemented in a variety of settings with important lessons learned. Future evaluation studies are needed to assess the impact of transition interventions that incorporate transition planning, transfer of care, and integration into adult care and that take into account population health, consumer and provider experience, and service utilization and costs of care. Focusing special attention on youth and young adults with chronic medical conditions and psychiatric comorbidities would fill a major gap in the transition research field.

REFERENCES

1. Perrin JM, Anderson LE, VanCleave J. The rise in chronic conditions among infants, children and youth can be met with continued health system innovations. Health Aff 2014;33:2099–105.

2. Perrin JM, Bloom SR, Gortmaker SL. The increase of childhood chronic conditions in the United States. JAMA 2007;297:2755–6.

3. Estimate prepared by authors based on calculation of 4.5 million 18 year olds, as reported in the 2010 Census, multiplied by the prevalence rate of special needs among 12-17 year olds (25.1%), from the 2011/12 National Survey of Children's Health.

4. Cohen P, Pine D, Must A, et al. Prospective associations between somatic illness and mental illness from childhood to adulthood. Am J Epidemiol 1998;147:232–9.

5. Combs-Orme T, Heflinger A, Simpkins CG. Comorbidity of mental health problems and chronic health conditions in children. J Emotional Behav Disord 2002; 10:116–25.

6. Hysing M, Elgen I, Gillberg C, et al. Chronic physical illness and mental health conditions in children. Results from a large-scale population study. J Child Psychol Psychiatry 2007;48:785–92.

7. Lavigne JV, Faier-Routman J. Psychological adjustment to pediatric physical disorders. A meta-analytic review. J Pediatr Psychol 1992;17:133–57.

8. Spady DW, Schopflocker DP, Swenson LW, et al. Medical and psychiatric comorbidity and health care use among children 6 to 17 years old. Arch Pediatr Adolesc Med 2005;159:231–7.

9. Druss BG, Walker ER. Mental disorders and medical co-morbidity. Research synthesis report No. 21. Princeton (NJ): Robert Wood Johnson Foundation; 2011.

10. Prevalence estimate for youth ages 12 through 17. Available at: childhealthdata. org/browse/survey/results?q=2625&r=1&g=448. Accessed October 1, 2016.

11. McManus MA, Pollack LR, Cooley WC, et al. Current status of transition preparation among youth with special needs in the United States. Pediatrics 2013;131: 1090–7.

12. Children with Special Health Care Needs Screener. Baltimore (MD): Data Resource Center for Child and Adolescent Health.

13. Betz CL, Lobo ML, Nehring WM, et al. Voices not heard: a systematic review of adolescents' and emerging adults' perspectives of health care transition. Nurs Outlook 2013;61(5):311–36.

14. Bindels-de Heus KGCB, van Staa A, van Vliet I, et al. Transferring young people with profound intellectual and multiple disabilities from pediatric to adult medical care: parents' experiences and recommendations. Intellect Developmental Disabilities 2013;51:176–89.

15. Cheak-Zamora NC, Teti M. "You think it's hard now...It gets much harder for our children": youth with autism and their caregiver's perspectives of health care transition services. Autism 2015;19(8):992–1001.

16. Fegran L, Hall EOC, Uhrenfeldt L, et al. Adolescent and young adults' transition experiences when transferring from paediatric to adult care: a qualitative meta synthesis. Int J Nurs Stud 2014;51:123–35.

17. Fernandes SM, O'Sullivan-Oliviera J, Landzberg MJ, et al. Transition and transfer of adolescents and young adults with pediatric onset chronic disease: the patient and parent perspective. J Pediatr Rehabil Med 2014;7:43–51.

18. Heery E, Sheehan AM, While AE, et al. Experiences and outcomes of transition from pediatric to adult health care services for young people with congenital heart disease: a systematic review. Congenit Heart Dis 2014;10:413–27.

19. Van Staa A, Sattoe JNT. Young adults' experiences and satisfaction with the transfer of care. J Adolesc Health 2014;55:796–803.

20. Nehring WM, Betz CL, Lobo ML. Uncharted territory: a systematic review of providers' roles, understanding, and views pertaining to health care transition. J Pediatr Nurs 2015;30:732–47.

21. Davidson LF, Chhabra R, Cohen HW, et al. Pediatricians transitioning practices for youth with special health care needs in New York State. Clin Pediatr 2015; 54:1051–8.

22. Embrett MC, Randall GE, Longo CJ, et al. Effectiveness of health system services and programs for youth to adult transitions in mental health care: a systematic review of academic literature. Administrative Policy Ment Health J 2016;43:259–65.

23. Fishman LN, DiFazio R, Miller P, et al. Pediatric orthopeadic providers' views on transition from pediatric to adult care. J Pediatr Orthopedics 2015;0:1–6.

24. Gray WN, Monaghan MC, Marchak JG, et al. Psychologists and the transition from pediatrics to adult health care. J Adolesc Health 2015;15:468–74.

25. Gray WN, Resmini AR, Baker KD, et al. Concerns, barriers, and recommendations to improve transition from pediatric to adult IBD care: perspectives of patients, parents, and health professionals. Inflamm Bowel Dis 2015;21:1641–51.

26. Kuhlthau KA, Warfield ME, Husson J, et al. Pediatric providers' perspectives on the transition to adult health care for youth with autism spectrum disorder: current strategies and promising new directions. Autism 2015;19:262–71.

27. Lindgren E, Soderberg S, Skar L. The gap in transition between child and adolescent psychiatry and general adult psychiatry. J Child Adolesc Psychiatr Nurs 2013;26:103–9.

28. Lyons SK, Helgeson VS, Witchel SF, et al. Physicians' self-perceptions of care for emerging adults with type 1 diabetes. Endocrinol Pract 2015;21:903–9.

29. Paul M, Street C, Wheeler N, et al. Transition to adult services for young people with mental health needs: a systematic review. Clin Child Psychol 2015;20: 436–57.

30. Singh SP, Tuomainen H. Transition from child to adult mental health services: needs, barriers, experiences, and new models of care. World Psychiatry 2015; 14:358–61.

31. Healthy People 2020 transition goal. Available at: healthypeople.gov/node/3501/ objectives #4153. Accessed October 3, 2016.

32. Lu MC, Lauver CB, Dykton C, et al. Transformation of the title V maternal and child health services block grant. Matern Child Health J 2015;19:927–31.

33. McManus M, Beck D, White P. State title V health care transition performance objectives and strategies: current snapshot and suggestions. Washington, DC: Got Transition; 2016.

34. American Academy of Pediatrics, American Academy of Family Physicians, American College of Physicians, Transitions Clinical Report Authoring Group. Clinical report—supporting the health care transition from adolescence to adulthood in the medical home. Pediatrics 2011;128:182–200.

35. National Institute for Health and Care Excellence. Transition from children's to adult's services for young people using health or social care services. London: NICE; 2016.

36. Six Core Elements of Health Care Transition. Available at: www.gottransition.org. Accessed October 7, 2016.

37. Information about the American College of Physicians Pediatric to Adult Transition Initiatives. Available at: acponline.org/clinical-information/high-value-care/ resources-for-clinicians/pediatric-to-adult-care transitions-initiative. Accessed October 10, 2016.

38. Wood DL, Sawicki GS, Miller MD, et al. The transition readiness assessment questionnaire (TRAQ): its factor structure, reliability, and validity. Acad Pediatr 2014;14:415–22.

39. Martel A, Derenne J, Chan V. Teaching a systematic approach for transitioning patients to college: an interactive continuing medical education program. Acad Psychiatry 2015;39:549–54.

40. The breakthrough series: IHI's collaborative model for achieving breakthrough improvement. Cambridge (MA): Institute for Healthcare Improvement; 2003.

41. McManus M, White P, Barbour A, et al. Pediatric to adult transition: a quality improvement model for primary care. J Adolesc Health 2015;56:73–8.

42. McManus M, White P, Pirtle R, et al. Incorporating the six core elements of health care transition into a Medicaid managed care plan: lessons learned from a pilot project. J Pediatr Nurs 2015;30:700–13.

43. White P, Cooley WC, McAllister J. Starting a quality improvement process using the six core elements of health care transition. Washington, DC: Got Transition; 2015.

44. Prior M, McManus M, White P, et al. Measuring the "triple aim" in transition care: a systematic review. Pediatrics 2014;134:e1648–61.
45. Bonnie RJ, Stroud C, Breiner H, editors. Investing in the health and well-being of young adults. Washington, DC: The National Academies Press; 2014.
46. Six Core Elements measurement tools. Available at: www.gottransition.org. Accessed October 10, 2016.

Neuroscience-Inspired, Behavioral Change Program for University Students

James J. Hudziak, MD[a],*, Gesa L. Tiemeier, MD/PhD Program[b]

KEYWORDS

- Health promotion ● Behavioral change ● Transitional age brain development
- Critical period ● Developmental mismatch

KEY POINTS

- Transitional age youth (TAY) with their associated transitional age brains (TAB) are at high risk for negative health outcomes, high rates of psychiatric illness, suicide attempts, and morbidity and mortality.
- In the context of the TAB, the high-risk living environments sometimes found in college combined with little or no external regulatory support are associated in some cases with profoundly negative statistics on alcohol and drug use, emotional behavioral health, and perhaps low 6-year graduation rates.
- These statistics led to the design, development, and implementation of a neuroscience-inspired, incentivized behavioral change program at the University of Vermont called the Wellness Environment (WE).
- WE argues that the prescription of an incentive-based, behavioral change, contingency management program with brain-building activities simply makes good scientific, programmatic, and financial sense for colleges and universities as they attempt to support TAY to graduation.

TRANSITIONAL AGE BRAIN GOES TO COLLEGE: WHY THIS IS A PERFECT STORM

In this issue, Chung and Hudziak describe the process of neurodevelopment during the transitional age brain (TAB) epoch and summarize the argument that because of the neurodevelopmental mismatch of different parts of the brain, TAY are at high risk for engaging in behaviors that can lead to negative outcomes, morbidity, and mortality. As conveyed in the article by Winston W. Chung and James J. Hudziak,

The authors have nothing to disclose.
[a] University of Vermont College of Medicine and Medical Center, FAHC-UHC Campus, Box 364SJ3, Room 3213 St. Joseph, Burlington, VT 05401-3456, USA; [b] Leiden University Medical Center, Albinusdreef 2, Leiden, 2333 ZA, The Netherlands
* Corresponding author.
E-mail address: james.hudziak@uvm.edu

Child Adolesc Psychiatric Clin N Am 26 (2017) 381–394
http://dx.doi.org/10.1016/j.chc.2016.12.016
childpsych.theclinics.com

"The Transitional Age Brain: The Best of Times and the Worst of Times," in this issue, the central hypothesis is that the TAB has fully matured risk-taking hardware (because of early maturation of subcortical brain regions amygdalae, nucleus accumbens, and so forth) but not yet matured regulatory hardware (prefrontal cortical regions). The early years (13–17) of the TAB epoch occur within the context of external structure provided by parents, other family members as well as educational institutions and other social structures. Thus, some of the high-risk behavior of early TAY is moderated by parental rules and expectations. These external controls and expectations do not completely negate the risk for morbidity and mortality associated with suicide, substance use and misuse, psychiatric illness, and accidents in TAY.

In almost every measurable domain, adolescence is a developmental period of strength and resilience. The aim of this article is to draw added attention to the special case of why the student with a TAB at college represents a perfect storm; novelty, risk, stress, pressure, substance use and substance abuse are present at the same time the external regulatory system (parents and others) has been removed. The authors focus on the potential outcome when there is an intersection between the high rates and easy access to alcohol and drugs, high-risk social and living environments, and the lack of supervision and regulatory support at a critical period of neurodevelopment in which the regulatory regions of the brain are going through the critical process of maturation (pruning). The authors end by presenting one possible model solution to this critical problem: the prescription of a neuroscience-inspired, incentivized behavioral change program developed at the University of Vermont (UVM).

TRANSITIONAL AGE BRAIN GOES TO COLLEGE: THE FACTS

The TAB, and the resultant thoughts, actions, and behaviors of the TAY, represents one key to understanding the causal relations to the spike in morbidity and mortality in this age group. Where is the evidence? Recent evidence of the rates and consequences of high-risk alcohol and drug use, accidents, and psychiatric illness is presented in the context of the TAB.

About 1 in 4 college students report academic consequences from drinking, including missing class, falling behind in class, doing poorly on examinations or papers, and receiving lower grades overall. Furthermore, about 20% of college students meet the criteria for an alcohol use disorder (AUD). Drinking often causes inappropriate or impulsive behavior among college students. Approximately 900,000 students are injured simply because of being intoxicated. About 696,000 students between the ages of 18 and 24 are assaulted by another student who has been drinking. About 97,000 students between the ages of 18 and 24 report experiencing alcohol-related sexual assault or date rape.[1] A full 28.5% of female students reported having experienced an attempted or completed sexual assault either before or since entering college.[2] As mentioned earlier, suicide and depression are strongly emerging in adolescence.

Suicide is the second-leading cause of death among 20 to 24 year olds, and 1 in 12 US college students makes a suicide plan. More teenagers and young adults die from suicide than from all medical illnesses combined. This period is also notable for the high rates of accidents and health problems related to risky sexual behaviors.[3] In addition, adolescence is the peak time of emergence for several types of mental illnesses, including anxiety disorders, bipolar disorder, depression, eating disorders, psychosis, and substance abuse. As reported in the National Comorbidity Survey

Replication Study by Kessler and colleagues,[4] 50% of most mental illnesses people experience emerge by age 14 and 75% start by age 24.[5,6]

Addiction is seen as a developmental disease, starting in adolescence and young adulthood. In fact, addiction is perhaps best conceptualized as epiphenomena of the environment's effect on the TAB. Eighteen to 25 year olds have the highest past month and past year use percentages of *all* substances, except inhalants. Exposure to drugs during pruning leads to heightened susceptibility to abuse and dependence disorders. Several population- and clinical-based studies have documented that drug use during youth contributes to an elevated risk for developing a substance use disorder. The risk of cannabis dependence is the highest in the early to late adolescent age groups (age 12–18 –year old), with the highest rate at around the 14- to 15-year-old range. For teenagers with cannabis onset, the risk of dependence is 4 to 7 times higher than the estimated risk to recent cannabis onset users aged 22 to 26. The risk of AUD with alcohol onset in teenage years is twice the risk compared with recent alcohol onset users aged 22 to 26.[1,7] The older youth who delays drug use for the first time when the brain is more mature may be more resilient to neurobiological processes that contribute to abuse and dependence.[8]

Neuropsychological studies of adults with AUD have consistently revealed visuospatial, executive functioning, psychomotor, and memory impairments. Greater cumulative lifetime alcohol experiences predicted poorer attention.[9] One brain structure that has consistently demonstrated sensitivity to alcohol-related neurotoxicity is the hippocampus—a structure crucial to intact learning and memory formation.

TAB with AUD have reduced left hippocampal volume compared with nonabusing controls.[7] Furthermore, drinking heavily during adolescence showed significantly diminished frontal and parietal functional MRI (fMRI) response as well as less accurate performance during a spatial working memory task relative to demographically similar controls. The toll of reduced hippocampal volume and poor performance on working memory tasks suggests that heavy alcohol involvement during college is associated with cognitive deficits that may worsen as heavy drinking continues.[9]

3,4-Methylenedioxymethamphetamine (MDMA) damages central serotonergic nerve fibers in human primates after 2 weeks of use and significant damage of neurons 7 years later without ongoing use of MDMA. This lack of serotonin activity may lead to depression, anxiety, and movement abnormalities. In addition, MDMA has been shown to produce pathologic changes in nerve cell bodies in the dorsal raphe nucleus, which can cause sleep problems.[10]

In summary, the TAB is exquisitely sensitive to the effects of alcohol and drugs. The vicious cycle that results from a brain that is primed to make impulsive, risk-taking, pleasure-seeking decisions contributes to the potential for highly dangerous alcohol and drug use, increased academic problems, sleep problems, and higher rates of common psychiatric symptoms and suicide. All of these in turn (both directly and indirectly) negatively affect neurodevelopment, during the highly critical period of pruning/cortical organization, of the key regulatory regions of the brain.

WHAT IS THE COST OF IGNORING THE UNIQUE PROBLEMS OF THE TRANSITIONAL AGE BRAIN AT COLLEGE?

Few businesses could survive with the statistics surrounding success rates at US colleges. The US Department of Education in their 2016 report[11] reveals that the "6-year graduation rate for first-time, full-time undergraduate students who began their pursuit of a bachelor's degree at a 4-year degree-granting institution in fall 2008 varied according to institutional selectivity," ranging from 36% to 89% with an overall rate of

60%. "That is, 60 percent of first-time, full-time students who began seeking a bachelor's degree at a 4-year institution in fall 2008 completed the degree at that institution by 2014." Although it is clear that there are many contributing factors to these data, such as pre-existing emotional behavioral problems, lack of preparation for the college life, socioeconomic obstacles to completing college, and individual differences in resiliency, the data point to the fact that completing a college education is not an easy task.

Although there is no literature on the direct correlation between the dynamic problems of the developmental mismatch of the TAB, with high-risk AUD behaviors and failure to graduate, what is clear is that increased understanding of neurobiology introduces the potential to make a great deal of progress in assisting high-risk students with TABs to safely achieve their goal of a college degree.

WHY UNIVERSITY OF VERMONT WELLNESS ENVIRONMENT?

Taken together, the high-risk epoch of TAB development, the high risk of living in a college environment with limited external regulatory support, the profoundly negative statistics on alcohol, drug, and emotional behavioral health plus the low 6-year graduation rates are concerning. In response, the authors designed, developed, implemented, and tested a neuroscience-inspired, incentivized behavioral change program at the UVM called the Wellness Environment (WE).

UVM WE was designed and developed by one of the authors (J.H.), a child and adolescent psychiatrist, in order to test whether health promotion and illness prevention strategies could be implemented in college settings. The goal was relatively straightforward: design a model college experience based on what is known about TAB development, the negative impact of high-risk behaviors in a high-risk environment (eg, free of parental supervision and guidance), and emerging behavioral change and neuroimaging research. WE is based on the hypothesis that such a program would result in more positive choices regarding health-promoting activities in a university setting. The overarching hypothesis is that TAB students would respond to health-promoting, brain-building activities through lifestyle changes if they were presented in an incentive-based framework.

UVM WE is an incentive-based behavioral change program aimed at developing healthy brains and healthy bodies in a college setting. Students who live in WE residential halls receive incentivized exercise, mindfulness, yoga, nutrition, hydration, mentoring, and community opportunities. They receive all of these free of charge with only one requirement: no alcohol or drugs are allowed in the environment. Students are admitted on a first-come, first-serve basis. Over the first 2 years, the authors have tracked bias pathways and can report that although many of the students who live in WE have come to college without pre-existing alcohol and drug problems and are attracted to the health promotion aspects and the WE code, others have specifically signed up to live in WE because they have pre-existing struggles with alcohol, drugs, and emotional or behavioral problems.

The authors have argued that in the same way daily exercise, working out in the gym, or lifting weights could lead to achieving the goal of building a healthy body, it is now evident that a series of brain-building activities is emerging in the literature that provide evidence that TAY (in fact, all ages) could engage in brain-building activities. From behavioral change research comes the second foundation of WE. Incentive-based behavioral change is at the heart of all health care, and college life is no different. The WE design is based on the argument that moving students with

TABs, from high-risk damaging behaviors into health-promoting brain-building behaviors, would require incentivization.

Based on this template, Hudziak proposed the UVM WE to university leaders (President, Provost, Vice Provost of Student Affairs, Director of Student Health, Residential Life, Admissions, and many other key stakeholders), who unanimously approved an implementation project. The design included a model system based on the creation of a course, *Healthy Brains, Healthy Bodies: Surviving and Thriving in College*, in which students would be taught the impact of specific behaviors on genomic and brain health in a nonjudgmental context. The second feature of UVM WE was a proposed residential community based on 4 pillars of brain-building wellness activities, in which students are incentivized to exercise daily with personal trainers, engage in mindfulness and yoga with certified instructors, and participate in healthy dietary practices with a nutrition coach inspired by recent advances in gut-brain neuroscience.[12] Last, a mentoring program was built (wementor.org) to encourage participating students, TAY, to engage in mentoring programs aimed at advancing personal wellness through teaching younger less fortunate youth. All of these activities would be (and have been) incentivized (and are free of additional cost). A key feature of UVM WE is faculty engagement through coursework, in residence halls and campus-wide programming. Students who live in WE are required to sign a contract that indicates they understand if they have alcohol or drugs, or are grossly intoxicated in the WE, they will be removed from the program (and live elsewhere on campus). UVM leadership enthusiastically accepted the proposal. A leadership team was developed; necessary additional personnel were hired, and UVM WE opened during the 2015 to 2016 school year with 120 students. The program grew to 480 students for the 2016 to 2017 academic year, including new students and returning students, and is anticipated to house 1200 students in the 2017 to 2018 year.

Although very preliminary, as WE has only completed one pilot year, there is emerging evidence that the program has achieved its central goals, having students engaged in brain-building activities, understanding the implications of decisions on their brain health, and creating and maintaining communities with lower rates of AUD problems. Universities and colleges around the country are currently working on designing similar programs. Hudziak has also been awarded a grant from the Conrad Hilton Foundation to assist him in the development of the UVM WE App, an iOS-based health promotion, illness prevention App built on the goals and pillars of the WE program. In addition, UVM WE has drawn the attention of national print and news outlets as well as in local media stories. Each of these news stories as well as a detailed representation of UVM WE, the App, and plans for the future of WE can be viewed at: https://www.uvm.edu/we.

What follows is a primer on Behavioral Change science and the importance of contingency management (CM) to the TAB. The authors then present the neuroscience evidence for several brain-building activities that are incentivized in the WE program.

WHAT CAN BE DONE? BEHAVIORAL CHANGE GOES TO COLLEGE

It has been argued elsewhere[11] that all health emerges from emotional behavioral health. Why an individual decides to drink alcohol, use drugs, assault another, or commit acts of self-harm is an emotional behavioral decision. In the same way, why an individual chooses not to engage in the above but rather pursues healthy, brain-building activities such as daily fitness, meditation, yoga, music, mentoring, or healthy dietary choices is also a brain-based emotional moment. Similarly, the authors have published elsewhere that health care reform is simply the business of behavioral change,[13] moving an individual from engagement in unhealthy behavioral decisions to healthy ones. The science of behavioral change is perfectly positioned to help TAY negotiate the high-risk neurodevelopmental and environmental task of going to college.

UNDERSTANDING BEHAVIORAL CHANGE SCIENCE

Behavior change refers to a modification of human behavior or a change in public health approaches, which "focus on the individual, community, and environmental influences on behavior." Behavioral change models have been successfully applied as a way to better understand, and treat, addictive disorders such as smoking, and later, alcohol abuse.[14] Over the past 4 decades, the model has been applied to a wide range of health behaviors ranging from substance abuse to overeating and physical inactivity with the goal to help health professionals to design, implement, and evaluate health-promoting interventions.[15] The concept of applying behavior change models as a way to promote healthy brain development during the TAB epoch in college settings is the core of the approach at the UVM WE program.

Incentivized-Based Behavior Change (Contingency Management)

In order to most effectively apply behavioral change models in a college environment, the authors have added the science of CM. CM is most widely used in the field of substance-related disorders and refers to the application of a contingency to influence behavior change. Incentive-based behavior change can simply be understood as paying for behavior change. The payment might come in the form of a valuable reenforcer (money, privileges, prizes) that a participant ultimately finds more rewarding than the drug or alcohol use. A large body of literature supports the use of CM for health-promoting behavior with participants given rewards for not engaging in negative or high-risk behaviors.[16]

BRAIN-BUILDING ROUTINES/HABITS

Using the methods and strategies of incentive-based behavioral change with CM has shown great value in the treatment of substance-related and addictive disorders. In the UVM WE program, the authors have "teetered the totter" and argued that one can incentivize positive health-promoting brain-building behavior for TABs at a time when TAY need it most. In the service of that goal, the authors present in later discussion some of the neuroscience evidence for 4 of the brain-building activities that are incentivized in the WE program.

PRACTICE MINDFULNESS, BUILD YOUR COLLEGE BRAIN

Mindfulness, as described by Dr Jon Kabat-Zinn,[17] "cultivates present moment awareness" and "involves attending to relevant aspects of experience in a nonjudgmental manner."

Mindfulness meditation, by paying full attention to present-moment experience, results in "disengaging oneself from strong attachment to beliefs, thoughts, or emotions, thereby developing a greater sense of emotional balance and well-being."

Research shows that with mindfulness treatment there are significant reductions in mood disturbance (65%) and symptoms of stress (31%).[18] An 8-week mindfulness program resulted in significant reductions in anxiety and depression scores after treatment according to both self-report and interviewer report.[19] Furthermore, there is some evidence that meditation may also influence recovery from or prevention of disease. A Chinese study showed that after mindfulness intervention students had lower salivary cortisol and higher salivary immunoglobulin A concentration in response to psychological stress compared with control students.[20]

Finally, mindfulness practice has a profound effect on brain function. Neuroimaging studies using fMRI found that mindfulness meditation was associated with activation in attention and emotion-regulating areas, such as prefrontal cortex and anterior cingulate cortex (ACC),[21] whereas the amygdala, an important region for emotion modulation and amplification, showed decreased activation.[22,23]

Mindful individuals are shown to have smaller right amygdala volumes, associated with reduced stress reactivity and lower negative affect in daily life. The amygdala has been shown to contribute significantly to mental and emotional health, with abnormal amygdala function identified in depression, anxiety, posttraumatic stress disorder, phobias, and panic disorders.[24] Moreover, mindful individuals have been shown to have smaller left and right caudate volumes, which are involved in processing negative affect and the neural response to sadness.[25] Mindfulness increases gray matter volume, similar to treatment with selective serotonin reuptake inhibitors, gray matter concentration within the left hippocampus, which also plays a crucial role in the regulation of emotion and cognition.[26]

It has been demonstrated that the effects of mindfulness train the brain to decrease the activation of spontaneous self-generated mental activity; that is, the default mode networks, and downregulation of emotional reactivity.[27–29] Activation in the default mode network is observable in streams of thoughts or episodic memories and mental time traveling.[30,31] Furthermore, the default mode network has been related to monitoring the reliability of internal and external information, often a source of worry and anxiety.[32] A goal of meditation is to train the brain to switch from this default mode network of emotions to test the positive network of cognition. The authors determined that this form of meditation can be used as the basis for an effective behavioral program in self-regulation.[19]

Mindfulness and Wellness Environment

With the above in mind, WE students meditate at the beginning and end of all *Healthy Brain, Healthy Body* classes and have specialized mindfulness and yoga instruction in the WE residential halls. WE Mindfulness Based Health Promotion (MBHP) instructors complete a one-credit-hour training selected from MBHP classes, and the WE App has dozens of guided meditations designed for the TAB college student.

TAKE A (DAILY) HIKE: THE IMPORTANCE OF DAILY PHYSICAL ACTIVITY TO TRANSITIONAL AGE BRAINS

Despite mounting evidence for the importance of physical activity, 74% of adults in the United States do not meet the recommended guideline of at least 30 minutes of moderate-intensity physical activity most days of the week.[33] The economic cost of this sedentary lifestyle is enormous, with estimates indicating that inactivity was associated with $76 billion in medical costs in the year 2000.[34]

Physical activity is not exclusively beneficial for physical health; research has shown profound effects of exercise on mental and emotional health. Animal research has shown that chronic exercise results in antidepressant-like effects and can reduce anxiety-related behavior, similar to responses of antidepressant drug–treated animals.[35]

In human research, exercisers are on average more satisfied with their lives and happier than nonexercisers, demonstrating less anxiety and depression.[36] Cross-sectional research has indicated that reduced levels of exercise are associated with depression among young adults.[37]

A recent meta-analysis determined a positive relation between physical activity and cognitive performance in school-aged children (aged 4–18 years). Time spent in physical activity programs does not hinder academic performance, and it is hypothesized that it could indeed improve performance.[38] The authors' group has published that TAY who exercised more frequently (4–5 days or 6–7 days) had significantly lower odds of sadness, suicidal ideation, or suicide attempt than students who exercised less frequently. Furthermore, these relationships extended to students who were victims of bullying. In particular, these data demonstrate that being physically active on 4 or more days per week was related to an approximate 23% reduction in the odds of both suicidal ideation and suicide attempt in bullied adolescents.[39]

In a large study of young Dutch children, being active in sports at least once a week was associated with reduced externalizing and internalizing problems.[40] Aerobic fitness training has also been found to induce changes in patterns of functional activation using fMRI. In humans, aerobic fitness training has been correlated with larger volumes of anterior white matter and prefrontal and temporal gray matter[41,42] as well as increased cerebral blood volume in the dentate gyrus of the hippocampus[43] and decreases in activation in the ACC.[44,45] Specifically, children with higher aerobic fitness levels showed less behavioral interference to misleading and irrelevant cues, coupled with a larger dorsal striatum (ie, left caudate nucleus and bilateral putamen).[46–48] In addition, children with higher aerobic fitness levels also have larger hippocampal volumes compared with children with lower-fitness levels. These larger hippocampal volumes were associated with superior relational memory task performance. The results are consistent with animal models that indicate aerobic activity positively impacts hippocampal structure and function.[46–48]

Finally, recent data continue to show a positive relationship between grades and visits to the sports center. Among (https://www.eab.com/daily-briefing/2014/11/13/gym-data-shows-gpa-bump-for-fitness-inclined-students?WT.mc_id=Email%7CDaily+Briefing+Headline%7CDBA%7CDB%7CAug-19-2016%7CArchive%7C%7C%7C%7C&elq_cid=2240438&x_id=003C0000021F87sIAC) all undergraduates of Purdue University, students who visited the gym on average 16 times per month averaged a 3.2 GPA, compared with a 3.1 GPA for nonusers. It is unclear if these data are statistically significant. Among new students in the fall of 2013, students who visited the gym at least 15 times that semester averaged a 3.08 GPA, compared with 2.81 for nonusers.[49] Earlier this year, Michigan State University (MSU) conducted a similar study and found that gym visits correlated not only with higher grades but also with better retention. The group of students with gym memberships had a 3.5% higher 2-year retention rate (a difference of about 1575 students on MSU's campus) and held GPAs that were 0.13 points higher. The study saw 74% sophomore retention compared with 60% for those without gym memberships.

Fitness and Wellness Environment

With the above in mind, WE students are invited to voluntarily complete a fitness evaluation and have access individually to a personalized fitness coach. WE residence halls all have state-of-the-art workout facilities to incentivize daily workouts. In the WE halls, they also have "Fitness on Demand," allowing the students 24/7 access to world class individual and group fitness instructors. Daily fitness is incentivized by earning WE points toward rewards such as WE hoodies, hats, and other positive contingencies. There is also a one-credit WE-Les Mills–accredited Fitness Training laboratory in which graduates are certified to become WE fitness trainers. On the WE App is a fitness pillar that includes instructions and incentives to engage in exercise 7 days a week.

THE GUT-BRAIN AXIS AT COLLEGE: WHY NUTRITION MATTERS

Research on both animal and human models strongly suggests an important role of nutrition and the microbiota in the regulation of the brain and behavior.[12] The microbiota-gut-brain axis represents a bidirectional network of communication between the intestinal microbiota and the brain. The gut microbiota is required for development of the hypothalamic-pituitary-adrenal (HPA) axis, optimal stress responsivity, and social cognition. Dysregulation of the microbiota-gut-brain axis may contribute to the development of psychiatric and gastrointestinal diseases, a link supported by the comorbidity found between anxiety disorders and irritable bowel syndrome[50] as well as the abnormal composition of gut microbiota in patients with autism.[51]

Animal research shows that mice lacking a gut microbiota have enlarged amygdala and hippocampus, without a difference in total brain volume between germ-free (GF) and control mice, ruling out the possibility that these enlargements were due to whole-brain expansion. The absence of a gut microbiota in mice induced dendritic atrophy, with 32% fewer synaptic connections on the hippocampal pyramidal neurons. Changes in amygdala and hippocampal size have also been documented in rodents subjected to stressors. Furthermore, GF mice exhibit exaggerated HPA axis responses to acute stressors and deficits in social cognition.[52] Similar results were found in rats after chronic antibiotic treatment. The depletion of the gut microbiota of rats during adulthood resulted in deficits in spatial memory, increased visceral sensitivity, and a greater display of depressive-like behaviors. In addition to these clear behavioral alterations, the authors found changes in altered central nervous system serotonin concentration along with changes in the messenger RNA levels of corticotrophin-releasing hormone receptor 1 and glucocorticoid receptor.[53]

Nutrition and Wellness Environment: Eat Well, Study Well, Sleep Well, Live Well

With the above in mind, WE partnered with the Nutrition Department at UVM as well as leading gut-brain scientists around the world and developed WE dietary programs. All students are offered one-on-one dietary consultations with master level dietetics graduate students at UVM. In addition, colleagues at UVM Dining provide tours to all WE students to connect their education in healthy nutrition to real-time direction on how and where to get the food they want. Students are incentivized to engage in probiotic education and healthy dietary planning and eating. On the WE app, there is a scanning pillar that allows WE students to design their dietary goals and then scan their dietary choices to track their ability to meet their own goals. In addition, there is a one-credit laboratory in WE Nutrition Training in which graduates become WE Nutrition trainers.

Music and Wellness Environment: play, practice, and regulate

Research has shown that practicing a musical instrument was associated with higher performance on tests of reasoning, processing speed, attentional and working memory networks, as well as mathematics.[54] After 2 years of group music training, the speech-in-noise perception has been shown to improve, resulting in better school performance and attention. Furthermore, music training was associated with a reduction in the word gap of children raised in poverty.[55] The rich overlap between neural systems devoted to language and music is hypothesized to underlie the benefits music training confers on reading and its neural correlates across multiple timescales of auditory processing.[56–58] In addition, musical intervention is shown to reduce pediatric pain, anxiety, and distress and has an especially large effect on cognitive skills and social behavior in autistic children.[59]

Music training has been shown to affect the anatomy of the brain, with greater gray matter volumes observed in motor-related areas,[60–62] auditory discrimination areas, corpus callosum,[62,63] as well as greater white matter volumes in motor tracts.[64] In addition, the behavioral and functionality improvements after music training were correlated with the structural brain changes of the specific areas.[62]

Research with children and adolescents who play musical instruments showed brain changes in motor areas, the corpus callosum, and the right primary auditory region, all areas important for music performance and auditory processing. In addition, unexpected areas increased in volume compared with those of the controls; these included various frontal areas, the left posterior pericingulate, and the left middle occipital region. Music training is associated with the rate of cortical thickness maturation in several brain areas distributed throughout the right premotor and primary cortices, namely the left primary and supplementary motor cortices, bilateral parietal cortices, bilateral orbitofrontal cortices, as well as bilateral parahippocampal gyri.[65]

Thus, music training may accelerate cortical development. Music training leads to greater gains in auditory and motor function when begun in young childhood. Nevertheless, the results establish that music training impacts the auditory system even when it is begun in adolescence, suggesting the possibility that a modest amount of training begun later in life can affect neural function.[56–58]

Music Training and Wellness Environment

In addition to the core education described above, WE students are invited to participate in sponsored music training programs. WE offers violins and violin instruction to students who live in the resident halls. These programs are highly subscribed. In addition, WE students participate in campus-wide activities such as "WE has Talent" in which they are able to perform their musical and singing skills. The WE music program is being further developed with a goal of offering lessons in a variety of instruments.

SUMMARY

TAY with their associated TABs are at high risk for negative health outcomes, high rates of psychiatric illness, suicide attempts, and morbidity and mortality. In the context of the TAB, the high-risk living environments sometimes found in college combined with little or no external regulatory support are associated in some cases with profoundly negative statistics on alcohol and drug use emotional behavioral health, and perhaps low 6-year graduation rates. These statistics led to the design, development, and implementation of a neuroscience-inspired, incentivized behavioral change program at the UVM called the Wellness Environment.

WE argues that the prescription of an incentive-based, behavioral change, CM program with brain-building activities simply makes good scientific, programmatic, and financial sense for colleges and universities as they attempt to support TAY to graduation.

REFERENCES

1. Hingson R, Heeren T, Winter M, et al. Magnitude of alcohol-related mortality and morbidity among U.S. college students ages 18-24: changes from 1998 to 2001. Annu Rev Public Health 2005;26:259–79.

2. Krebs CP, Lindquist CH, Warner TD, et al. College women's experiences with physically forced, alcohol- or other drug-enabled, and drug-facilitated sexual assault before and since entering college. J Am Coll Health 2009;57(6):639–47.

3. May JC, Delgado MR, Dahl RE, et al. Event-related functional magnetic resonance imaging of reward-related brain circuitry in children and adolescents. Biol Psychiatry 2004;55(4):359–66.

4. Kessler RC, Berglund P, Demler O, et al. Lifetime prevalence and age-of-onset distribution of DSM-IV disorders in the National Comorbidity Survey Replication. Arch Gen Psychiatry 2005;62:593–603.

5. Hankin BL, Abramson LY, Moffitt TE, et al. Development of depression from pre-adolescence to young adulthood: emerging gender differences in a 10-year longitudinal study. J Abnorm Psychol 1998;107(1):128–40.

6. Giedd JN. The amazing teen brain. Sci Am 2015;312(6):32–7.

7. Winters KC, Lee CY. Likelihood of developing an alcohol and cannabis use disorder during youth: association with recent use and age. Drug Alcohol Depend 2008;92(1–3):239–47.

8. Nagel BJ, Schweinsburg AD, Phan V, et al. Reduced hippocampal volume among adolescents with alcohol use disorders without psychiatric comorbidity. Psychiatry Res 2005;139(3):181–90.

9. Tapert SF, Schweinsburg AD. The human adolescent brain and alcohol use disorders. Recent Dev Alcohol 2005;17:177–97.

10. Ricaurte GA, Forno LS, Wilson MA, et al. (+/−)3,4-Methylenedioxymethamphetamine selectively damages central serotonergic neurons in nonhuman primates. JAMA 1988;260(1):51–5.

11. U.S. Department of Education, National Center for Education Statistics. (2016). The condition of education 2016 (NCES 2016-144), undergraduate retention and graduation rates.

12. Sandhu KV, Sherwin E, Schellekens H, et al. Feeding the microbiota-gut-brain axis: diet, microbiome, and neuropsychiatry. Transl Res 2016;179:223–44.

13. Hudziak J, Ivanova MY. The Vermont family based approach: family based health promotion, illness prevention, and intervention. Child Adolesc Psychiatr Clin N Am 2016;25(2):167–78.

14. Stonerock GL, Blumenthal JA. Role of counseling to promote adherence in healthy lifestyle medicine: strategies to improve exercise adherence and enhance physical activity. Prog Cardiovasc Dis 2016. [Epub ahead of print].

15. Prochaska JO, Velicer WF. The transtheoretical model of health behavior change. Am J Health Promot 1997;12(1):38–48.

16. Stitzer M, Petry N. Contingency management for treatment of substance abuse. Annu Rev Clin Psychol 2006;2:411–34.

17. Ludwig DS, Kabat-Zinn J. Mindfulness in medicine. JAMA 2008;300(11):1350–2.

18. Speca M, Carlson LE, Goodey E, et al. A randomized, wait-list controlled clinical trial: the effect of a mindfulness meditation-based stress reduction program on mood and symptoms of stress in cancer outpatients. Psychosom Med 2000; 62(5):613–22.

19. Kabat-Zinn J, Massion AO, Kristeller J, et al. Effectiveness of a meditation-based stress reduction program in the treatment of anxiety disorders. Am J Psychiatry 1992;149(7):936–43.

20. Tang YY, Ma Y, Wang J, et al. Short-term meditation training improves attention and self-regulation. Proc Natl Acad Sci U S A 2007;104(43):17152–6.

21. Chiesa A, Serretti A. Mindfulness-based stress reduction for stress management in healthy people: a review and meta-analysis. J Altern Complement Med 2009; 15(5):593–600.

22. Lutz J, Herwig U, Opialla S, et al. Mindfulness and emotion regulation–an fMRI study. Soc Cogn Affect Neurosci 2014;9(6):776–85.

23. Creswell JD, Way BM, Eisenberger NI, et al. Neural correlates of dispositional mindfulness during affect labeling. Psychosom Med 2007;69(6):560–5.

24. Haase L, Thom NJ, Shukla A, et al. Mindfulness-based training attenuates insula response to an aversive interoceptive challenge. Soc Cogn Affect Neurosci 2016; 11(1):182–90.

25. Taren AA, Creswell JD, Gianaros PJ. Dispositional mindfulness co-varies with smaller amygdala and caudate volumes in community adults. PLoS One 2013; 8(5):e64574.

26. Hölzel BK, Carmody J, Vangel M, et al. Mindfulness practice leads to increases in regional brain gray matter density. Psychiatry Res 2011;191(1):36–43.

27. Goldin PR, Gross JJ. Effects of mindfulness-based stress reduction (MBSR) on emotion regulation in social anxiety disorder. Emotion 2010;10(1):83–91.

28. Tomasino B, Fabbro F. Increases in the right dorsolateral prefrontal cortex and decreases the rostral prefrontal cortex activation after-8 weeks of focused attention based mindfulness meditation. Brain Cogn 2016;102:46–54.

29. Dickenson J, Berkman ET, Arch J, et al. Neural correlates of focused attention during a brief mindfulness induction. Soc Cogn Affect Neurosci 2013;8(1):40–7.

30. Addis DR, Knapp K, Roberts RP, et al. Routes to the past: neural substrates of direct and generative autobiographical memory retrieval. Neuroimage 2012; 59(3):2908–22.

31. Schacter DL, Addis DR, Buckner RL. Remembering the past to imagine the future: the prospective brain. Nat Rev Neurosci 2007;8(9):657–61.

32. Dehaene S, Charles L, King JR, et al. Toward a computational theory of conscious processing. Curr Opin Neurobiol 2014;25:76–84.

33. Centers for Disease Control and Prevention. Prevalence of physical activity, including lifestyle activities among adults—United States, 2000–2001.

34. Pratt M, Macera MA, Wang G. Higher direct medical costs associated with physical inactivity. Phys Sportsmed 2000;28:63–70.

35. Duman CH, Schlesinger L, Russell DS, et al. Voluntary exercise produces antidepressant and anxiolytic behavioral effects in mice. Brain Res 2008;1199:148–58.

36. De Moor MH, Beem AL, Stubbe JH, et al. Regular exercise, anxiety, depression and personality: a population-based study. Prev Med 2006;42(4):273–9.

37. Farmer ME, Locke BZ, Mościcki EK, et al. Physical activity and depressive symptoms: the NHANES I epidemiologic follow-up study. Am J Epidemiol 1988;128(6): 1340–51.

38. Sibley BA, Etnier JL. The relationship between physical activity and cognition in children: a meta-analysis. Pediatr Exerc Sci 2003;(3):243–56.

39. Sibold J, Edwards E, Murray-Close D, et al. Physical activity, sadness, and suicidality in bullied US adolescents. J Am Acad Child Adolesc Psychiatry 2015; 54(10):808–15.

40. Tiemeier GL, Tiemeier H, Hudziak JJ. Bullying externalizing problems team sports. New Research Poster. AACAP Annual Meeting 2016.

41. McAuley E, Kramer AF, Colcombe SJ. Cardiovascular fitness and neurocognitive function in older adults: a brief review. Brain Behav Immun 2004;18(3):214–20.

42. Colcombe SJ, Erickson KI, Scalf PE, et al. Aerobic exercise training increases brain volume in aging humans. J Gerontol A Biol Sci Med Sci 2006;61(11): 1166–70.

43. Pereira AC, Huddleston DE, Brickman AM, et al. An in vivo correlate of exercise-induced neurogenesis in the adult dentate gyrus. Proc Natl Acad Sci U S A 2007; 104(13):5638–43.

44. Themanson JR, Pontifex MB, Hillman CH. Fitness and action monitoring: evidence for improved cognitive flexibility in young adults. Neuroscience 2008; 157(2):319–28.

45. Chaddock L, Erickson KI, Prakash RS, et al. Basal ganglia volume is associated with aerobic fitness in preadolescent children. Dev Neurosci 2010;32(3):249–56.

46. Chaddock L, Erickson KI, Prakash RS, et al. A neuroimaging investigation of the association between aerobic fitness, hippocampal volume, and memory performance in preadolescent children. Brain Res 2010;1358:172–83.

47. Erickson KI, Voss MW, Prakash RS, et al. Exercise training increases size of hippocampus and improves memory. Proc Natl Acad Sci U S A 2011;108(7): 3017–22.

48. Weinstein AM, Voss MW, Prakash RS, et al. The association between aerobic fitness and executive function is mediated by prefrontal cortex volume. Brain Behav Immun 2012;26(5):811–9.

49. Amy Patterson Neubert, Purdue University, 765-494-9723.

50. Luczynski P, Whelan SO, O'Sullivan C, et al. Adult microbiota-deficient mice have distinct dendritic morphological changes: differential effects in the amygdala and hippocampus. Eur J Neurosci 2016;44(9):2654–66.

51. Mayer EA, Padua D, Tillisch K. Altered brain-gut axis in autism: comorbidity or causative mechanisms? Bioessays 2014;36:933–9.

52. Fond G, Loundou A, Hamdani N, et al. Anxiety and depression comorbidities in irritable bowel syndrome (IBS): a systematic review and meta-analysis. Eur Arch Psychiatry Clin Neurosci 2014;264:651–60.

53. Hoban AE, Moloney RD, Golubeva AV, et al. Behavioral and neurochemical consequences of chronic gut microbiota depletion during adulthood in the rat. Neuroscience 2016;339:463–77.

54. Bergman Nutley S, Darki F, Klingberg T. Music practice is associated with development of working memory during childhood and adolescence. Front Hum Neurosci 2014;7:926.

55. Fitzroy AB, Krizman J, Tierney A, et al. Longitudinal maturation of auditory cortical function during adolescence. Front Hum Neurosci 2015;9:530.

56. Slater J, Strait DL, Skoe E, et al. Longitudinal effects of group music instruction on literacy skills in low-income children. PLoS One 2014;9(11):e113383.

57. Kraus N, Slater J, Thompson EC, et al. Music enrichment programs improve the neural encoding of speech in at-risk children. J Neurosci 2014;34(36):11913–8.

58. Strait DL, Slater J, O'Connell S, et al. Music training relates to the development of neural mechanisms of selective auditory attention. Dev Cogn Neurosci 2015;12: 94–104.

59. Treurnicht Naylor K, Kingsnorth S, Lamont A, et al. The effectiveness of music in pediatric healthcare: a systematic review of randomized controlled trials. Evid Based Complement Alternat Med 2011;2011:464759.

60. Elbert T, Pantev C, Wienbruch C, et al. Increased cortical representation of the fingers of the left hand in string players. Science 1995;270(5234):305–7.

61. Pascual-Leone A. The brain that plays music and is changed by it. Ann N Y Acad Sci 2001;930:315–29.

62. Hyde KL, Lerch J, Norton A, et al. Musical training shapes structural brain development. J Neurosci 2009;29(10):3019–25.
63. Gaser C, Schlaug G. Brain structures differ between musicians and non-musicians. J Neurosci 2003;23(27):9240–5.
64. Bengtsson SL, Nagy Z, Skare S, et al. Extensive piano practicing has regionally specific effects on white matter development. Nat Neurosci 2005;8(9):1148–50.
65. Hudziak JJ, Albaugh MD, Ducharme S, et al, Brain Development Cooperative Group. Cortical thickness maturation and duration of music training: health-promoting activities shape brain development. J Am Acad Child Adolesc Psychiatry 2014;53(11):1153–61, 1161.e1–e2.

Summary

Successful Transition to Young Adulthood with Mental Illness

Common Themes and Future Directions

D. Catherine Fuchs, MD[a], Adele Martel, MD, PhD[b],*

The transitional age youth (TAY) demographic (as defined in the Preface), representing a unique developmental period in life, has recently garnered the interest of clinicians, researchers, educators, governmental agencies, and policymakers. Historically this age group has been considered late adolescents and early adults rather than a subgroup of its own. The implications of categorization are significant in terms of understanding of these individuals and the ability to support them. Attention to this group has been prompted by increasing the knowledge base in neurodevelopment, epigenetics, epidemiology, prevention, overall young adult health, and functional outcomes, particularly in regard to mental health. Addressing the mental health needs of TAY has become a national priority and there is increasing recognition of the potential for productive interventions in this complex and important developmental period.

Mental illness may present in childhood, adolescence, or young adulthood, with influences on psychosocial, emotional, and brain development that vary with the age and context of illness presentation. Temperament and genetics are baseline factors contributing to individual responses to life experiences. Developmental experiences can be protective and build resilience or convey risk to expression of illness or to negative outcomes. In combination, these factors influence developmental trajectories and developmental branch points, contributing to variable expression of health and illness.

The authors in this issue have identified many common themes. One overarching theme is the importance of culturally competent care. There continue to be health disparities related to race, ethnicity, and other diversity. Culture influences how mental health is defined and viewed by individuals. TAY are often in transition, which can introduce a variety of cultural attitudes, challenging familiar norms and introducing, at times, an unanticipated level of stress. It is imperative to develop more sophisticated awareness of our own ethnocentric views and possible ethnocentric graduate medical education training. It is equally imperative to orient training of child and adolescent psychiatry and general psychiatry residents toward cultural understanding within the TAY population. Rivas-Drake and Stein (this issue) state it well: "Researchers and practitioners must strive to build their capacity to keep pace with the demographic shifts of the US youth population."

[a] Psychological and Counseling Center, Vanderbilt University, 2015 Terrace Place, Nashville, TN 37203, USA; [b] Department of Psychiatry and Behavioral Sciences, Northwestern University Feinberg School of Medicine, Ann & Robert H. Lurie Children's Hospital of Chicago, Child and Adolescent Psychiatry, 225 E Chicago Avenue, Box 10, Chicago, IL 60611, USA
* Corresponding author.
E-mail address: adele.martel@gmail.com

Child Adolesc Psychiatric Clin N Am 26 (2017) 395–396
http://dx.doi.org/10.1016/j.chc.2016.12.015
1056-4993/17/© 2016 Elsevier Inc. All rights reserved.

childpsych.theclinics.com

Another theme is the paucity of evidence-based mental health treatments specifically targeting the TAY age group. Research on adults includes a wide range of ages (often 18 and older), developmental stages of the brain, and environmental influences; often, these results are not stratified into age groupings. Likewise, early adolescents may be included in studies with older adolescents. It is necessary to perform research specific to TAY, spanning the midadolescent to late adolescent and the young adult age range, so that clinicians can more accurately determine appropriate care models for this age group. The contributors offer information on evidence-based practices where they exist. Some of the research that is available focuses on college students, in part due to the ability to capture the student population for review of data and development of research studies. Researchers and clinicians should consider this information but must remember that there are many other TAY subgroups for which the information may not extrapolate. Although the evidence base is being developed, the contributors encourage the use of promising practices and best practices as derived from studies, such as case reports, cohort studies, and so forth and those that are built on solid theoretic grounding, such as the public health model or the systems of care approach.

A critical theme is the prime importance of developing treatment approaches to engage and maintain TAY in treatment. In the spirit of offering developmentally attuned care, the contributing authors agree that focusing on strengths, shared decision making, collaborative treatment planning, using peer supports or peer mentors, and offering multidimensional supports are useful approaches. Another area of agreement is the importance of integrating the family, broadly defined, into the treatment of TAY at a level commensurate with individuation and with a cultural lens. The authors highlight that developmentally focused care necessitates factoring in evolving brain development with the associated shifting balance between executive function and emotions. This contributes to the challenges in dealing with substance use, both in terms of early experimentation and addiction in TAY.

Another theme is that successful transition to adulthood is not defined by the presence or absence of disease but by self-determination and successful management of illness when present. The authors discuss the meaning of success in the context of the individual, the family, and the system of care, all while considering TAY at risk for or dealing with mental illness. Concepts around education, environmental support, and individual resilience consistently indicate that patients' knowledge of their own mental illness, treatment, and the availability of a support network or community are all factors that contribute to success. Aligning individual strengths with TAY environmental contexts and experiences can also improve outcomes and enhance an individual's trajectory along lines of development. The authors suggest that creating a developmentally appropriate transition plan for the individual, the family or caregivers, and the system may provide a structure that can help TAY with mental illness succeed in their transition to young adulthood. Consideration of normal development, environmental challenges, and the balance between critical thinking, emotions, and behavior must be done in the context of the baseline biology, the vulnerabilities, and the protective factors of each person. This is already a complex process. There is a growing appreciation of how the environment influences gene expression, neural circuitry, emotions, and behaviors; this increase in knowledge challenges understanding of mental illness. Furthermore, age and stage of life invariably influence cultural factors. As recognition of unique aspects of the TAY stage of life grows, it is critical to incorporate this understanding into research, education, and clinical work. Development of evidence-based practices regarding TAY will help expand the concepts required to teach the necessary knowledge, skills, and attitudes for effective mental health care for TAY.

Index

Note: Page numbers of article titles are in **boldface** type.

A

Acculturative stress
    in undermining health adaptation
        resilience in TAY related to, 273
ADA. *See* Americans with Disabilities Act (ADA)
Adaptive skills
    of TAY with autism spectrum disorders, 333
ADHD. *See* Attention-deficit/hyperactivity disorder (ADHD)
Adolescence
    defined, 235
Adolescent(s)
    late
        developmental stage and needs of
            aligned with mental health treatments, **177–190** *See also* Mental health
                treatments, developmental stage and needs of late adolescents and young
                adults aligned with
Adult health care services
    transition to
        for young adults with chronic medical illness and psychiatric comorbidity, **367–380**
            See also Transition to adult health care services, for young adults with chronic
            medical illness and psychiatric comorbidity
Adulthood
    pathways to
        temporary trends in, 148–149
Age of vulnerability, 149–150
Alcohol eCHECKUP TO GO
    for substance use problems in TAY, 259
Alcohol use
    among transitional age LGBTQ youth, 300
Americans with Disabilities Act (ADA)
    in postsecondary education and employment, 321–323
Anxiety
    SM and
        among young adults, 223
Anxiety disorders
    in transitional age LGBTQ youth, 300
Attention-deficit/hyperactivity disorder (ADHD)
    schizophrenia with, 346
    in TAY, 316
        outcome effects of, 316–318
Autism spectrum disorders, **329–339**
    schizophrenia with, 346

Child Adolesc Psychiatric Clin N Am 26 (2017) 397–410
http://dx.doi.org/10.1016/S1056-4993(17)30025-1
1056-4993/17

Printed and bound by CPI Group (UK) Ltd, Croydon, CR0 4YY

03/10/2024

01040392-0013